ULTRASOUND IMAGING – MEDICAL APPLICATIONS

Edited by **Igor Minin** and **Oleg Minin**

Ultrasound Imaging – Medical Applications
Edited by Igor Minin and Oleg Minin

Published by InTech
Janeza Trdine 9, 51000 Rijeka, Croatia

Publishing Process Manager Romina Krebel

Technical Editor Teodora Smiljanic

Cover Designer InTech Design Team

Additional hard copies can be obtained from orders@intechopen.com

Ultrasound Imaging – Medical Applications, Edited by Igor Minin and Oleg Minin
p. cm.
ISBN 978-953-307-279-1

For EU product safety concerns:
IN TECH d.o.o., Prolaz Marije Krucifikse Kozulić 3, 51000 Rijeka, Croatia, info@intechopen.com or visit our website at intechopen.com.

Meet the editors

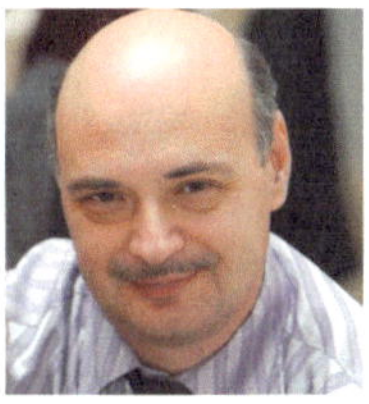

Igor V. Minin is a full Professor in the Department of Information Protection at Novosibirsk State Technical University (NSTU), Russia. Dr. Minin received a B.A. in Physics from the Novosibirsk State University, a Ph.D. in Physics from Leningrad Electro-Technical University in 1986 and a Doctor of science from NSTU in 2002. Dr. Minin has over twenty years of international industrial and academic experience and has played key roles in a number of projects including 3D millimeter wave real-time imaging and antiterrorism applications. He is the author or coauthor of approximately 350 research articles, seven monographs (including Diffractive optics of millimeter waves (IOP Publisher, Boston-London, 2004), Basic Principles of Fresnel Antenna Arrays (Springer, 2008)), and has been awarded 24 patents and inventions. He is the author of several books and book chapters in technical publications and has been the Editor of several books including Microwave and Millimeter Wave Technologies Modern UWB antennas and equipment (InTech Open Access Publisher, 2010) and Microwave and Millimeter Wave Technologies from Photonic Bandgap Devices to Antenna and Applications (InTech Open Access Publisher, 2010).

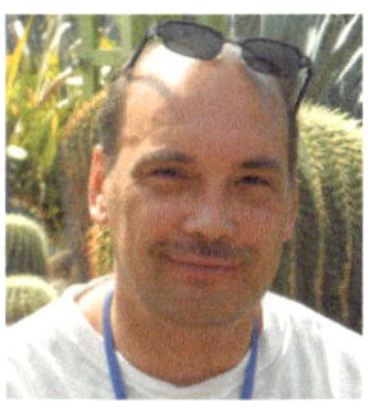

Oleg V. Minin received a B.A. in Physics from the Novosibirsk State University, a Ph.D. in Physics from Tomsk State University in 1987 and a Doctor of science from NSTU in 2002. He is currently a full Professor in the Department of Information Protection at Novosibirsk State Technical University (NSTU), Russia. From 1982 to 2001 he was Chief Research Scientist at the Institute of Applied Physics, Novosibirsk, Russia. Dr. Minin's research interests are in the areas of diffractive optics and antenna experiment (including explosive plasma antenna), millimeter wave and THz photonics and nanophotonics, information security, detection of hidden weapons as well as development of antiterrorism devices, experiment technologies, explosive physics. He is a member of SPIE, COST-284 and COST-ic0603 and he is the author of several books and book chapters in technical publications. For his work Dr. Minin was awarded the Commendation for Excellence in Technical Communications (LaserFocusWorld, 2003) and commendation by the Minister of Defense of Russia, 2000.

Contents

Preface

Despite that ultrasound has been in existence for more than 100 years and is considered a mature technology by many, the field is constantly evolving. The history of ultrasound can be traced to L.Spallanzani. In 1790 he experimented with bats and found that they maneuvered through the air using their hearing rather than sight. In 1880, Pierre and Jacques Curie discovered the piezoelectric effect using natural quartz. Later physicist Paul Langevin attempted to develop piezoelectric materials as senders and receivers of high-frequency mechanical disturbances (ultrasound waves) through materials. His specific application was the use of ultrasound to detect submarines during World War I. Industrial uses of ultrasound began in 1928 with the suggestion of Soviet Physicist Dr.Sokolov that it could be used to detect hidden flaws in materials. Medical uses of ultrasound through the 1930s were confined to therapeutic applications such as cancer treatments and physical therapy for various ailments. The potential of ultrasound as an imaging modality was realized as early as in late 1940's when several groups of investigators around the world utilizing sonar and radar technology developed during World War II started exploring diagnostic capabilities of ultrasound. he publication by Dr. Dussik (Austria) in 1942 on their work on transmission ultrasound investigation of the brain was the first published medical ultrasonic application. Since then, with the development of the computer technology, ultrasound sensors technology, and the use of micro gas-bubble based contrast agents enable the resolution and quality of the ultrasound imaging to improve substantially. In 1955 S.Satomura and Y.Nimura were credited for the earliest development of ultrasonic Doppler devices for monitoring tissue motion and blood flow. In 1985 color Doppler flow mapping system that combined Doppler flow imaging in color with B-mode imaging in gray scale was introduced by Aloka.

Ultrasonic imaging is one of the most important tools in diagnostic medicine and nondestructive testing today. The objective of this book is to provide graduate students, researchers, engineers and physicists involved in Ultrasound Imaging the latest information on state-of-the-art work in the development and application of Ultrasound Imaging.

This reference book is a collection of 17 chapters characterized in 3 parts: ultrasonic imaging, medical applications and clinical applications of ultrasonic.

This book provides an overview of ultrafast ultrasound imaging, 3D high-quality ultrasonic imaging, correction of phase aberrations in medical ultrasound images, etc.

Several interesting medical and clinical applications area are also discusses in the book like use of three dimensional ultrasound imaging in evaluation of Asherman's syndrome, the role of 3D ultrasound in assessment of endometrial receptivity and follicular vascularity to predict the quality oocyte, ultrasound imaging in vascular diseases and the fetal palate, clinical application of ultrasound molecular imaging, Doppler abdominal ultrasound in small animals and so on.

Prof. Dr. Igor Minin
Prof. Dr. Oleg Minin
Novosibirsk State Technical University
Russia

Part 1

Ultrasonic Imaging

1

Ultrafast Ultrasound Imaging

Jeremy Bercoff
SuperSonic Imagine
France

1. Introduction

Ultrasound can be considered as a disruptive technology in the medical device arena (Christensen, 2003). A disruptive technology has the potential to break the rules of existing markets. Thanks to its real time capabilities, its non ionizing properties and its cost - much lower than any other medical modality - ultrasound has significantly impacted clinical segments within radiology, obstetrics, vascular or cardiology and created new markets of emergency medicine and intervention. It could, in the future, change the rules for screening (where whole breast ultrasound devices are entering the market of breast imaging), diagnosis (with the standardization of elastography techniques in the prostate) and surgery (with HIFU – High Intensity Focused Ultrasound –, histotripsy devices and therapy monitoring tools).

In this context, innovations in the ultrasound field always have enormous potential. In the history of ultrasound, many innovations have been developed since its establishment as a medical imaging device in the 1960s, roughly one or two per decade (Szabo, 2004). The key innovation that launched the modality in the 1960s, is the real time imaging capability through mechanical scanning. Multichannel systems with electronic control of transducer arrays were developed in the 1970s. In the 1980s, flow analysis tools came to maturity through color flow imaging and quantitative Doppler modes (Pulse Wave Doppler - PWD). In the 1990's significant improvements in image quality were made possible with the introduction of real time compounding techniques and harmonic imaging. Although many of these concepts were studied in research laboratories years before the commercial dates cited above, it is systematically the maturity of a new technology that trigger the introduction of the innovations on commercially available platforms: for example, real time imaging was triggered by microprocessors development, Doppler modes were prompted by digital signal processing chips with enough dynamics to detect, at the same time, very weak blood signal and strong tissue echoes. The introduction of low cost Analog to Digital (A/D) converters has led to fully digital systems, significantly increasing the quality of the information delivered. Harmonic imaging was triggered by large bandwidth transducers, allowing reception of the signal at twice the transmit frequency.

In the first decade of the 21st century, technology moved towards extensive miniaturization leading to the introduction of high performances portable devices. Portable devices have created new markets for ultrasound - the emergency market for example, underlying again the disruptive potential of the modality. Today portable devices are the primary sources of

market growth in the industry and miniaturization can be considered as a global trend of the ultrasound industry: available technologies and innovations are progressively integrated in portable systems.
The figure below summarizes the evolution of ultrasound in the last decades.

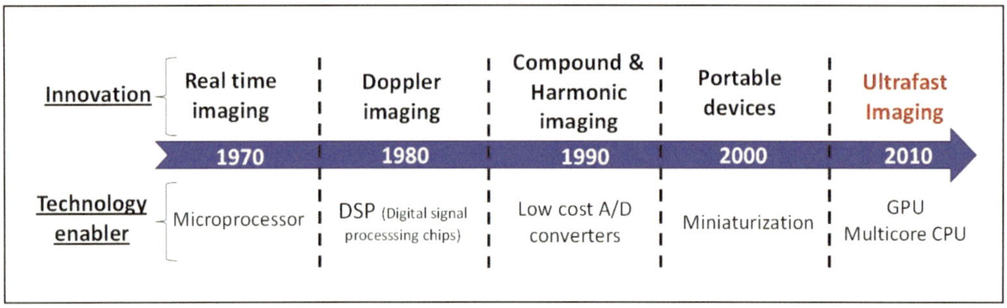

Fig. 1. A few important innovations in ultrasound imaging and their corresponding technology enablers.

Today a new technological breakthrough is ongoing with the advent of massive parallel computing capabilities. This results from the incredible demand in processing and display performances needed in the videogame industry. In addition to multicore architecure CPU's, new graphical processing units (GPU) allow parallel processing on thousands of channels simultaneously. This technology is available for the ultrasound industry and is the enabler to full software-based architecture systems. In 2009, SuperSonic Imagine introduced the first full software-based ultrasound system (Aixplorer®): instead of increasing integrated hardware processing channels, all the processing is performed by the software unit (CPU and GPUs). The concept of processing channels disappears - the system is able to compute in parallel as many channels as required by the acquisition.
This architecture paves a new way to perform ultrasound imaging: ultrafast ultrasound imaging. This is the focus of this chapter: what is ultrafast imaging (section 2), what new information can be assessed using it (section 3), how can we revisit standard ultrasound modes using ultrafast capabilities and enhance performances of current ultrasound devices (sections 4) and what innovations could it bring in the future (section 5) ?

2. Ultrafast ultrasound imaging: definition and example

2.1 Conventional ultrasound imaging

Ultrasound imaging is usually performed by sequential insonification of the medium using focused beams. Each focused beam allows the reconstruction of one image line. A typical 2D image is made of a few tens of lines (64 to 512). The overall sequence is illustrated on Fig. 2. The frame rate of the imaging mode is set by the time required to transmit a beam, receive and process the backscattered echoes from the medium and repeat that for all the lines of the image.
For a conventional 2D image, the time to build an image is:

$$T_{image} = \frac{N_{lines} * 2 * Z}{c} \tag{1}$$

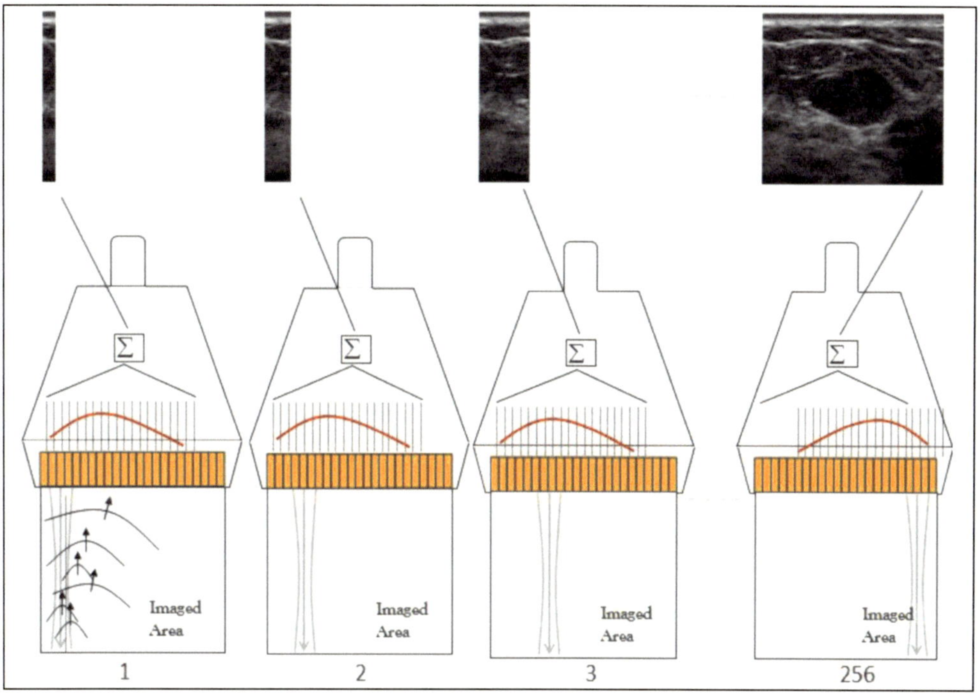

Fig. 2. Conventional imaging acquisition process

Where Z is the image depth, c the speed of ultrasound waves assumed constant (1540 m/s) and Nlines the number of lines in the image.
The maximum frame rate that can be reached with this technique is:

$$FR_{\max} = \frac{1}{T_{image}} \tag{2}$$

For example, an image of 5cm in depth and 256 lines in width would have the following frame rate:

$$FR_{\max} = 60Hz \tag{3}$$

Ultrasound system architectures were designed to process one image line at a time.

2.2 Increasing ultrasound imaging frame rate

Limitations of the conventional approach appears as soon as higher frame rates are required, typically in echocardiography for the heart motion analysis, as well as in 3D/4D imaging where the number of lines become significant (~ a few thousands).
Parallelization schemes have been considered to overcome these limitations. In the academic area this has been reported as soon as the late 70's (Delannoy, 1979; Shattuck, 1984; Von Ramm, 1991). Most current systems have multiline capabilities: for each transmit beam, several lines (typically from 2 to 16) are computed. Multiline processing can be used either to increase the frame rate (for echocardiography for example) either to increase the number of lines computed per image (for 3D imaging).

2.3 Ultrafast imaging

With or without multiline capabilities, current ultrasound systems are built on a serialized architecture and images are reconstructed sequentially from several equivalent transmits.
Ultrafast imaging breaks this paradigm. An ultrafast imaging system is able to compute in parallel as many lines as requested and is therefore capable of computing a full image from one single transmit whatever the size and the characteristics of the image. In such a system the image frame rate is no longer limited by the number of lines reconstructed but by the time of flight of a single pulse to propagate in the medium and get back to the transducer. Table 1 gives typical frame rates for different ultrasound clinical applications using conventional and ultrafast architectures.

Application	Typical imaging depth	Conventional architecture	Ultrafast architecture
Abdominal imaging	20 cm	20 Hz	3800Hz
Cardiac Imaging	15 cm	150 Hz	5000Hz
Breast imaging	5 cm	60 Hz	15000 Hz

Table 1. Example of typical frame rates in different clinical applications for conventional and ultrafast architectures.

New applications of ultrafast systems have been reported in the literature. Fink demonstrated for the first time that transient shear waves, never visualized before on an ultrasound scanner, can be imaged (Sandrin, 2000). Jensen used an ultrafast device to implement synthetic imaging techniques and derive vectorial estimation of flow motion (Jensen 2005). Ultrafast prototypes reported in those works allowed the storage of acquisitions in a digital memory stack and then the transfer to a PC. Processing was then performed offline on the stored data.
Although the concept of ultrafast imaging has been explored in academics during the last decade, it is only recently that this technology has entered the commercial realm due to major technological barriers that had to be overcome.
For example, to achieve ultrafast imaging, the image computation must be performed on a fully parallelized platform, typically a software-based platform.
There are two technologically challenging aspects to building a fully software-based platform:

- the data transfer rate from the acquisition module to the processing unit. As raw (non beamformed) Radio Frequency (RF) signals are directly transferred to the PC, the data rate required to perform real time imaging is huge: several GigaBytes/s.
- the processing unit needs to be powerful enough to ensure real time imaging. As an example, conventional gray scale imaging requires 1 to 2 Gigaflops (multiplication + addition) per second.

New powerful processing units (GPUs) have reached a satisfactory level of performance at the end of the 2000s. Consequently, GPU's are more and more used in the medical field to speed up processing algorithms (Schiwietz, 2006; Xu, 2007; Rosenzweig, 2011). The ultrafast architecture leverages this processing power by combining it with fast numerical links (PCI express technology) capable of transferring huge volume of data to these units. This combination allows the shift of the beamforming process - the most demanding processing step of an ultrasound system - from hardware to software, enabling full parallelization of ultrasound image computation.
Fig. 3 represents the architecture of an ultrafast system compared to a conventional one.

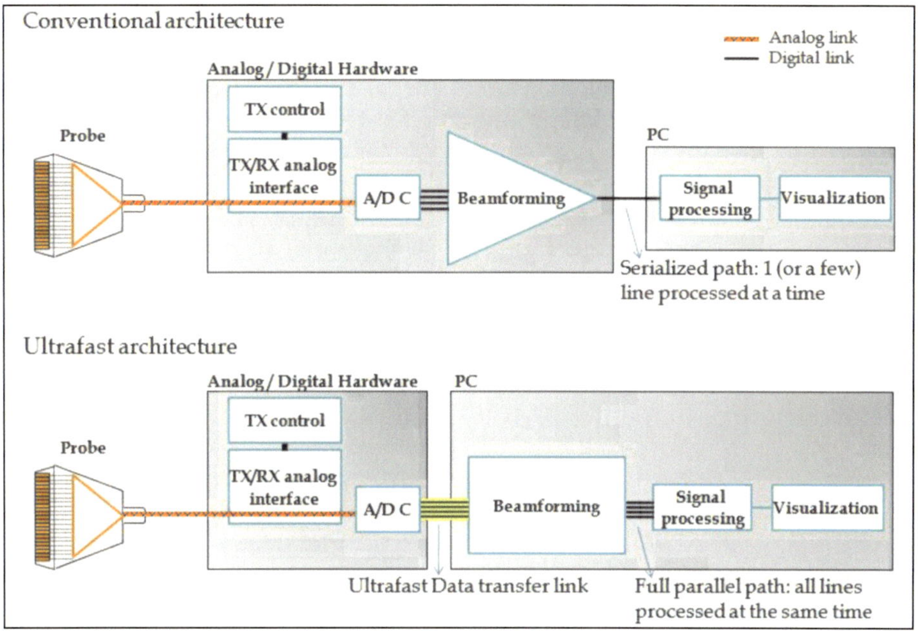

Fig. 3. As beamforming is performed in software, full parallelization of image formation can be performed. Each insonification can therefore lead to a full image. (TX refers to Transmit and RX to Receive).

2.4 Ultrafast imaging using coherent plane wave compound

There are many ways to leverage an Ultrafast imaging architecture (Lu, 1998; Jensen 2005). SuperSonic Imagine's approach is based on the use of plane wave insonifications. A plane wave is generated by applying flat delays on the transmit elements of the ultrasound probe as illustrated on Fig. 4. The generated wave will insonify the whole area of interest.

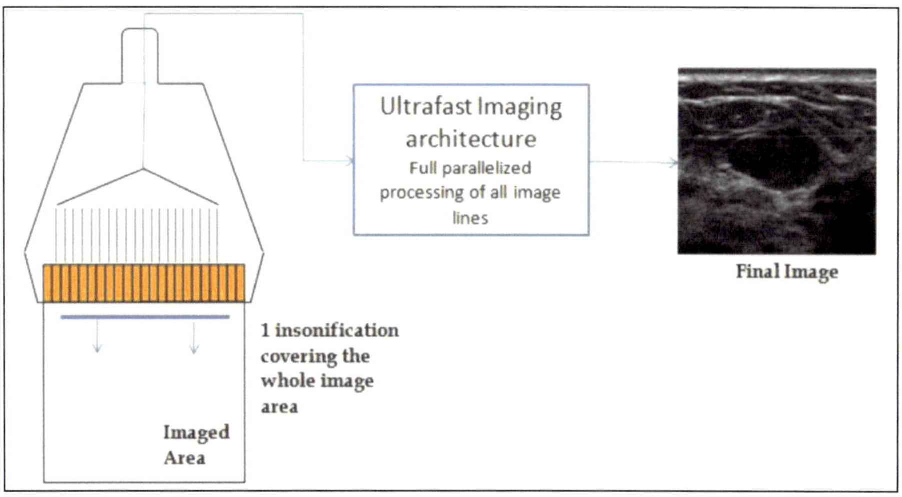

Fig. 4. A plane wave is sent by a linear transducer and insonifies the whole region of interest. An ultrasound image is computed from this single insonification.

The backscattered echoes are then recorded and processed by the ultrafast scanner to compute an image of the insonified area.
Plane wave imaging allows the computation of one full ultrasound image per transmit at the expense of the image quality. As the transmit focalization step is removed, the image contrast and resolution are reduced, as illustrated in the figure below:

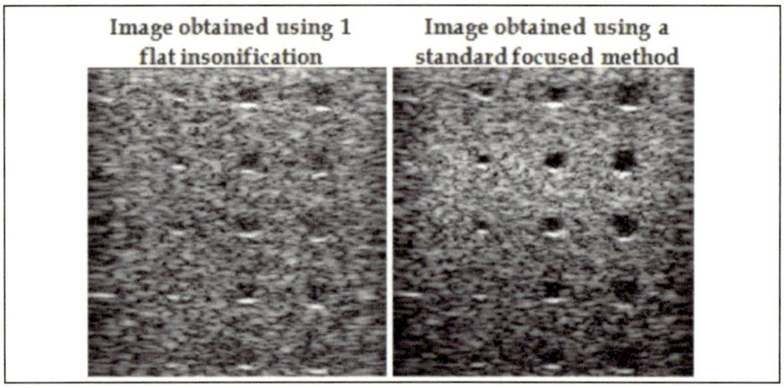

Fig. 5. Image of a phantom with anechoic inclusion of different sizes with plane wave insonification (left) and standard focused method (right). The images were acquired with a 5 MHz linear probe.

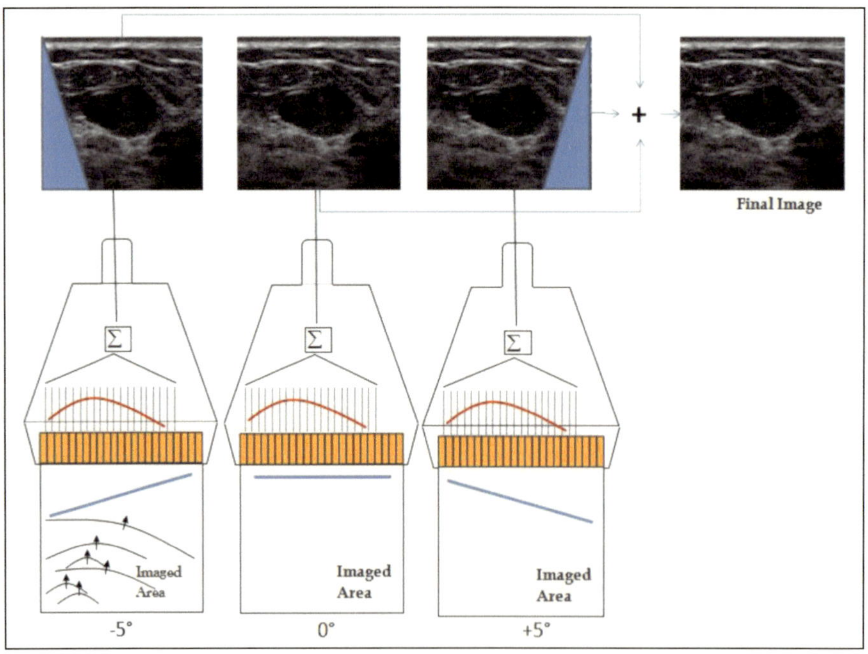

Fig. 6. Ultrasound image obtained using ultrafast coherent plane wave compound

To overcome this limitation, several tilted plane waves are sent into the medium (Montaldo, 2009) and coherently summed to compute a full image. Using this method the transmit focalization step is retrospectively done by this summation (Fig. 6). The quality of the final

image is therefore dependent on the number of angles used to reconstruct it as illustrated on Fig. 7.
There is a trade off between the maximum ultrafast frame rate achievable by the mode and the image quality: the higher the number of angles, the better the image quality.

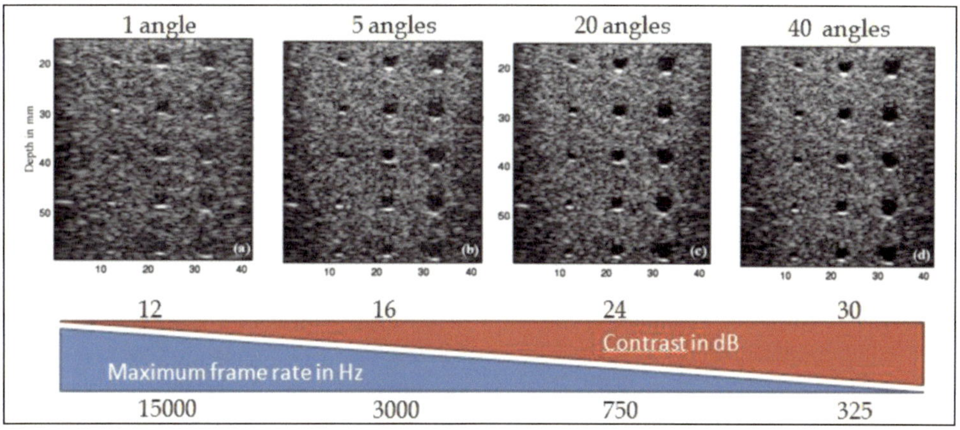

Fig. 7. Image quality as a function of the number of angles used to compute the final ultrasound image for a 40mm depth image.

The ultrafast compounded acquisition sequence presents several advantages:
- Firstly, the retrospective transmit focalization can be done dynamically for each pixel of the image increasing the homogeneity of the final image compared to physical insonification.
- Secondly, the number of firings required to obtain an image of a quality equivalent to a focused mode (in terms of contrast and resolution) is around 5 to 10 times lower (Montaldo, 2009). As a consequence, frame rates of ultrasound imaging can be increased by the same factor using coherent plane wave strategies on an ultrafast system. Fig. 8 shows an example of equivalent quality ultrasound images using the coherent plane wave approach and the focused one. Maximum reachable frame rates increase from 30 Hz to more than 300 Hz.
- Finally by cleverly trading off the compromises in the image quality, imaging frame rates of a few thousands of Hz can be reached and allow a full new range of applications and innovations.

This chapter presents two innovations that leverage ultrafast imaging on an ultrasound system: the first one is a new imaging mode called Shear Wave Elastography that provides quantitative visco-elastic analysis of tissues. The second one is a new way to perform Doppler flow analysis changing the performances and workflow paradigms of current available Color and PW modes.

3. Shear wave elastography

3.1 Transient shear waves for tissue mechanical investigation

Ultrasound imaging provides both morphological (gray scale images) and functional imaging (flow imaging) of soft tissue. Using ultrafast capabilities, a third dimension can be added to ultrasound: physio-pathological information through the assessment of tissue

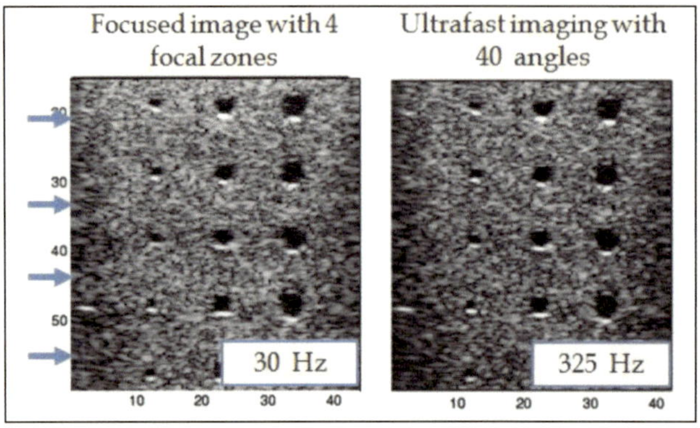

Fig. 8. 2 images of equivalent quality using focused (left) and ultrafast (right) techniques. Maximum achievable frame rates are respectively 30 and 325 Hz.

viscoelasticity. Ultrafast imaging can be used to capture phenomena that have never been imaged on commercial ultrasound devices: transient shear waves propagating in soft tissue. Shear wave imaging leads to quantification of tissue mechanical properties.

3.1.1 Shear waves in soft tissues

Two types of mechanical waves propagate in soft tissue: compressional waves (ultrasound waves are compressional waves in a given frequency range) and shear waves. Compressional waves travel much faster than shear waves in soft tissue: typically 1 to 1500m/s compared to 10m/s for shear waves. In other words, the bulk modulus (K) of soft tissue is much larger than the shear modulus (μ) (a factor 10^6 higher).

$$K >> \mu \tag{4}$$

This has two important consequences:

- Tissue viscoelasticity is only dependent on the shear modulus. The Young's modulus, that quantifies tissue viscoelasticity, can be written :

$$E = \frac{9 * K * \mu}{3K + \mu} \approx 3\mu \tag{5}$$

- The difference in propagation speed is so large that shear wave motion can be considered as negligible during the propagation time of a compressional wave. Imaging methods relying on compressional waves such as ultrasound can therefore be used to record propagation of shear waves. Note that this is not true in other solids such as metals or rocks (in seismology for example, bulk waves cannot image shear waves)

In summary, shear waves reflect tissue viscoelasticity properties and they can be imaged using ultrasound.

3.1.2 Imaging shear waves: need for ultrafast imaging

If compressional waves can propagate within tissue on a very large frequency range [up to the GHz), shear waves suffer from much stronger viscous/attenuation effects. Maximum shear wave frequencies propagating in human tissue are organ-dependent and typically vary between 500 Hz and 2000 Hz. As a consequence the minimum frame rate required to

correctly sample transient waves are of a few thousands Hertz (from 1000 Hz to 4000Hz taking the Nyquist limit).
Those frame rates are only achievable using ultrafast imaging.
In order to image shear waves, the system must be tuned to maximize the imaging frame rate. Typically a single flat wave is sent to compute a full image (Fig. 4), allowing to reach the required frame rates (a few thousands Hz), the maximum value only depending on the considered image depth (time of flight of the wave back and forth from the maximum depth imaged).

3.1.3 Generating transient shear waves

There are three different types of source of transient shear waves in the body.
The first type is natural body vibrations: heart beating, arterial pulses or voice are examples of vibrating sources that induce shear waves. It is a free source of information but the assessment of reliable information is challenging outside of the vicinity of the vibrating organ.
To better control the generation of the vibration, external vibrators that create controlled transient pulses have been proposed. The first report of externally generated transient shear wave analysis was published in the 1990s (Catheline, 1999). A that time, ultrafast imaging was not used and shear wave propagation was analyzed along a single ultrasound line. The work was extended to 2D shear wave imaging using the first ultrafast imaging prototype (Sandrin, 2000) and the first quantitative elasticity image was shown.
Also in the late 1990s, Sarvazyan proposed a third way to generate transient shear waves in the body (Sarvazyan, 1998): the acoustic radiation force induced by ultrasound beams. If sufficient energy if applied at the focus of an ultrasound beam, tissue can be remotely pushed in the direction of the ultrasound wave propagation. A transient shear wave that propagates transversally is generated as illustrated on Fig. 9.

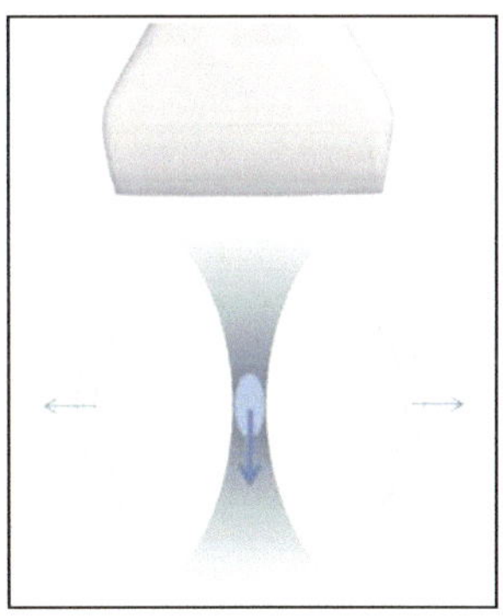

Fig. 9. Radiation force from an ultrasound focused beam generates a transverse bipolar shear wave.

In Sarvazyan's setup, the shear wave was induced with a specific transducer and the motion was recorded using a separate conventional scanner and iterative methods.
In 2004, a new imaging mode has been introduced coupling radiation force induced transient shear waves and ultrafast imaging called Supersonic Shear Imaging (Bercoff, 2004). In this approach, the shear wave is generated and imaged with the same ultrasound probe. The generation method was based on the induction of a shear wave source that moves into

the body at a supersonic speed, allowing, through the equivalent of a sonic boom, the creation of high amplitude shear waves in human organs.

3.1.4 Measuring tissue viscoelasticity

Once properly generated and imaged, a transient shear wave can provide many insights on the mechanical properties of the imaged tissue. Fig. 10 illustrates the propagation of a shear wave in a tissue-mimicking phantom using Supersonic Shear Imaging. The wave is captured on a 2D imaging plane thanks to ultrafast imaging.

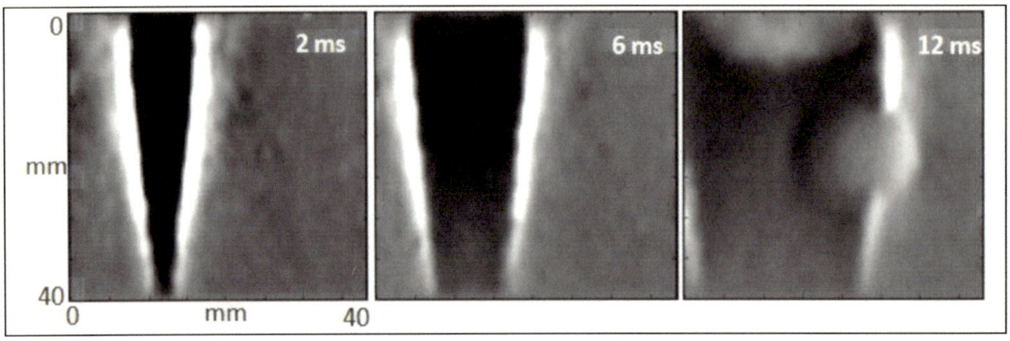

Fig. 10. 3 snapshots of a shear wavefront propagating in a phantom. The gray level indicates amplitude of the displacements generated by the shear in the tissue. The wavefront is distorted when passing through a harder inclusion (right image) as the shear wave propagates faster in the inclusion.

The phase velocity as a function of the frequency as well as the group velocity can be calculated locally.

Fig. 11 shows a group velocity map derived from the ultrafast imaging scanner in the same mimicking phantom.

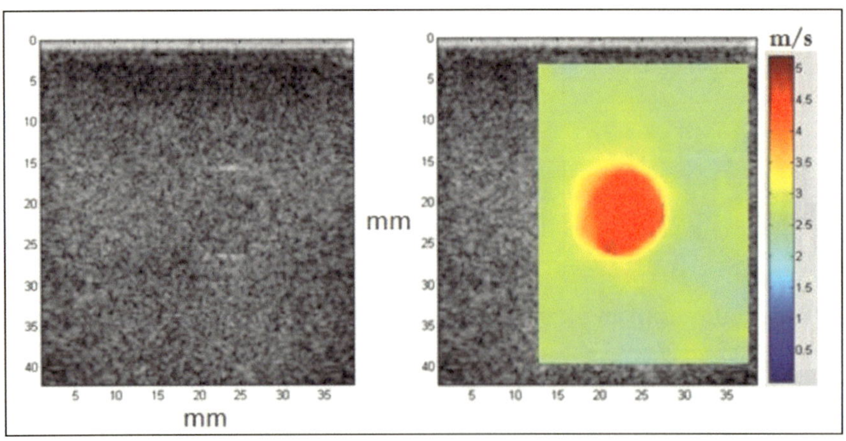

Fig. 11. Shear wave velocity map superimposed on the ultrasound image of the phantom. The harder spherical inclusion appears on the velocity map in red while it is barely visible on the ultrasound image. This enhances the fact that the contrast given by both imaging modes are uncorrelated.

Because the shear wave is imaged inside the medium, all wave components can be assessed and used for velocity estimation including evanescent waves. The resolution of the shear wave velocity image is therefore not limited by the shear wavelength but by the wavelength of the imaging method, i.e. ultrasound. In the above example, the resolution of the image is 1mm while the shear wavelength is around 15 mm.

Depending on the organ, different rheological models can be used to derive tissue mechanical characteristics from the shear wave propagation map.

- In a purely elastic medium, phase velocity does not vary as a function of frequency (Royer, 2000) and is equal to the group velocity. The velocity is directly linked to tissue Young's modulus E through the formula where c is the shear wave speed and ρ the tissue density.

$$E = 3\rho c^2 \tag{6}$$

- In a viscoelastic medium such as breast or liver, the phase velocity increases as a function of frequency. Many rheological models can be considered such as the Voigt or the thermoviscous models. Most of them appear to be consistent only in a limited frequency range (Orescanin, 2010). A well-established model for compressional waves is the time causal model (Szabo, 2004) which shows a power law dependence of the attenuation and phase velocity as a function of frequency and works on the full frequency range. It can also be applied to shear waves:

$$\frac{1}{c(f)} = \frac{1}{c(f_0)} + \alpha \tan\left(\frac{\pi y}{2}\right)\left[|f|^{y-1} - |f_0|^{y-1}\right] \tag{7}$$

  f and fo represents frequencies of analysis, α and y the two parameters modelizing the power law dependence of the attenuation. Analysis of the shear wave propagation allows deduction of c(fo), α and y enabling full rheological characterization of the tissue. In such cases, the estimation of group velocity values gives a representation of medium viscoelasticity at the central frequency of the wave spectral content.

- In a thin medium that has geometrical characteristics much smaller than the shear wavelength, such as arteries, guidance of the shear waves through medium leads to geometrical dispersion effects. Depending on the medium external environment and its geometrical characteristics, shear wave velocity propagation can be modeled and Young modulus can be deduced. The formula for a cylindrical artery can be written (Couade, 2010):

$$v = \sqrt{K \frac{\omega h c}{\sqrt{3}}} \tag{8}$$

Where c is the shear wave speed in an infinite medium, ω the frequency, h the height of the artery and K a correction factor. Young's modulus can then be deduced using the formula (6).

3.2 A new imaging mode in ultrasound imaging

3.2.1 Presentation

Basic concepts introduced in the Supersonic Shear Imaging technique (Bercoff, 2004) have been used to create a real time imaging mode, called ShearWave Elastography (SWE), on a commercially available system. Two key aspects have made this innovation transfer possible:

- An new technology (multicore CPU, GPUs, as explained above) for the building of a ultrafast imaging system able to image transient shear waves.

- A user workflow enabler: using this approach, the generation and imaging of the shear wave is performed with the same ultrasound probe as the one conventionally used for other imaging modes. No additional material is necessary to perform elasticity imaging. Acceptance of the mode in the clinical workflow is easier and the learning curve for the new mode is minimized.

The SWE mode is an additional real-time imaging mode that provides tissue elasticity estimation in kiloPascal (Fig. 12).

In its primary implementation, the mode estimates the shear wave group velocity locally and deduces the value in kPa assuming the medium is purely elastic (eq 6). This is done in real time on a 2D image plane as illustrated on figure below.

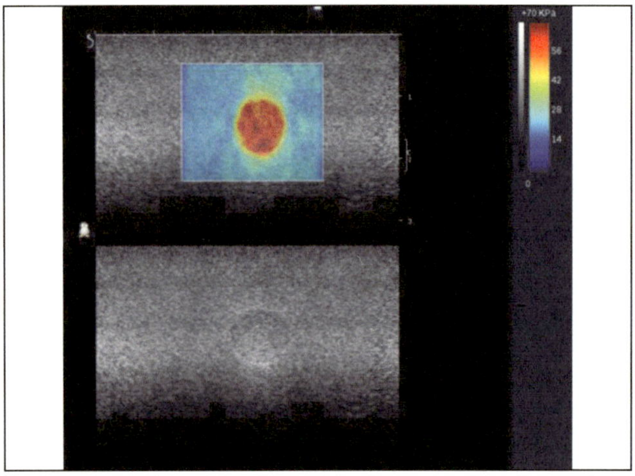

Fig. 12. ShearWave Elastography mode: Elasticity Information is displayed in real time in a box with color coded values.

Recently, the mode has been implemented on a specific probe providing volumetric imaging. In addition to axial view, transverse and coronal views of lesions elasticity distribution can be assessed as illustrated on figure below:

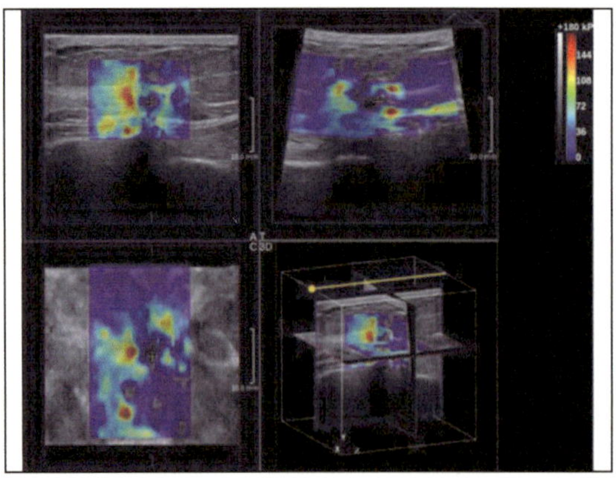

Fig. 13. 3D ShearWave Elastography. 3 planes can be viewed. By navigating within the volume the displayed imaging plane can be chosen.

Volume assessment can be performed allowing more accurate visualization and quantification of elastic distribution. 3D SWE may be extremely useful in the framework of therapy monitoring.

Indeed complementary information of tissue stiffness changes can increase information on response to therapy compared to simple tumor volume size. Additional modules for specific applications requiring more complex rheological modelizations can be envisioned. In the example below, it is possible to measure and display the phase velocity as a function of the wave frequency in a region of interest of the liver. In addition to the group velocity, the slope of the phase velocity variation can be assessed. This full assessment of the liver viscoelasticity could be of great interest for diffuse liver disease diagnostics and staging.

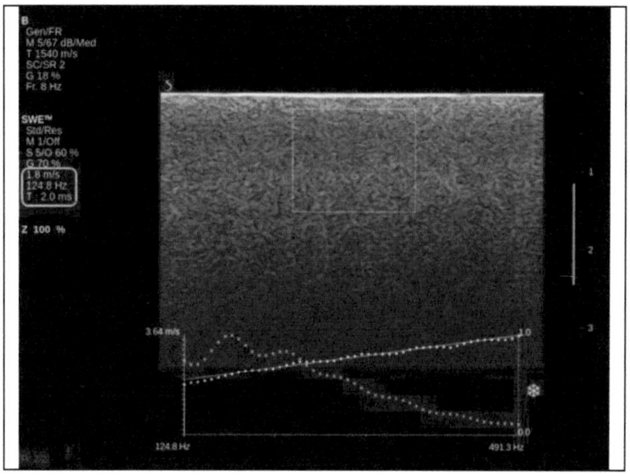

Fig. 14. Dispersion of shear waves in liver assessed by ShearWave Elastography. The white curve represents the shear wave phase velocity as a function of the frequency calculated in the square box displayed on the gray scale image. The yellow one is the spectrum amplitude of the transient wave. The group velocity, the central frequency of the shear wave and the relaxation time (in ms) corresponding to the slope of the curve are displayed to the left of the image.

The same principle can be applied to reconstruct the arterial Young's modulus by combining the group velocity measurement and the thickness of the artery as described in (8).

3.2.2 Clinical value

The ShearWave Elastography (SWE) mode has recently been implemented for different organs. Fig. 15 shows elasticity images in the breast, tendons, liver and prostate.

Multicentric studies to assess the clinical value of the mode are currently ongoing:

- Breast: SWE could potentially help improve the diagnosis of breast lesions by increasing the overall accuracy of the BI-RADS® (Mendelson, 2001) classification. Recent studies have shown promising results for breast cancer diagnostic (Evans, 2010). SWE could help correctly reclassify malignant lesions that would have been missed with ultrasound alone and declassify benign lesions that would have been biopsied. From a global perspective this could lead to a reduction of the number of unnecessary biopsies and an increase in positive biopsy rate reducing healthcare cost and patient's stressful experience.

A multicentric study on 1800 patients and 17 clinical sites is ongoing to confirm these preliminary results.

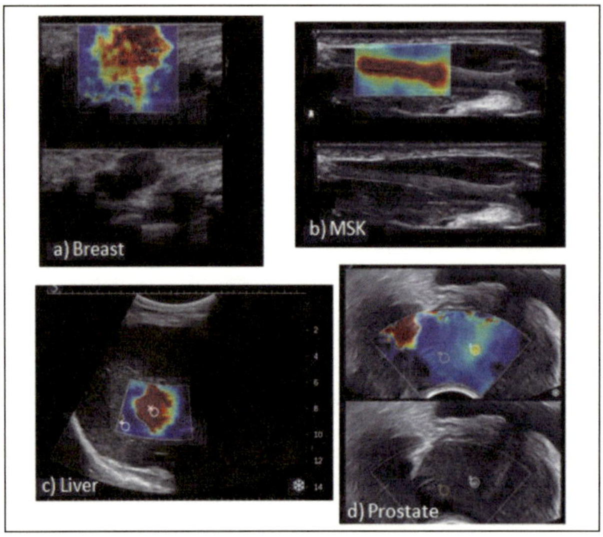

Fig. 15. SWE images in a) breast , b) MSK, c) liver, d) prostate

- Liver: SWE is currently being evaluated in the framework of diffuse liver disease staging and on its ability to improve the diagnosis of focal lesions. A preliminary study on 113 patients (Bavu, 2011) demonstrated high accuracy of fibrosis staging using SWE.
- Thyroid: As for breast, SWE could increase the diagnosis accuracy . The number of benign nodules that are undergoing Fine Needle Aspiration is currently extremely high. A preliminary study (Sebag, 2010) demonstrated very promising results on the pertinence of elasticity images for nodule characterization. More importantly, the specific case of follicular neoplasm raises an important issue as 85% of surgeries of this type of lesions are done for benign lesions.
- Prostate: SWE could be of great interest for improved detection rate of prostate cancer, through localization of prostate lesions, monitor localized treatments. Ongoing studies intend to demonstrate the value of SWE for increased positive biopsy rate in the prostate diagnostic workflow.

3.2.3 Perspectives for SWE

Today, SWE is mainly positioned in the disease diagnosis of specific static organs (cited above). However, given its specificities, other domains could benefit from the mode:

- Its resolution (up to 1mm in superficial organs) and sensitivity (elastic contrasts of 20 % can be detected) could improve screening for specific organs.
- Its quantitative aspect, implemented on a 3D imaging system, can target the emerging field of localized and minimally (or non) invasive therapy monitoring (RF, Cryoablation, HIFU).
- Its ability to acquire the elasticity information on a wide region of interest in a few tens of milliseconds allows elasticity imaging of moving organs and the analysis of elasticity variation in time. Cardiology is one of the areas where SWE could bring tremendous clinical value. Preliminary studies demonstrated that SWE could be a reliable and easy tool to assess heart myocardial stiffening (Couade, 2011).

4. Changing the paradigm in blood flow analysis using ultrafast imaging

We demonstrated how ultrafast imaging could bring new information to the medical community by imaging fast transient phenomena such as shear waves. Ultrafast imaging can also be used to re-think conventional ultrasound modes. We will investigate in this section the potential of ultrafast imaging for flow analysis.

Doppler analysis is one of the most demanding features in ultrasound from a technical standpoint - the number and complexity of firings to acquire the information is huge - and from a performance standpoint - quantitative measurements are expected, raising the requirements of the mode in term of accuracy and reproducibility. Due to this complexity, Doppler tools suffer from technical limitations that impact the user in a significant way. It is shown here how ultrafast imaging can overcome those limitations and open new perspectives in Doppler analysis both in terms of performance and user workflow.

4.1 Ultrafast sequence for Doppler imaging

The same type of ultrafast sequences as the ones described above for B-mode (2.4) are used in Doppler imaging. Several tilted plane waves are sent into the medium and backscattered echoes are coherently summed to reconstruct ultrasound images. Then Doppler processing can be performed as on conventional images.

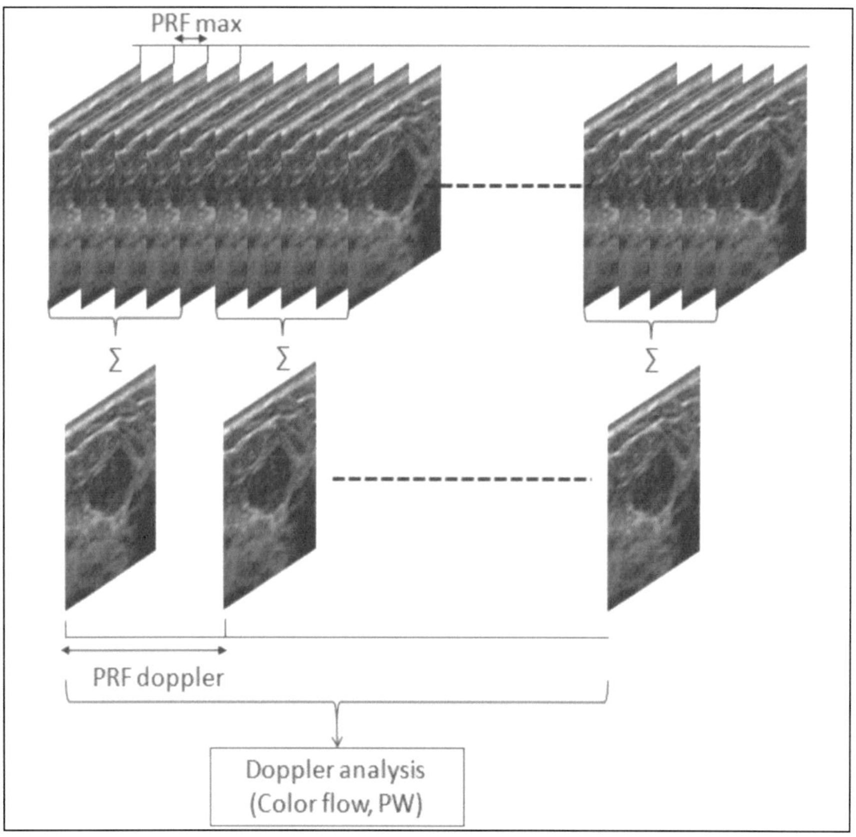

Fig. 16. Ultrafast compound imaging for Doppler analysis of flow.

The maximum number of angles that can be used to compute an image is limited by the acquisition Pulse Repetition Frequency ($PRF_{doppler}$) needed to measure the desired Doppler velocity scale (usually this value is set by the user).

$$Nangles = \frac{PRF_{\max}}{PRF_{doppler}} \tag{9}$$

Where PRFmax is the maximal PRF reachable given the imaging depth considered.
Interestingly, it has been shown, in Color flow imaging, that resolution and sensitivity equivalent to classical schemes can be obtained using only 9 different angles (Bercoff, 2011). This indicates that Doppler images can be acquired 10 to 15 times faster than with conventional approaches (For a typical 20 to 30 mm color box, around 100 lines are acquired). Such a huge gain in acquisition time can be used in several ways:

- Increase Doppler imaging modes performance: we demonstrate below increases in temporal resolution and sensitivity (4.2).
- Improve user workflow: this gain in time can be used to perform other acquisition types such as PW, potentially increasing performances of highly demanding modes such as triple mode (Bmode, Color flow imaging and PW simultaneously).
- Change Doppler mode paradigm by merging Color flow imaging and PW Doppler modes in a single acquisition and with this, increase the accuracy of the examination and reduce its overall time (4.3).

The use of several tilted plane compounded waves as described above is essential for the performance of the mode in terms of sensitivity and accuracy (Udesen, 2008).

4.2 Improving color flow imaging (CFI)

Conventional schemes offer limited frame rates for color flow imaging (typically 20 Hz) and suffer from severe trade-offs between image size and frame rate (that can go down to a few Hertz for boxes covering the whole image area). Ultrafast compound based Doppler imaging provides flow images with a temporal resolution never reached before on ultrasound systems whatever the box size. Complex and fast flows can be visualized in a much finer way potentially leading to a more reliable diagnosis of cardiovascular diseases such as stenoses.

The figure below shows images of a color flow clip acquired at 200 Hz (around 10 times faster than the conventional mode). A histogram of the velocities in one sample volume is provided as a function of time. It demonstrates the ability to quantify flow with very high temporal resolution.

With such high frame rates as demonstrated above (100- 200Hz), the visualization of the color clip can be done after acquisition through a slow motion movie.

For slower flow imaging, high frame rates are not necessary. Ultrafast sequences can therefore be tuned to increase spatial resolution and sensitivity. In a sensitive ultrafast acquisition, as the PRF required to measure slow flows is lower, the number of angles to compute a color image is increased to calculate the Doppler frequency shift. Sensitive color images acquired on the thyroid of a healthy volunteer is shown below and compared to classical color flow imaging. Deep small vessels are detected only on the ultrafast compounded image.

Increasing the ensemble length can even further optimize sensitivity. The number of samples used to calculate the flow per pixel can be increased up to a factor 15. Ultrasensitive images can be obtained like the ones reported by Institut Langevin on the rat brain (Macé, 2010) and may be of great interest in many applications: functional imaging of the brain, imaging of tumor vascularization, obstetrics....

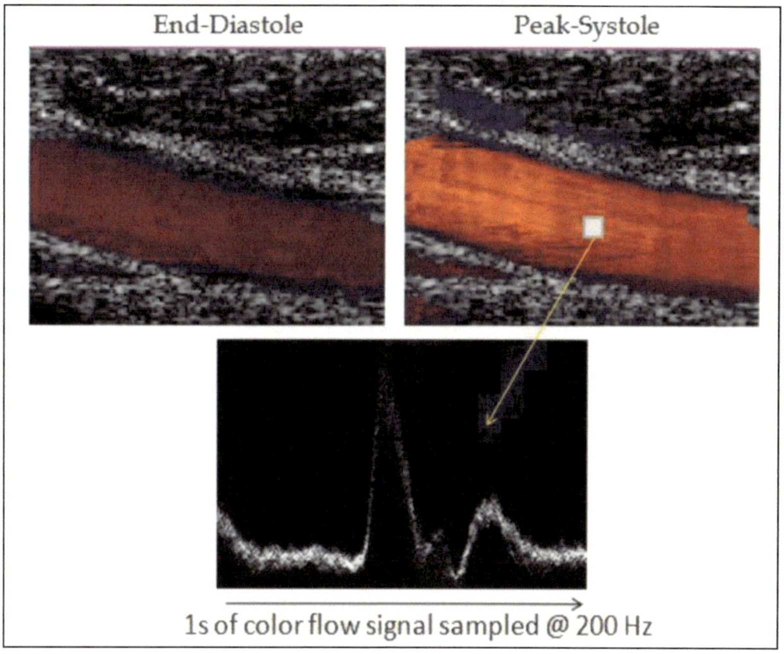

Fig. 17. Ultrafast color flow imaging provides very fine temporal resolution. The plot is computed by displaying a histogram of the velocity on the small ROI indicated as a function of time.

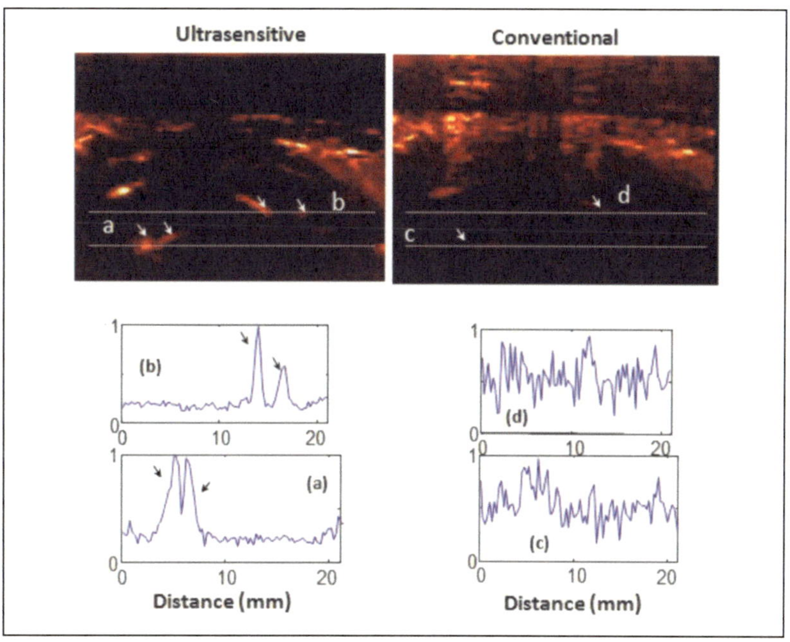

Fig. 18. Sensitive flow images based on ultrafast plane wave acquisition on the thyroid. Images have been acquired using 16 angles to compute ultrasound images and an ensemble length of 16 to deduce flow images.

From a general perspective, ultrafast imaging breaks usual limitations and compromises of color flow imaging:

- Clips of color data can be generated with higher sensitivity and frame rate than on conventional systems.
- The increase quality is maintained whatever the box size. Usual schemes suffer from trade-offs between frame rate and color box size. Using plane waves, the whole area of interest can be filled with color Doppler information without any drop in frame rate.

The information is consistent and synchronous all over the imaged area. Doppler pixels have been assessed at the same time on the contrary of focused strategies where lines are sequentially acquired. In a classical approach, the Doppler signals on the sides of the box are therefore acquired with a time lag that can reach several hundreds of milliseconds.

4.3 Quantitative ultrafast Doppler imaging

Conventional Doppler analysis is usually performed using in two ultrasound modes:

- the color flow imaging mode to spatially locate a region of interest
- the Pulsed Wave mode to perform quantitative measurements at the region of interest depicted by color flow imaging. PW mode is a local assessment of quantitative information - information is assessed at one single location at a time.

In clinical exams, the user constantly goes back and forth between those two modes and successively analyzes with the PW the locations pointed out by the color flow imaging mode. Triple mode (simultaneous color and PW) has been introduced to improve the user workflow. Despite some compromises on the PW spectrum quality, it facilitates the acquisition of information in many cases.

Using an ultrafast architecture, Doppler can be envisioned in a completely different manner: quantitative information is acquired at the same time in all pixels of the color box breaking the incompatibility between imaging and quantitative measurements. In a typical implementation, a one shot acquisition can be launched from the conventional color flow imaging mode. A full clip of Doppler data is acquired (typically 2 to 6 s) and the system is frozen. The user can then review the color flow imaging clip, locate the frame of interest that better depicts flow properties and perform PW measurements at several locations, allowing for the first time a comparison of spectra from different regions of interest from the same cardiac cycle.

The quantitative ultrafast Doppler acquisition workflow is illustrated on the figure 19.

Using the retrospective review of ultrafast data, many automatic tools can be added to help physician diagnosis:

- Comparison of flow data from several locations (as described above)
- Automatic localization of peak velocities within the image for accurate flow quantification
- Calculation and display of the mean and peak velocities all over the image
- Automatic calculation and compensation of the Doppler angle.

Ultrafast imaging opens perspectives to Doppler imaging by enhancing its performances, allowing visualization of very fast flow characteristics, perform accurate quantification and comparison of flow velocities through the whole image area and provide new types of visualization and automation tools. It will probably allow a significant reduction of the vascular exam duration as all data necessary for the diagnosis of a given area is acquired in a few seconds.. In the future, ultrafast Doppler could be used to derive new information such as the shear stress on the arterial wall, perform accurate vortex analysis and quantification

5. Conclusion

ShearWave Elastography and Ultrafast Doppler are two important innovations that are made possible thanks to ultrafast imaging. They are the first demonstrations of many other benefits that an ultrafast architecture can bring to the clinical world. Cardiovascular is one of the fields that could tremendously benefit from this technology. Ultrafast imaging can change the way moving organs are imaged. Recent works demonstrated, for example, the ability to locally measure Pulse Wave Velocity in the artery in less than one second (Couade 2010). Other publications reported dynamic analysis of heart mechanics using SWE for higher performance and more accurate detection of cardiovascular diseases. Elasticity of myocardium has been assessed locally as a function of time through a whole heart cycle (Couade 2011). Ultrafast imaging can also provide analysis of other transient phenomena that have not been extensively explored such as the dissolution of ultrasound contrast agents (Couture 2009) or the monitoring of brain activity (Macé 2010) through ultrasensitive flow images - positioning for the first time ultrasound in the field of functional brain imaging.

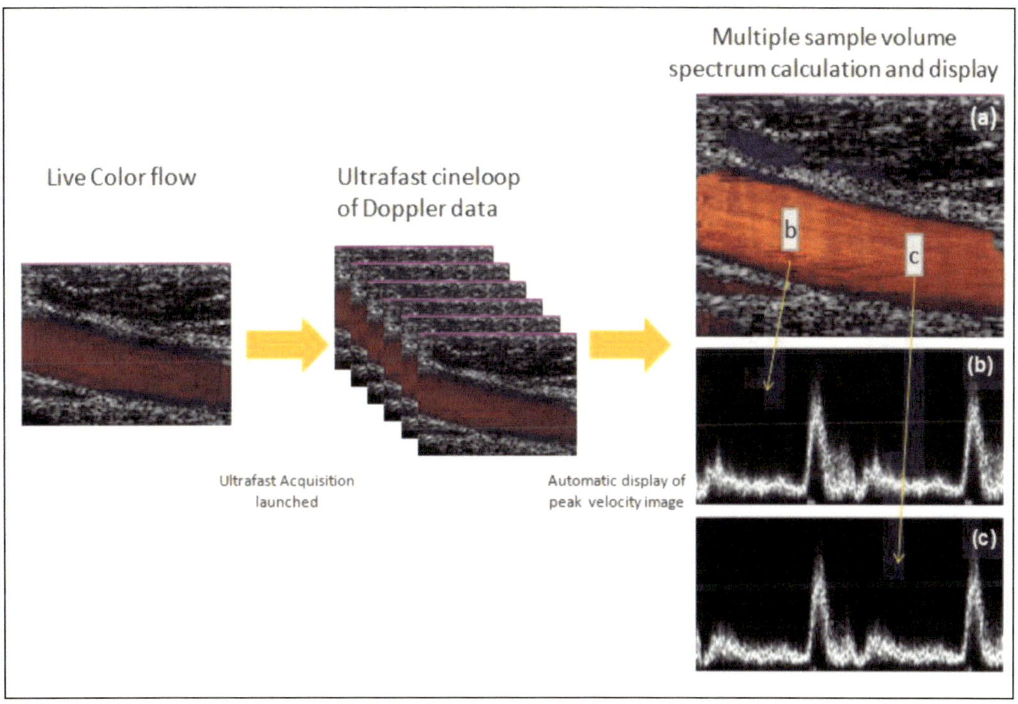

Fig. 19. Doppler analysis workflow.

There is no doubt that such ultrafast imaging based academic works will create new standards in ultrasound imaging in the next coming years - in 2D, as well as, on a longer perspective, in 4D.

6. Acknowledgment

I would like to thank Jessica Bercoff, Claude Cohen-Bacrie, Aline Criton, Michèle Debain and Jacques Souquet for their support, feedback and enthusiasm on this chapter as well as all scientific contributors of the reported work (Matt Bruce, Mathieu Couade, Nicolas Felix, Mathias Fink, Christophe Fraschini, Jean Luc Gennisson, Fabien Mezière, Emilie Macé, Gabriel Montaldo, Thanasis Loupas, Mathieu Pernot, David Savéry, Mickael Tanter ....)

7. References

Bavu, E.; Gennisson,J.L.; Couade, M.; Bercoff, J.; Mallet, V.; Fink, M.; Nalpasc, B.; Tanter, M.; Pol, S. (2011). *Non-invasive in-vivo Liver Fibrosis evaluation using Supersonic Shear Imaging: a clinical Study on 113 Hepatitis C Virus patients.* accepted for publication in Ultrasound in Medicine and Biology.

Bercoff, J.; Tanter, M.; Fink, M. (April 2004). *Supersonic shear imaging: A new technique for soft tissues elasticity mapping,* IEEE Transactions on Ultrasonics, Ferroelectrics and Frequency Control, vol. 51, no. 4, pp. 396–409.

Bercoff, J.; Montaldo, G.; Loupas, T.; Savery, D.; Mézière, F.; Fink, M.; Tanter, M. (January 2011). *Ultrafast compound Doppler imaging: providing full blood flow characterization,* IEEE Transactions on Ultrasonics, Ferroelectrics and Frequency Control, 58(1), pp. 134-47.

Catheline, S.; Wu, F.; Fink M. (May 1999). *A solution to diffraction biases in sonoelasticity: the acoustic impulse technique.* J Acoust Soc Am, 105(5), pp. 2941-50.

Christensen, C. M. (2003). *The Innovator's Dilemma,* HarperBusiness Essentials, 2003

Couade, M.; Pernot, M.; Prada, C.; Messas, E.; Emmerich, J.; Bruneval, P.; Criton, A.; Fink, M.; Tanter, M. (October 2010). *Quantitative assessment of arterial wall biomechanical properties using shear wave imaging,* Ultrasound Med Biol., 36(10), pp. 1662-76.

Couade, M.; Pernot, M.; Messas, E.; Bel, A.; Ba, M.; Hagege, A.; Fink, M.; Tanter, M. (February 2011). *In vivo quantitative mapping of myocardial stiffening and transmural anisotropy during the cardiac cycle.* IEEE Trans Med Imaging. 2011 Feb, 30(2), pp. 295-305.

Couture, O.; Bannouf, S.; Montaldo, G.; Aubry, J.F.; Fink, M.; Tanter, M. (November 2009). Ultrafast imaging of ultrasound contrast agents. Ultrasound Med Biol, 35(11), pp. 1908-16.

Delannoy, B.; Torgue, R.; Bruneel, C.; Bridou, E. (1979). Ultrafast electronic image reconstruction device, Echocardiology, Vol. 1, C. T. Lancee, Ed., ch. 3, pp 447-450.

Evans, A.; Whelehan, P.; Thomson, K.; McLean, D.; Brauer, K.; Purdie, C.; Jordan, L.; Baker, L.; Thompson, A. (2010). *Quantitative shear wave ultrasound elastography: initial experience in solid breast masses.* Breast Cancer Res. 12(6).

Jensen, J.A.; Holm, O.; Jerisen, L.J.; Bendsen, H.; Nikolov, S.I.; Tomov, B.G.; Munk, P.; Hansen, M.; Salomonsen, K.; Hansen, J.; Gormsen, K.; Pedersen, H.M.; Gammelmark, K.L. (May 2005). *Ultrasound research scanner for real-time synthetic aperture data acquisition,* IEEE Transactions on Ultrasonics, Ferroelectrics and Frequency Control, Volume 52, Issue 5, pp. 881 - 891

Lu, J-Y. (January 1998). *Experimental study of high frame rate imaging with limited diffraction beams,* IEEE Transactions on Ultrasonics, Ferroelectrics and Frequency Control, Volume 45, Issue 1, pp. 84 - 97

Macé, E.; Montaldo, G.; Bercoff, J.; Cohen, I.; Fink, M.; Tanter, M. (2010). *Ultrafast Doppler Imaging and its application to high sensitivity brain angiography.* IEEE UFFC conference.

Mendelson, E.B.; Berg, W.A.; Merritt, C.R. (July 2001). *Toward a standardized breast ultrasound lexicon, BI-RADS: ultrasound.* Semin Roentgenol. 36(3), pp. 217-25.

Montaldo, G.; Tanter, M.; Bercoff, J.; Benech, N.; Fink, M. (March 2009). *Coherent plane-wave compounding for very high frame rate ultrasonography and transient elastography,* IEEE Transactions on Ultrasonics, Ferroelectrics and Frequency Control, 56(3), pp. 489-506.

Orescanin, M.; Qayyum, M.A.; Toohey, K.S.; Insana, M.F. (October 2011) *Dispersion and shear modulus measurements of porcine liver.* Ultrasonic Imaging, 32(4), pp. 255-66.

Rosenzweig, S.; Palmeri, M.; Nightingale, K. (February 2011). *GPU-Based Real-Time Small Displacement Estimation With Ultrasound,* IEEE Transactions on Ultrasonics, Ferroelectrics and Frequency Control, 58(2), pp. 399-405.

Royer, D.; Dieulesaint, E. (2000). *Elastic Waves in Solids: Free and guided propagation*, Springer.

Sandrin, L.; Catheline, S.; Tanter, M.; Vinçonneau, C.; Fink, M. (2000), *2D transient elastography,* Acoust. Imaging, vol 25, pp. 485-492

Sarvazyan, A.P.; Rudenko, O.V.; Swanson, S.D.; Fowlkes, J.B.; Emelianov, S.Y. (November 1998). *Shear wave elasticity imaging: a new ultrasonic technology of medical diagnostics.* Ultrasound Med Biol. 24(9), pp. 1419-35.

Schiwietz, T.; Chang, T.; Speier, P.; Westermann, R. (2006). *Mr image reconstruction using the GPU,* Proc. SPIE, vol. 6142, no. 1.

Sebag, F.; Vaillant-Lombard, J.; Berbis, J.; Griset, V.; Henry, J.F.; Petit, P.; Oliver, C. (December 2010). *Shear wave elastography: a new ultrasound imaging mode for the differential diagnosis of benign and malignant thyroid nodules.* J Clin Endocrinol Metab. 95(12), pp. 5281-8.

Shattuck, D. P.; Weinshenker, M. D.; Smith, S. W.; Von Ramm, O. T. (April 1984). *Explososcan: A parallel processing technique for high speed ultrasound imaging with linear phased arrays,* The Journal of the Acoustical Society of America, Volume 75, Issue 4, pp.1273-1282

Szabo, T. L. (2004). Diagnostic ultrasound imaging: inside out, Elsevier Academic Press. Von Ramm, O.T.; Smith, S.W.; Pavy, H.G., Jr. (March 1991), *High-speed ultrasound volumetric imaging system. II. Parallel processing and image display Ultrasonics,* Ferroelectrics and Frequency Control, IEEE Transactions on Volume 38, Issue 2, pp.109 - 115

Szabo, T.L. (1994). *Time domain wave equations for lossy media obeying a frequency power law,* J. Acoust. Soc. Am. Volume 96, Issue 1, pp. 491-500.Xu, F.; Mueller, K. (2007). *Real-time 3d computed tomographic reconstruction using commodity graphics hardware,* Phys. Med. Biol., vol. 52, no. 12, pp. 3405–3419.

Udesen, J.; Gran, F.; Hansen, K. L.; Jensen, J. A.; Thomsen, C.; Nielsen, M. B. (August 2008). *High Frame-Rate Blood Vector Velocity Imaging Using Plane Waves: Simulations and Preliminary Experiments,* IEEE Transactions on Ultrasonics, Ferroelectrics and Frequency Control, vol. 55, no. 8, pp. 1729-1743

Xu, F.; Mueller, K. (2007). *Real-time 3d computed tomographic reconstruction using commodity graphics hardware* Phys. Med. Biol., vol. 52, no. 12, pp. 3405–3419

2

3D High-Quality Ultrasonic Imaging

I.V. Minin and O.V. Minin
Novosibirsk State Technical University
Russia

1. Introduction

Methods of direct quasioptical vision and holography can be used in systems of ultrasonic vision to form high-quality images of objects (V. A. Zvereva, I. N. Stepanova, 1979). The formation of images in the ultrasonic wavelength bands has certain specific features, namely: the sizes of the image-forming systems and of the objects of observation are comparable with wavelength, so that the diffraction nature of the image must be taken into account in calculating the structure of the image.

Both in the ultrasonic and optical wave bands, dielectric lenses and mirror antennas are used to format images of objects (Zelkin E. T., Petrova R. A., 1974). The application of these focusing elements does not solve the problem completely since objective lenses with very large apertures - on the order of several meters - are needed to obtain high-quality ultrasonic images. Fabrication of such lenses involves considerable technological problems because the more practical ones are lenses with a small refractive coefficient and focal length equal to the aperture (Minin I.V., Minin O.V., 1992).

The thickness of the lens is several tens of percent of aperture size. Therefore the mass of such a ultrasonic objective is considerable. Energy losses connected with absorption of the transmitted radiation in the lens material are high. Using mirrors to generate ultrasound images is constrained by the fact that the object and the image area on the same side of the focusing system.

Promising analogues of lenses in the ultrasonic band are objectives based on diffractive elements (Minin I.V., Minin O.V., 1992. Minin I. V., Minin O. V. , 1988. Minin I. V., Minin O. V., 1989).

When building a real system for generating ultrasonic images of objects with the resolution depth greater than given by a conventional image, one must scan the object in three coordinates. For instance, using a mechanical scanning into the depth of the object makes it difficult, and sometimes impossible, to obtain the entire radio image of the object in real time.

A realistic system of visualization of three-dimensional objects in the ultrasound wave band must provide scanning of a volume of space of at least $(10^5 - 10^8)\lambda^3$, and it is required that objects whose characteristic sizes come to several wavelength must be reliably identified in this volume. Therefore, the system of visualization must provide resolving power in the object space of about 5-6 mm. In classical systems of image generation, that is, in systems that use lenses and mirrors as image formatting elements, high transversal resolution (relative to the optical axis of the objective lens) is achieved at high values of numerical aperture. However, as the resolution on the object increases, the resolution depth of the lens (and therefore, the longitudinal resolution) decreases, and if we take into account that

$$\delta_{longit} \sim 2\lambda(F/D)^2 \quad \text{and} \quad \delta_{transv} \sim 1.22\lambda(F/D),$$

it is not difficult to arrive at the following estimate:

$$\delta_{longit} \sim 1.3\delta^2_{transv}/\lambda\ .$$

A contradiction thus arises: trying to increase resolution on the object in the transverse direction, the resolution depth of the image-formatting systems decreases following square law, that is, the problem of generating a ultrasonic image of a three-dimensional object whose extension in the longitudinal direction is several tens of wavelengths, becomes practically unresolvable in this approach because of the high spatial resolution.

Generation of quasioptical ultrasonic images of objects

We shall consider now how to obtain images of objects with resolution depth greater than that provided by the quasioptical system.

The problem may be solved in this case by applying the so-called layer-by-layer scanning of the object. The essence of this technique is that at each given moment of time a flat two-dimensional radio image is constructed of one layer of the object or of an individual point within the resolution depth of the transmitting lens with high transversal resolution. The total image of a three-dimensional object is then reconstructed by summing up individual layer images with assigned weight coefficients. A layer-by-layer scanning of a three-dimensional object can be implemented, for instance, using the method pointed to in (Pat. FRG 1762, 406, 2301800, 26555257).

For instance, three-dimensional information is reconstructed in several spatial zones arranged stepwise into 3D space. The zones are then displayed sequentially one after another for a short interval on the controlling video device. Therefore, the observer is offered not only the general view of an object observed in a single plane of image - as we have in cinema or television - but also information on spatial depth which is used as additional information by quantizing over depth. It is expedient to choose the time sequence of the displayed two-dimensional flat images in such a way that the observer (owing to the inertia of eye vision) perceives the sequence as one total image.

In a continuous process of creating a large number of images with various positions of layers, an object is created and poorly defined details are suppressed by filtering through a filter with predominantly high-frequency characteristics. By adding up these filtered signals, the total image of a three-dimensional object is created and the corresponding non-filtered image is added to the filtered one. Filtration here can be implemented with a filter with a linearly growing frequency curve - because it is assumed that in continuous focusing and summation (integration). For instance, if a distribution of intensity of light dots over black background is processed and then this image is integrated, a pointlike image with a wide halo appears.

A change in the focal distance of the quasi-optical system that uses diffractive elements is implemented by changing the frequency of radiation emitted by the irradiator. To implement spatial selection of the signal reflection by the object and the signal sent by the irradiator, and for automatic "tracing" of the region of focusing along one of the coordinates, for instance, along the optical axis, it is advisable to use either off-axis diffractive elements or diffractive elements with off-axis position of the focusing region. The former option is preferable for the radio vision because diffractive elements then retain their focusing ability in a wider frequency band than elements with off-axis position of the focal point.

Formation of images using partially coherent radiation

We will consider the problem of suppressing interference fringes in the optical system for formatting the image, with the irradiator being a small-size thermal source of quasi-monochromatic radiation $\Delta\nu/\nu << 1$, where $\Delta\nu$ and ν are the effective frequency and the irradiator's frequency band, respectively.
According to (Perina J., 1972. Tarlykov V. A., Magurin V. G., 2002) we can observe here interference fringes, provided

$$\Delta\nu\Delta a < \bar{\lambda},$$

where $\bar{\lambda} = c/\bar{\nu}$ is the effective wavelength, c is the velocity of light and Δa is the size of the source (Kaliteevskii N. I., 1971).
If a thermal source of quasi-harmonic radiation is used as irradiator, the interference fringes on the image is removed if the ratio of numerical apertures of the source and the receiver $\rho_s/\rho_0 >> 1$ and the resulting resolution corresponds to the diffraction limit of receiver optics with non-coherent illumination.
When an object with specularly reflecting surface is observed, its image contains sparkling that suppresses the fine structure of the image. At the same time sparkling from external sources are superimposed onto the original images.
It is possible to remove this distorting noise without changes in illuminating sources, for instance, by placing in front of a flat object a nonuniform transparent scattering (refracting) plate. The possibility of removing the sparkling is determined by the scattering diagram of the plate and by the optical power of noise.
The illumination of the object in systems of direct vision in the ultrasound band is done with coherent radiation. The image of the object is constructed in reflected radiation using special high-aperture objectives (lenses). An interference image is formed when layer images are added up. Furthermore, most objects have specular surface in this wavelength band. This occurs because the wavelength λ_0 at which vision systems work is much longer than the visible light wavelength λ_c used to visualize an object $\lambda_0/\lambda_c \sim 10^4$. Therefore the surface structure of visualized objects is smoother (more specular) with respect to ultrasonic than it is for light by a factor of (λ_0/λ_c); hence, an interpretation of the resulting image becomes ambiguous. For instance, the image of a sphere is a point.
Method of isotropic construction of images of three-dimensional objects (Minin I. V., Minin O. V., 1998)
As it well known reflection coefficients of objects for ultrasound waves are generally random complex value. Hence the conventional coherent imaging systems have suffered to some extent from speckle noise. Speckle occurs when scattered radiation from objects or rough surfaces randomly destructively interferes and degrades image smoothness. So speckle noise and weak edges make the image difficult to identify the object in the ultrasound image. And the analysis of ultrasound image is more challenging one. But if we can generate at each point on the object sufficient large number of sample wave fields with the same magnitude and random phases and the image of the average intensity of the field can be derived, then a desired imaging which is free from speckle noises must be realized (Takayoshi Yokota, Takuso Sato, and Makoto Hirama, 1985).

The "spaced-apart reception" techniques can be used to suppress interference noise in ultrasonic images.
Let us consider an object model consisting of two pointlike reflectors. With two-frequency illumination, the best suppression of interference noise is achieved if

$$\Delta\lambda/\lambda \sim 1/2m,$$

where $m = d/\lambda$ and d is the distance between the reflectors.
In the case where there is only one wavelength and we have two receivers whose signals are added up, the following condition can be obtained for the angular separation Ω between two receivers:

$$\Omega = \arctan[(4m - 1)^{1/2}/(2m - 1)] . \quad (1)$$

Similarly, we can derive for n-frequencies illumination and a string of n receivers the formulas

$$\Delta\lambda/\lambda = (n - 1)/mn,$$

$$\Omega_\kappa = \arctan[(2mn\kappa - \kappa^2)/(mn - \kappa)], \quad n = 2, \dots ,$$

$$\kappa = 0, \dots , (n - 1).$$

The interval $\Delta\lambda$ corresponds to the difference between the maximum and the minimum of wavelengths of n-frequencies irradiation and Ω_κ corresponds to the angular separation between the first and the Kth receiver of the linear string.
Consider the placement of several receivers optimized for suppressing interference noise in a finite field of view.
To suppress interference noise in a finite field of view we distribute n receivers in such a way that for each point there would be two receivers whose signals are in antiphase. We define the number of receivers as the ratio of the solid angle covering the system of receivers to the solid angle of a single receiver.
In order to maximally suppress interference effects at a point A on the axis (fig. 1) it is necessary to place the second receiver 2 at a distance given by formula (1). To suppress interference effects at the edge of the field of view at points BB′ it is necessary to install receivers 3 and 4 at such a distance from receiver 1 that the difference between the optical path lengths between receivers 3 and 4 and the point B equal 1/2 of the wavelength of the radiation used.

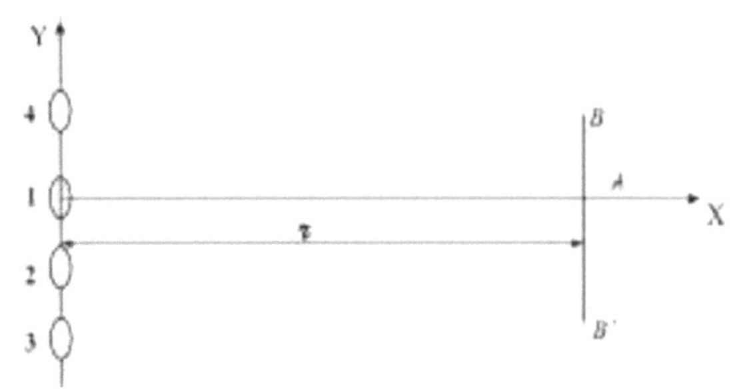

Fig. 1. Locations of radiation receivers for suppressing interference noise in a finite field of view.

Consequently, in a string of four receivers, two pairs of them are strictly in antiphase (at the centre and at the edge of the field of view). For n receivers, the number of such locations is n-1. We were looking so far at a one-dimensional case. To consider a two-dimensional case, the string of receivers has to be rotated K times around the X axis by an angle $\Delta\varphi$, so that $(K\Delta\varphi)=\pi$. The required number of receivers can be found as

$$N = \Omega/\Delta\Omega = \{2\pi(1 - \cos\theta/2)\}/\{(\pi/4)(D/4)^2\}.$$

Let us find the optimum location of two receivers for an arbitrary location of the object in the field of view. Let the object lie on the axis of the first receiver. The signals of the two receivers will be at opposite phases if

$$\frac{d(r_0+d)}{\sqrt{(r_0+d)^2+a^2}} - \frac{d(r_0+d)}{\sqrt{(r_0+d)^2+(a+y_0)^2}} = \frac{\lambda}{2}.$$

We conclude that for optimum suppression of interference noise the distance between the receivers must equal

$$y_0 = \left[\frac{r^2 d^2}{\left(\frac{rd}{\sqrt{r^2+a^2}} - \frac{\lambda}{2}\right)} - r^2\right]^{0.5} - a, r = r_0 + d.$$

Therefore, this method of forming radio images on the basis of an "isotropic" receiver (source) essentially consists in implementing the principle of spatial averaging. For instance, the object may be scanned by a focused beam of electromagnetic waves, the radiation scattered by the object being received by a systems of receivers located in space on the side of the irradiator, while the signals from them are added up non-coherently and are sent to the common system of reconstruction. The receivers are placed on the surface of a hemisphere whose centre lies on the object. As a result, it becomes possible to visualize objects using the difference between their reflection coefficient and the reflection coefficient for the background signal, that is, to visualize an image of a three-dimensional object. Non-coherent adding suppresses interference effects. When integrating narrow directed signals reflected from obstacles (the background signal), the received interference signal is proportional to the coefficient of reflection from the obstacle, and this is typically much lower than the coefficient of reflection from the object. On the whole, a system of N receivers proves to be more sensitive than a single receiver by a factor of $N^{1/2}$. Furthermore, averaging considerably reduces the dynamic range of signals recorded, which makes the requirements to systems reconstructing radio images less stringent.

Another important factor must be mentioned. In systems of direct vision, a receiving device is as a rule large and heavy which makes using this technique very difficult (for instance, the diameter of the objective is at least 200-300λ, so that even with a speed of 1 frame per second and the number of added layers $n \sim 30$, the objective that does mechanical scanning of the object over its depth must periodically move at a typical speed of about 350 m/s).

Attempts to use the conventional "optical" approach to constructing ultrasonic images of three-dimensional objects result in extremely unwieldy formulas. The resulting dimensions, weight and parameters of objective lenses fail to satisfy today's requirements.

Layer-by-layer construction of the image of a three-dimensional object without mechanical scanning over depth can be implemented by using the frequency characteristics of DOE in which the position of focusing area depends on the wavelength of the irradiating field. In this case the speed of the vision system improves considerably. It becomes possible to start with locating an object by scanning over the depth of the scene and then to carefully "scrutinize it" in detail.

Listed below are the main specifics of designing the ultrasonic vision system.

1. Row-by-row scanning for building the image of an object in real time is carried out by electronic scanning of the string of receivers.
2. Frame-by-frame scanning (column-by-column scanning) is implemented by mechanically moving the object controlled.
3. Mirror flashes in the image are removed and the images of the object in different orientations are obtained using quasi-isotropic illumination by a system of irradiators distributed in space.
4. Scanning of the controlled space is done by the electronically shifting the plane of focusing of the vision device (its focal length) by varying the irradiators' wavelength and using diffractive optics. The use of elements of diffractive optics on a non-flat surface makes it possible to extend the field of view of the vision device and improve the signal-to-noise ratio in the ultrasonic image.
5. Access to the object scanned is provided on one side only.

The vision set supports scrutinizing an object with a single frequency (scanning of a plane) or with a number of frequencies (scanning over the depth of the scene) in single-pass or continuous modes of recording the frames of image with an external coupling (to the motion sensor) or internal coupling to the motion of the object, and can also operate in adjustment mode to fine-tune individual components of the vision set.

The main component of any vision system of quasioptical type is an objective that must satisfy a number of requirements (Minin I. V., Minin O. V.,1986. Edward O.Belcher et al., 1999. Yuji Sato at al., 2009):

- to be multicomponent (to satisfy the requirements to field of view ($2\beta \sim 60^0$) and the number of resolved pixels on it ($N^2 \sim 100 \times 100$));
- to possess frequency characteristics adequate for inspecting three-dimensional scenes in real time;
- to have aperture ratio of at least 0.5 and lens aperture (D/λ) of at least 200 to provide high spatial resolution constrained by the diffraction limit over the entire field of view;
- to be fabricated of a material possessing low absorption of ultrasonic power, and be of minimal thickness.

In the active vision mode, when monochromatic radiation is used to illuminate the target object, it is possible to reshape the focusing surface by controlling the frequency of the illuminating radiation and scan the space over the depth of the scene by this surface (Minin I. V., Minin O. V., *et al.*1985). Therefore, frequency characteristics of diffractive objectives make it possible to remove limitations stemming from the small depth of definition of classical lenses. Such systems of image generation are capable of scanning space over depths exceeding the depth of definition by a factor of 10 to 20 without mechanical scanners (Minin I. V., Minin O. V. 1986. Baibulatov F. H., Minin I. V., Minin O. V. 1985.). Small thickness of diffractive objectives (on the order of radiation wavelength) allows designers to achieve high efficiency of using ultrasonic power.

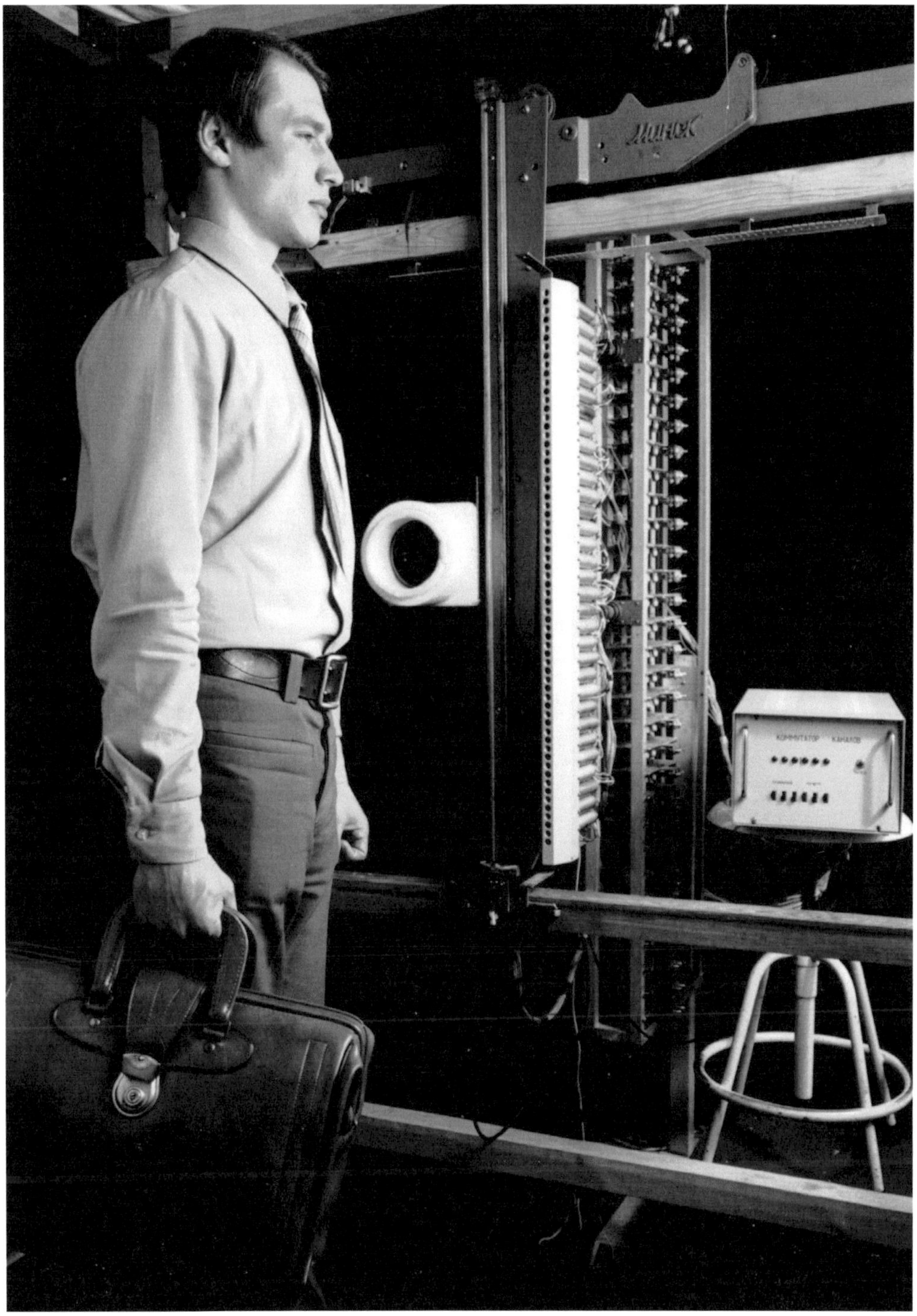

Fig. 2. The pilot version (1988) of 40 KHz real-time ultrasonic imaging system for concealed weapon detection, based on points 1,2,5 and developed under the scientific leadership of Professor V. F. Minin (Minin I.V., Minin O.V., 2003).

2. Fresnel lenses design by acoustic network

Fresnel zone plate (amplitude binary type) was designed by Shu Zhang (Shu Zhang., 2010) to pass only the odd (even) zones and obstructs the even (odd) zones. Fig.3 (left) shows the configuration of planar 1D Fresnel lens we designed. The lens is composed of an array of Helmholtz resonators. The resonators which resonate at 50 KHz in pass even zone are filled with water. The cells in odd zone are filled with air to induce large impedance mismatch, resulting large reflection to obstruct vibration.

Finite-element method was employed to study the focusing of the designed Fresnel plate lens. A collimated acoustic wave is incident on the plate, which is put inside water medium. More than 50dB pressure level difference is found between pass and obstruct zones in Fresnel zone plate based on acoustic network at 50 KHz. Compared with conventional Fresnel lens with the same thickness, the focus effect is more efficient through those based on acoustic network design .The focal length of the lens can be tuned at different frequency as well.

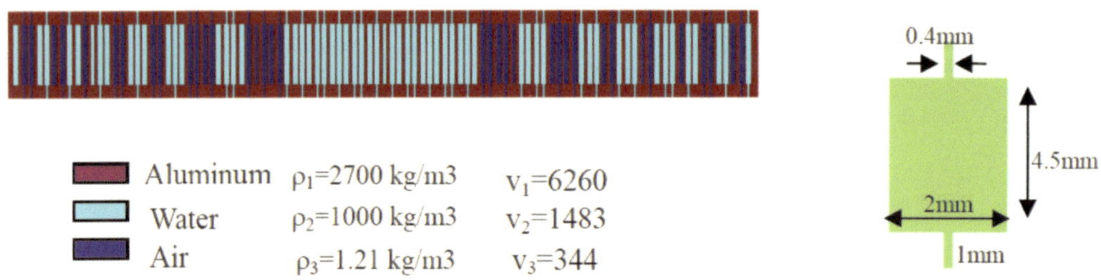

Fig. 3. Configuration of acoustic Fresnel lens (left) and the unit of Helmholtz resonator (right) (Shu Zhang., 2010)

3. Elementary principles of diffractive optics design in acoustics

Acoustic zone plates are used to demonstrate various physical processes (Kirilov V. A., Tverdohlebov V. I., Homenko V. I., 1964). Considerable difficulties are encountered, however, in creating acoustic zone plates that invert the phase of oscillations of one half of the zones. The reason is that the acoustic resistance ρu of any material is so high compared to the resistance of air that acoustic waves are nearly completely reflected. A phase zone plate can be produced using the method suggested by Kock (Kock W. 1965) for fabrication of microwave lenses. The method consists in forcing waves to move between tilted plates; the path length then increases by a factor of $1/\cos Q$ which corresponds to the effective index of reflection $n = 1/\cos Q$ for the propagation of waves in free space.

The strip width l is found from the conventional relation $d(n - 1) = \lambda/2$ or $d(n - 1) = \lambda$, which in this particular case of $n = 1/\cos Q$ and strip width $l = d/\cos Q$ takes the simplest and physically transparent form:

$$l - d = \lambda/2 .$$

Also the circular Fresnel zone transducers may be made, for example, of sandwiched structure with C-axis oriented ZnO piezoelectric film between two Au electrodes (QIAO DongHai, LI ShunZhou, WANG ChengHao. 2007).

3. Ultrasonic piezoelectric transducer based on diffractive optics

For active focusing systems the surface of a rigid plate makes bending oscillations, and allocation of their amplitudes of particle displacements along radius of a plate looks like standing waves. Each point oscillations surfaces radiate an ultrasonic wave in an air medium. As is well know, in condition of central exciting of thin flat disk, which radius is multiple to half of flexural waves (in disk material), distribution of oscillating displacement on the disk surface will look like stationary waves. The radial boundaries on the plate from centre of a plate calculating according to the formula from microwaves (Minin O.V., Minin I.V. 2003). In this case the waves radiated of each exact plate will come to a focal point in one phase. The Noise level in a focal point in that case reaches values 200-220 decibel and above, and around of focal point surfaces of equal phases where the noise level reaches values 140-170 decibel is formed. The vibration amplitude of a radiating surface is about 200 micron.

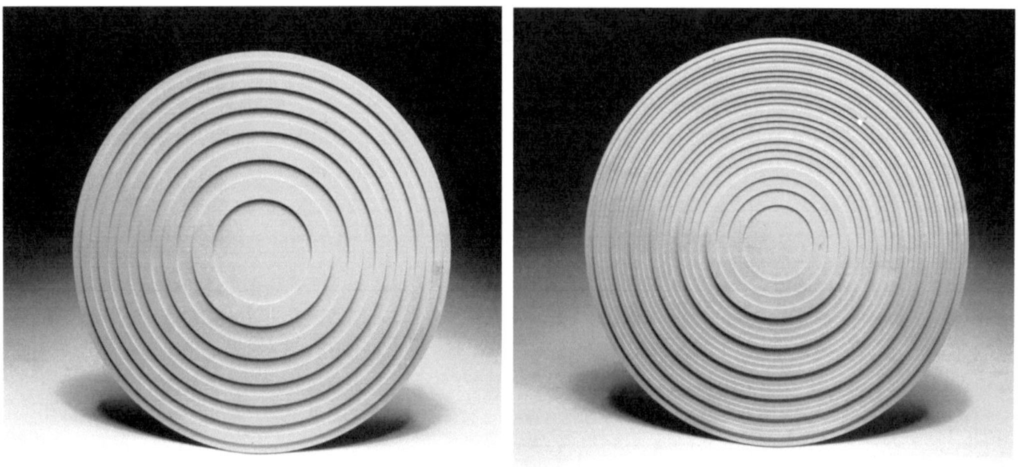

Fig. 4. The active ultrasonic diffractive transducers of half-wave (left) and four-level (right) types.

It could be noted that the advantages of diffractive plate-type emitters are: the possibility of forming ultrasonic vibrations of high power and provide frequency tuning of the radiation due to transition from one harmonic to another. The same diffractive plate-type emitter can create vibrations of different frequencies, operating at different harmonics.
For example, for the circular membrane in an common case we can use polar co-ordinates (r,θ). The spatial part of the wave function will be of the form $R(r)\Theta(\theta)$. The boundary conditions will act specifically on $R(r)$ which will be a Bessel function $J_m(kr)$ with zeros at well known (tabulated) values x_{mn} (m for the function and n for the nth zero). This leads to the relation $k_{mn}a=x_{mn}$ to force a zero at r=a, the radius of the membrane. These results in the following relation for computing the angular frequency associated with the different modes:

$$\omega_{mn} = \frac{x_{mn}v}{a},$$

where v is the velocity of the wave in the membrane. The solution of our problem for the mode (m,n) is, basically, of the form:

$$S(r,\theta,t) = J_m(k_{mn}r)\cos(m\theta)\cos(\omega_{mn}t)\,.$$

A dependence with sin(mθ) is also possible, giving rise to the existence of 2 degenerate modes for each m (except for m=0). In general, a linear combination of both modes will be excited.
For the case of a transducer we need only the modes with m=0. The distribution of oscillations amplitude on the first three oscillation modes of disk radiator is shown in Fig 5.

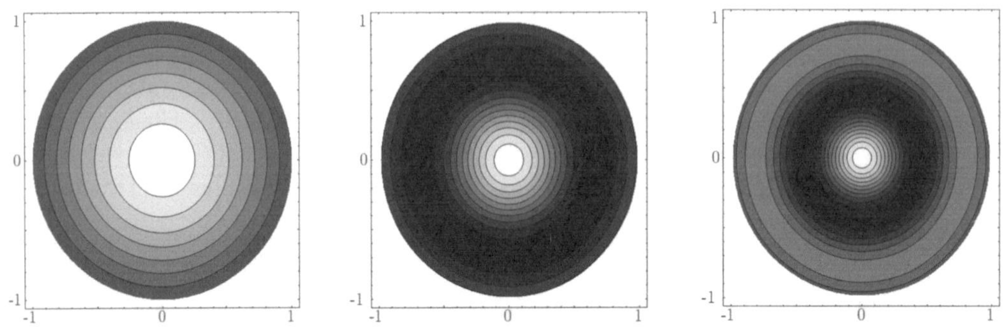

Fig. 5. The distribution of oscillation amplitude of diffractive radiator on the different oscillation modes: n=1, 2, 3.

4. Some other diffractive optical elements applications in acoustics

Fresnel zone plates can be used in audiovision (Greguss P. 1980) and nondestructive ultrasound testing (Stamnes J. J., Cravelsxter J., Bentsen O., 1982. Ermolaev I. N., Kanevskii I. N., Kofolev V. D. *et al.* 1980. Chernoverskii M. P. 1988), both in reception and emission modes. In reception mode, the zone plate consists of a sequence of alternating transparent and opaque zones. This zone plate behaves as a conventional acoustic lens.
If used as focusing emitter, the acoustic converter is fabricated as a zone plate. For instance, a binary zone plate with 10 zones made as a sequence of gold electrodes on the surface of a ceramic converter was described in (Stamnes J. J., Cravelsxter J., 1982). The other side of the converter has a common metal coating. When used to transform electric fields, only transparent zones emit. This means that the same zone plate can be used to generate both an "audio" picture and an image of an object.
Acoustically emitted diffractive focusing elements possess another very interesting and very promising property (Kock W., 1965. Greguss P., 1980). If zones made of gold electrodes are replaced with photoconducting layers and placed between a converter and an optically transparent electrode, this device can be controlled by light. If an optical image of a diffractive element is projected onto such a converter and is moved transversally, the point of acoustical focus will also move. Therefore, two-dimensional scanning can be realized.
The design and development of a low cost, electro-mechanical ultrasonic scanner for obtaining high resolution C-scan images of the friction skin ridge structure found on the digits of the hands or feet in order to create imagery of sufficient quality for use in automated personal identification systems were discussed in (J.K. Schneider, S.M. Gojevic. 2001). It has been shown the optical scanner is unable to image through the contamination, while the ultrasonic scanner is unaffected.
A breadboard ultrasound sensor has been developed for remotely detecting and imaging concealed weapons (Applied Technologies - Jaycor http://www.jaycor.com/eme_sens_

ultra.htm). The breadboard sensor can detect metallic and non-metallic weapons concealed on a human body under heavy clothing at ranges up to 8 m and can image concealed weapons at ranges up to 5 m.
This breadboard sensor has produced the only remote ultrasound images of concealed weapons, including lexan (plastic) knives and a handgun concealed under a heavy sweatshirt at 15 feet. The sensor includes a highly efficient source of high-power, tunable ultrasound radiation suitable for remote imaging in air. Together with millimeter-sized, highly sensitive ultrasound detectors and high-gain transceivers, these advances make possible the centimeter-resolution imaging of concealed weapons at ranges between 1 m and 5 m.
Ultrasound is also a "technology that uses high-pitched sound waves to create images of hidden internal anatomy" to detect a land-mine (C. P. Gooneratne, S. C. Mukhopahyay, G. Sen Gupta. 2004). Conventional ultrasound detection involves the emission of a sound wave with a frequency higher than 20 kHz into a medium. This sound wave reflects on boundaries between materials with different acoustical properties. A strong enough ultrasound signal could penetrate the ground and detect otherwise unobtainable signatures of buried mines. It is also capable of operating in wet ground. Ultrasound systems encounter problems at the interface of air and ground.
One of the classical applications of the ultrasonic imaging system is a nondestructive method of inspection. For example (SERDP PP-1134, Final Report, November 2001), the inspection of very thin metallic sheets (0.06 inches up to 0.125 inches thick) was shown to be difficult for the reflection method of ultrasound imaging to undertake; this was due to the extremely short time delay between the front and back surfaces of the thin sheets. By injecting the sound beam into the metallic sheet at an appreciable angle it was found to cause multiple reflections progressing along the sheet with the end result of illuminating a large region of the sample with sound energy. A prototype angle beam ultrasound camera was fabricated at the Becker Labs of the Naval Air Warfare Center Aircraft Division (Figure 6) and has proven that rapid ultrasound imaging of thin sheet is practicable and is unaffected by painted coatings.

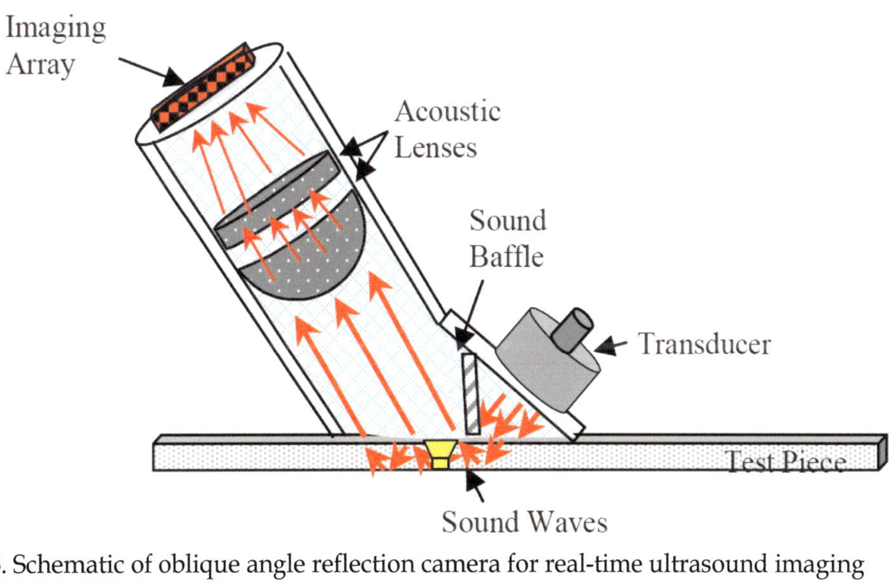

Fig. 6. Schematic of oblique angle reflection camera for real-time ultrasound imaging (SERDP PP-1134, Final Report, November 2001).

The Acoustocam system (Development of Innovative Nondestructive Evaluation Technologies for the Inspection of Cracking & Corrosion Under Coatings SERDP PP-1134, Final Report, November 2001) was shown to be able to respond to the dynamic range of the multiple bounces with an image very similar to that of a through transmission image with the exception that recurring images of a defect are observed in the oblique angle reflection mode owing to the fact that the sound beam continues to reflect (See Figure 7). The concept, however, has proven to be viable for the inspection of corrosion under painted coatings at high speed and with high sensitivity. Application has been made for the issuance of a patent based on the oblique angle beam system.

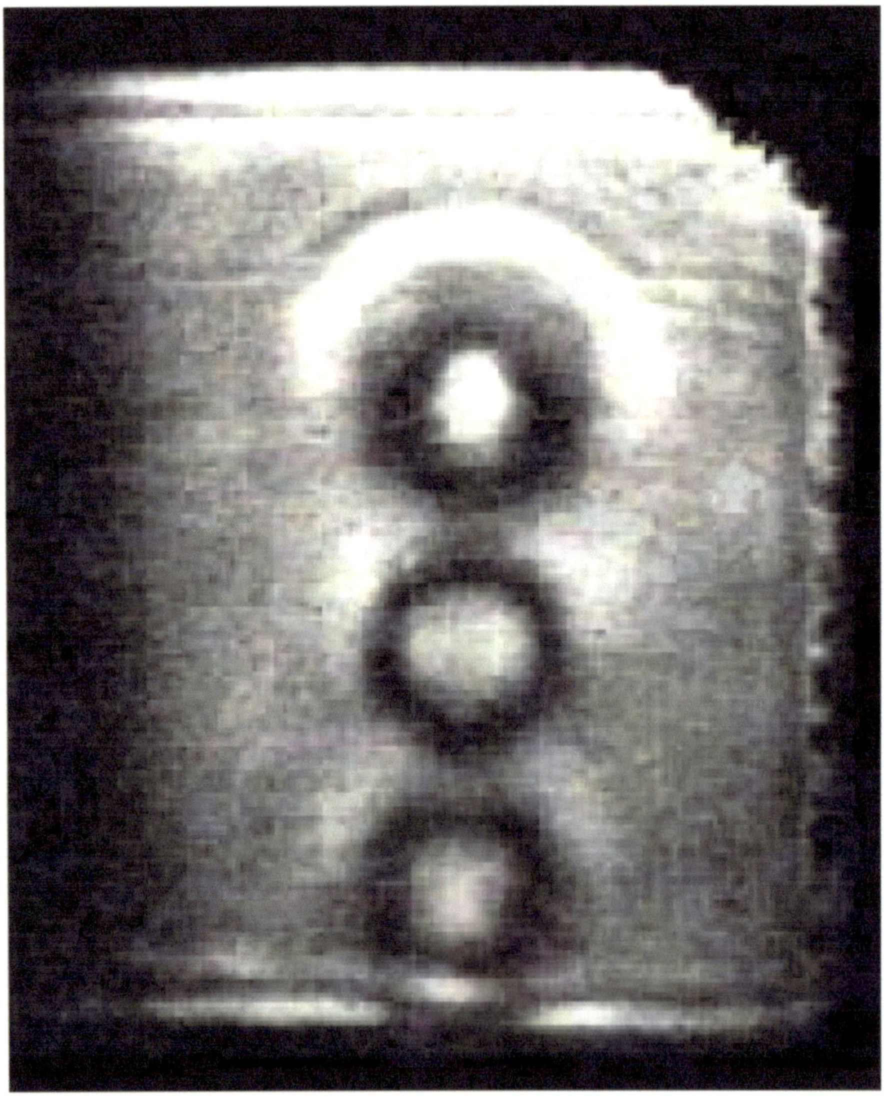

Fig. 7. Angle beam image of a flat bottom hole showing the multiple images that occur (C. P. Gooneratne, S. C. Mukhopahyay, G. Sen Gupta. 2004).

5. References

Experimental optics / Ed. V. A. Zvereva, I. N. Stepanova. M.: Nauka, 1979, p. 256

Zelkin E. T., Petrova R. A. Lens antennas. Moscow: Sov. radio, 1974, p. 279

Schukin I. I. Generation of radio images by phase inversion zone plates // Radiotehnika i elektronika. 1975, vol. 20, no 2. pp. 405-406

Minin I.V., Minin O.V. Diffractive Optics - Moscow: NPO InformTEI, 1992. -180 p. (in Russian)

Minin I. V., Minin O. V. Information properties of zone plates // Computer optics, 1988, no 3, pp. 15-22.

Minin I. V., Minin O. V. Diffractive radio optics systems: achievements and prospects: Abstracts of the USSR conference "Optical, radiowave and thermal methods of nondestructive monitoring". Mogilev, 1989, pp. 204-205.

Pat. FRG 1762, 406, 2301800, 2655525

Perina J, Coherence of light, Van Nostrand London 1972; Tarlykov V. A., Magurin V. G. Foundations of Coherent and Statistical Optics / Sankt-Peterburg, SPbGITMO, 2002 (in Russian)

Kaliteevskii N. I. Wave optics. M., Nauka, 1971 (in Russian)

Minin I. V., Minin O. V. Generation of radio images of 3D objects in the mm wavelength range // In: Proceedings of NVOKU, Novosibirsk, 1998, no 4, pp. 40-46.

Takayoshi Yokota, Takuso Sato, and Makoto Hirama. Active incoherent ultrasonic imaging through an inhomogeneous layer J. Acoust. Soc. Am. Volume 77, Issue 1, pp. 144-152 (January 1985)

Minin I.V., Minin O.V. Radiovision methods in terrorism struggle. - Novosibirsk, NSTU, 2003. - 192 p. (in Russian)

Minin I. V., Minin O. V. Wide-angle multicomponent diffractive microwave lens // Radiotehnika i elektronika. -1986. vol. 31, no 4. pp. 800-806.

Edward O.Belcher et al. Beamforming and imaging with acoustic lenses in small, high-frequency sonars. - The Proc. Of Oceans'99 conf., 13-16 Sept. 1999, Seattle WA, preprint,

Yuji Sato at al. Design for Aplanatic Fresnel Acoustic Lens for Underwater Imaging. Japanese Journal of Applied Physics 48 (2009) 07GL04, pp.1-7

Minin I. V., Minin O. V., Skarbo B. A. *et al* Application of microwave holographic radio lenses in nondestructive testing and plasma diagnostics. Abstracts of 5th USSR Conf. on Holography. Riga, 1985, pp. 233-234. (in Russian)

Baibulatov F. H., Minin I. V., Minin O. V. Focusing properties of Fresnel zone plate // Radiotehnika i elektronika. 1985. vol.30, no 9. pp. 1681-1688.

Shu Zhang. ACOUSTIC METAMATERIAL DESIGN AND APPLICATIONS. Dissertation Submitted in partial fulfillment of the requirements for the degree of Doctor of Philosophy in Mechanical Engineering in the Graduate College of the University of Illinois at Urbana-Champaign, 2010.

Kirilov V. A., Tverdohlebov V. I., Homenko V. I. Demonstration experiment with acoustic zone plate // UFN, 1964, vol. 70, no. 1, p. 166.

Kock W Sound waves and light waves, N.Y., 1965

QIAO DongHai, LI ShunZhou, WANG ChengHao. High frequency acoustic microscopy with Fresnel zoom lens, *Sci China-Phys Mech Astron.* Feb 2007, vol. 50, no. 1,pp. 41-52.

Minin O.V., Minin I.V. Diffractive optics of millimeter waves. - IOP publisher, Boston-London, 2003

Greguss P. Ultrasonic imaging. Focal Press Limited, London, N.Y., 1980

Stamnes J. J., Cravelsxter J., Bentsen O. Image quality and diffraction efficiency of a holographic lens for sound waves // Acoustical imaging / Ed. by P. Alais, A. F. Tetherell. N.Y.: Plenum Press, 1982. vol. 10. pp. 587-606.

Ermolaev I. N., Kanevskii I. N., Kofolev V. D. *et al* Focusing zoned finder for ultrasound non-destructive testing // Defektoskopiya. 1980, no 1. pp. 94-96.

Chernoverskii M. P. Focusing zoned converter with low electric capacitance // Defektoskopiya. 1988, no 2. p. 94.

J.K. Schneider, S.M. Gojevic. Ultrasonic Imaging Systems for Personal Identification. Proc. Of the Ultrasonics Symposium, 2001 IEEE, v.1, pages: 595 - 601.

Ultrasound Sensor for Remote Imaging: Concealed Weapons http://www.jaycor.com/eme_sens_ultra.htm

C. P. Gooneratne, S. C. Mukhopahyay, G. Sen Gupta. A Review of Sensing Technologies for Landmine Detection: Unmanned Vehicle Based Approach. Proc. 2nd International Conference on Autonomous Robots and Agents, December 13-15, 2004, Palmerston North, New Zealand, pp.401-407

Development of Innovative Nondestructive Evaluation Technologies for the Inspection of Cracking & Corrosion Under Coatings SERDP PP-1134, Final Report, November 2001

Part 2

Medical Applications of Ultrasonic Imaging

3

Use of Three Dimensional Ultrasound Imaging in Evaluation of Asherman's Syndrome

Catha Fischer and Alan Copperman
Mount Sinai School of Medicine in New York
USA

1. Introduction

Asherman's syndrome is defined as the presence of intrauterine adhesions or fibrosis within the uterine cavity that either partially or completely obliterate the cavity. It was initially described by Heinrich Fritsch in 1894 and then further characterized by Joseph Asherman in 1948. (1) The most common etiology of the disease is dilation and cutterage due to pregnancy complications such as incomplete abortion, postpartum hemorrhage, or retained placenta. (2, 3) While the disease is rare within the general population, it is commonly cited as a factor in pregnancy complications in the infertile population. (4) Clinical manifestations of the disease include recurrent pregnancy loss, infertility, menstrual abnormalities, and cyclic pelvic pain. (5) The extent of intrauterine adhesions is graded and the severity of disease classified by extent of cavity obliterated, location of adhesions within the cavity, and character of the adhesions. (6) The American Society of Reproductive Medicine recommends classification of disease based on extent of cavity obliterated (<1/3, 1/32/3, >2/3), quality of adhesions seen of hysteroscopy (filmy, filmy and dense, dense), and patient's menstrual pattern (normal, hypomenorrhea, amenorrhea).(7) At present, there are several modalities useful in the screening and diagnosis of Asherman's syndrome. In this chapter, we will discuss these modalities in detail, explaining the benefits and drawbacks of each. We also suggest that three dimensional sonography appears to enhance the physician's ability to provide an accurate diagnosis and prognosis to patients with Asherman's syndrome.

Traditionally, the diagnosis of Asherman's syndrome was made by history and physical examination. (1) Over time, direct visualization via hysteroscopy, hysterosalpingography, and sonography have all led to improved diagnostic accuracy. The hysterosalpingogram (HSG) is a procedure that provides an indirect means of evaluating the uterine cavity, since by injecting radio opaque dye transcervically, information can be gathered on the location and extent of adhesions. (8) Unfortunately, several studies have shown that hysterosalpingogram produces a large number of false positives, specifically in those whose cavities contain lesions other than intrauterine adhesions such as cervical stenosis, endometrial polyps, and myomas. (8, 9) Another drawback of this procedure is its inability to characterize the uterine cavity beyond where the radioopaque dye perfused, and thus potentially not identifying lower uterine segment outflow obstructions. Therefore, patients with normal cavities except for the presence of adhesions in the lower uterine segment will have hysterosalpingograms that appear similar to patients with severe disease, thus having their disease severity incorrectly classified and potentially leading to treatment errors. (10) Furthermore, even in patients who did not have lower tract obstruction, HSG over-estimated disease severity compared to three dimensional ultrasound due to decreased clarity. (10)

Sonohysterography is another modality used to survey the uterine cavity for adhesions. It is a simple procedure that involves injecting sterile saline into the uterus to distend the cavity. The saline outlines the cavity aiding the operator in identifying structural abnormalities on the two dimensional ultrasound. Unlike hysterosalpingography, sonohysterography does not use radiation and can be done in an office setting. Initially, in small studies and case reports sonohysterography was thought to have diagnostic superiority to hysterosalpingography. (11,12, 13) However, when a larger study was conducted, it showed that two dimensional sonohysterography and hysterosalpingography have similar sensitivities both with high false positive rates. (9) At this point, it was suggested by these authors that the use of three dimensional ultrasound may in fact improve sonohysterographic accuracy. (9)

The use of two dimensional transvaginal ultrasound to identify intrauterine adhesions is controversial. In two dimensional ultrasound, sound waves are sent straight and reflected back in a linear vector, allowing for an image to be constructed only from the x and y planes. This modality is very operator dependent making its efficacy at diagnosing and prognosticating Asherman's syndrome difficult to accurately assess. In small studies, sensitivities of 80 to 90 percent for diagnosing intrauterine adhesions have been reported, however these numbers have not been reproduced. (14, 15) Rather, in another small series, two dimensional transvaginal ultrasound failed to diagnose intrauterine adhesions in any of the 4 cases in the study and gave 3 false positive diagnoses. (11) In a larger study that included 209 patients, two dimensional transvaginal ultrasound had a 97% sensitivity and 11% specificity at identifying intrauterine adhesions.(9) Again suggesting that two dimensional transvaginal ultrasound has a high false positive rate but may be useful as a screening modality. However, it has been showed that hysterosalpingography is a more accurate screening test. (8)

In three dimensional ultrasound, sound waves are emitted across a sector. The intensity of these sounds waves is the same as two dimensional ultrasound. The returning echoes are processed by a sophisticated algorithm resulting in a reconstructed three dimensional volume image with x, y, and z planes. This process is very similar to a CT scan. Three dimensional ultrasound allows clinicians to see width, height, and depth of images. A Voluson Endocavity transducer S-VDW 5-8 (Kretztechnik AG, Austria) with a center frequency of 6.5 MHz connected to a Voluson 530D (Medison, USA) 3D ultrasound machine is applied for scanning. Every examination starts with a 2D evaluation of the endometrial cavity. After switching into 3D-mode, the region of interest is selected with the volume box and the volume is acquired. When possible, information regarding the scan is stored on a 540-MB removable hard disk for further evaluation and calculations One of the advantages of three dimensional ultrasound is the real time assessment of the uterine cavity. Unlike hysterosalpingography, three dimensional ultrasound uses no radiation and can be done during an office visit. In a study done by Knopman et al, 54 infertile patients with suspected Asherman's syndrome underwent both three dimensional ultrasound and hysterosalpingography prior to hysteroscopy. In this study, intrauterine adhesions were demonstrated on three dimensional ultrasound and hysterosalpingography in all cases. However, three dimensional ultrasound had a sensitivity of 100% and hysterosalpingography had a sensitivity of 66.7%. Furthermore, in 61.1% of cases in which hysterosalpingography results were inconsistent with hysteroscopy, lower uterine segment outflow tract obstruction was present and the hysterosalpingogram misclassified findings as severe disease with complete cavity obstruction. (10) Therefore, as prognosis in patients with Asherman's syndrome is based on severity of disease, it appears from this data that three dimensional ultrasound more accurately assesses prognosis, which has strong clinical applications.

Clinically, many women presenting with fertility problems are found to have Asherman's syndrome during routine infertility work-up. Knopman et al suggest that because the data obtained from three dimensional ultrasound correlates more closely with the character and extent of Asherman's disease, it could be a helpful tool in predicting fertility outcome postoperatively. Furthermore, the high pregnancy rates achieved in their clinic may in part be due to the excellent pre-operative information obtained from the three dimensional ultrasound, ensuring a well informed surgical procedure. Three dimensional ultrasound has many other uses in obstetrics, gynecology, and reproductive medicine. Three dimensional volumetry of the gestational sac in the first trimester has been suggested as a sensitive predictor of pregnancy outcome. (16) Additionally, three dimensional sonography has been suggested in case reports to be an accurate tool to identify multiple gestations in the first trimester. (17) Due to the high risk nature of multiple gestation pregnancies, an early assessment of amnionicity and chorionicity is an essential part of perinatal management. In summary, three dimensional ultrasound has many promising uses in infertility(18, 19, 20, 21), early pregnancy (22, 23, 24), and fetal malformations (25, 26). As the technology matures and treating physicians obtain more training, skills, and comfort with this technology, we anticipate more widespread acceptance and patient benefit to ensue.

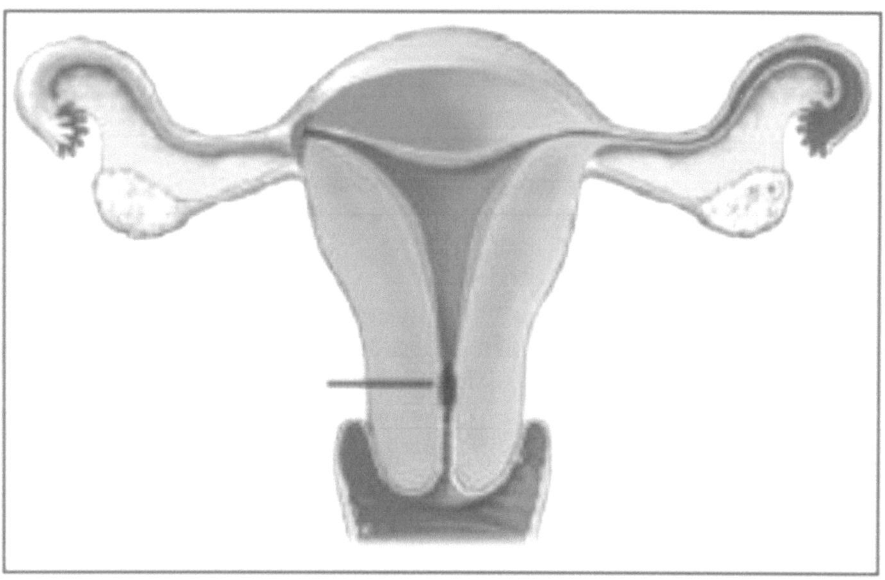

Fig. 1. Frontal plane demonstratinf a caviy with <10% scarring. Normal cavity with ouflow obstruction.

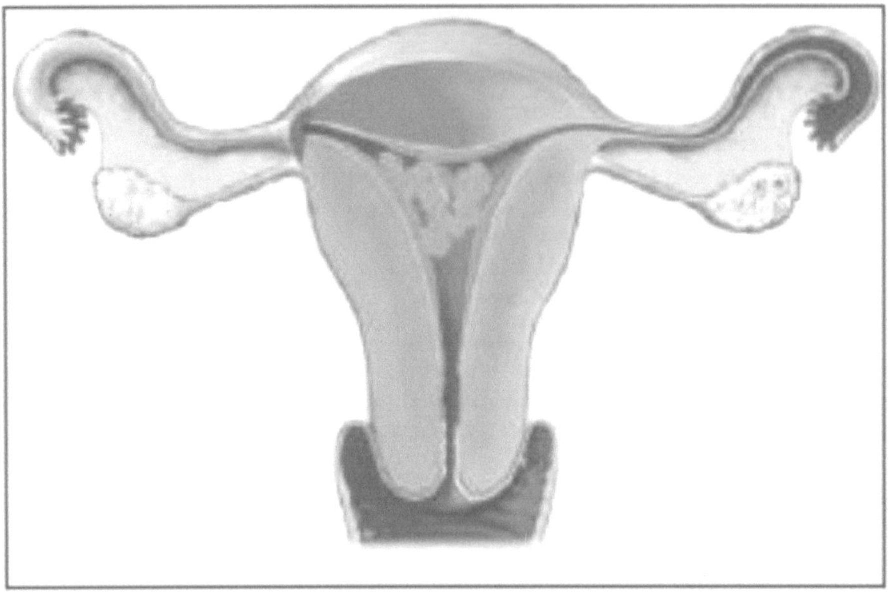

Fig. 2. Frontal plane demonstrating about 50% of cavity scarred. Abnoramal cavity without ouflow obstruction.

2. References

[1] Asherman JG. (1950). Traumatic intrauterine adhesions. *J Obstet Gynaecol Br Em.* Dec;57(6):892-6

[2] March CM. (1995). Intrauterine adhesions. *Obstet Gynecol Clin North Am.*22(3):491-505.

[3] Schenker JG . (1996). Etiology of and therapeutic approach to synechia uteri. *Eur J Obstet Gynecol Reprod Biol.*65(1):109-13.

[4] Al-Inany H. (2001). Intrauterine adhesions: An update. *Acta Obstet Gynecol Scand.*80:986-993.

[5] Magos A. (2002). Hysteroscopic treatment of asherman's syndrome. *Reprod BioMed Online.*4:46-51

[6] March CM, Israel R, March AD. (1978). Hysteroscopic management of intrauterine adhesions. Am J Obstet Gynecol.130:653-665

[7] The American Fertility Society classifications of adnexal adhesions, distal tubal occlusion, tubal occlusion secondary to tubal ligation, tubal pregnancies, mullerian anomalies and intrauterine adhesions.(1988).*Fertil Steril.*49(6): 944-55.

[8] Preutthipan S, Linasimita V. (2003). A prospective comparative study between hysterosalpingography and hysteroscopy in the detection of intrauterine pathology in patients with infertility. *J Obstet Gynaecol Res.*29:33-37

[9] Sylvestre C, Child T, Tulandi T, et al.(2003). A prospective study to evaluate the efficacy of two- and three-dimensional sonohysterography in women with intrauterine lesions. *Fertil Steril.*79:1222-1225

[10] Knopman J, Copperman AB. (2007). Value of 3D ultrasound in the management of suspected Asherman's syndrome.*J Reprod* Med. Nov;52(11):1016-22

[11] Soares S, Reis M, Camargos A. (2000). Diagnostic accuracy of sonohysterography, transvaginal sonography, and hysterosalpingography in patients with uterine cavity diseases. *Fertil Steril.*73:406-411

[12] Salle B, Gauchernad P, Hilaire P, et al.(1999). Transvaginal sonohysterographic evaluation of intrauterine adhesions. *J Clin Ultrasound.*27:131-134.

[13] Widrich T, Bradely LD, Mitchinson AR, et al. (1996). Comparison of saline infusion sonography with office hysteroscopy for the evaluation of the endometrium. *Am j Obstet Gynecol.*174:1327-1334

[14] Fedele L, Bianachi S, Dorta M, et al. (1996). Intrauterine adhesions: Detection with transvaginal ultrasound. *Radiology.*199:757-759

[15] Shalev J, Meizner I, Bar-Hava I, et al. (2000). Predictive value of transvaginal sonography performed before routine diagnostic hysteroscopy for evaluation of infertility. *Fertil Steril.*73:412-417

[16] Babinszki A, Nyari T, Jordan S, Nasseri A, Mukherjee T, Copperman AB. (2001). Three-dimensional measurement of gestational and yolk sac volumes as predictors of pregnancy outcome in the first trimester. *Am J Perinatol.* Jun;18(4):203-11.

[17] Babinszki A, Mukherjee T, Kerenyi T, Berkowitz RL, Copperman AB. (1999). Diagnosing amnionicity at 6 weeks of pregnancy with transvaginal three-dimensional ultrasonography: case report. *Fertil Steril.* Jun;71(6): 1161-4

[18] Lin MT, Chen GD, Lin LY, and Lee MS. (1991). Measurements of follicle size and the volume of follicular fluid by 3-dimensional ultrasound scanning compared with aspirated findings in IVF programs. *J. Obstet. Gynecol. Rep. China,* 30, 47-50

[19] Brunner M, Obruca A, Bauer P, and Feichtinger W. (1995) Clinical application of volume estimation based on three dimensional ultrasonography. *Ultrasound Obstet. Gynecol.*,6,358-61

[20] Kyei-Mensah A, Zaidi J, Pittrop R, Shaker AA, Campbell S, and Tan SL. (1996) Three-dimensional ultrasound: accuracy of follicular volume measurements. *Fertil. St*eril., 65, 371-6

[21] Bonilla-Musoles F, Raga F, Blanes J, Osborne N, and Siles CH. (1995) The use of three-dimensional ultrasound in reproduction: preliminary report. *Hum. Reprod.* Update.

[22] Gregg A, Steiner H, Bogner G, Staudach A, and Weiner CP. (1993) The gestational sac and 3-D volumetry. *Am. J. Obstet. Gynecol.*, 168, 348

[23] Kelly IM, Gardener JE, and Less WR. (1991) Three-dimensional fetal ultrasound. Lancet, 339, 1062-4

[24] Kelly IM, Gardener JE, Brett AD, Richards RR, and Less WR. (1994). Three-dimensional ultrasound of the fetus. *Radiology,* 192, 253-9

[25] Merz E, Bahlmann F, and Weber G. (1995) Volume scanning in the evaluation of fetal malformations: a new dimension in prenatal diagnosis. *Ultrasound Obstet. Gynecol.*, 5, 222-7
[26] Lee A, Kratochwil A, Deutinger J, and Bernaschek G. (1995) Three-dimensional ultrasound in diagnosing phocomelia. *Ultrasound Obstet. Gynecol.*, 5, 238-40

4

Correction of Phase Aberrations in Medical Ultrasound Images Using Signal Redundancy

Yue Li
Information and Communication Technologies Centre
Commonwealth Scientific and Industrial Research Organisation (CSIRO)
Australia

1. Introduction

The pulse-echo technique has been widely used in medical ultrasound imaging. This technique uses an array of transducer elements to transmit a focused beam into the body, and each element then becomes a receiver to collect the echoes. The received echoes from each element are dynamically focused to form an image. Focusing on transmission and reception is performed assuming that the wave propagation speed inside the body is the same everywhere. Unfortunately, the speed inside the body is not constant; it varies from 1470 m/s to greater than 1600 m/s. This speed variation will result in increased side lobes and degraded lateral resolution. Aberration phenomena and their extent in tissue have been evaluated in many works (O'Donnell & Flax 1988; Zhu & Steinberg, 1992; Shmulewitz et al., 1993; Robinson et al., 1994; Hinkelman et al., 1998). The degradation might be tolerable if the frequency is not very high and the aperture size of the array is not very large. However, higher frequencies and larger apertures have been used to improve lateral resolution of ultrasound images. But the resolution improvement cannot be achieved beyond a certain limit, because both larger aperture and higher frequency make the system more sensitive to propagation velocity variations in the body. For example, the four transverse abdominal scan images shown in the first row of Fig.1 were formed with a 64-element linear array using four different aperture sizes (9 mm, 12 mm, 18 mm, and 27 mm) to form each single beam in the image. The array pitch was 1.0 mm and the pulse had a 3.5 MHz centre frequency and 2 MHz bandwidth. The Superior-Mesenteric-Artery (SMA) and the Aorta (A) are the main objects in these images. Because of the shape of the rectus muscles (speed ~ 1580 m/s) and the fat layers (speed ~ 1450 m/s) at this position, the distortions caused by phase aberration in these images can be easily seen. In the 9-mm aperture image, the superior-mesenteric-artery is almost doubled but the artery wall can still be recognized. When the aperture size becomes larger, the distortion becomes worse.

Phase aberration is one of the most important factors that limit improvement to lateral resolution of ultrasound imaging systems. Successful correction of phase aberrations will make it possible to improve the lateral resolution of images. Phase aberration corrected images using the near-field-signal-redundancy algorithm (Li, 1997) are shown in the second row of Fig.1 and the lateral resolution is improved when the aperture size becomes larger. In this chapter, the near-field-signal-redundancy algorithm is described in details. But first, a review of some related methods developed for phase-aberration correction is given. The phase aberration problem is not unique to medical ultrasound imaging. It exists in almost all imaging areas, such as atmospheric effects in astronomical imaging (Jennison, 1958; Goodman et al., 1966; Ishiguro, 1974; Muller & Buffington, 1974; Buffington et al., 1977; Hamaker et al., 1977; Hogg, 1981; Tyson, 2010), antenna-position errors in radar and microwave imaging (Steinberg, 1991) and weathered-layer-effect in seismic imaging (Yilmaz & Doherty, 1987).

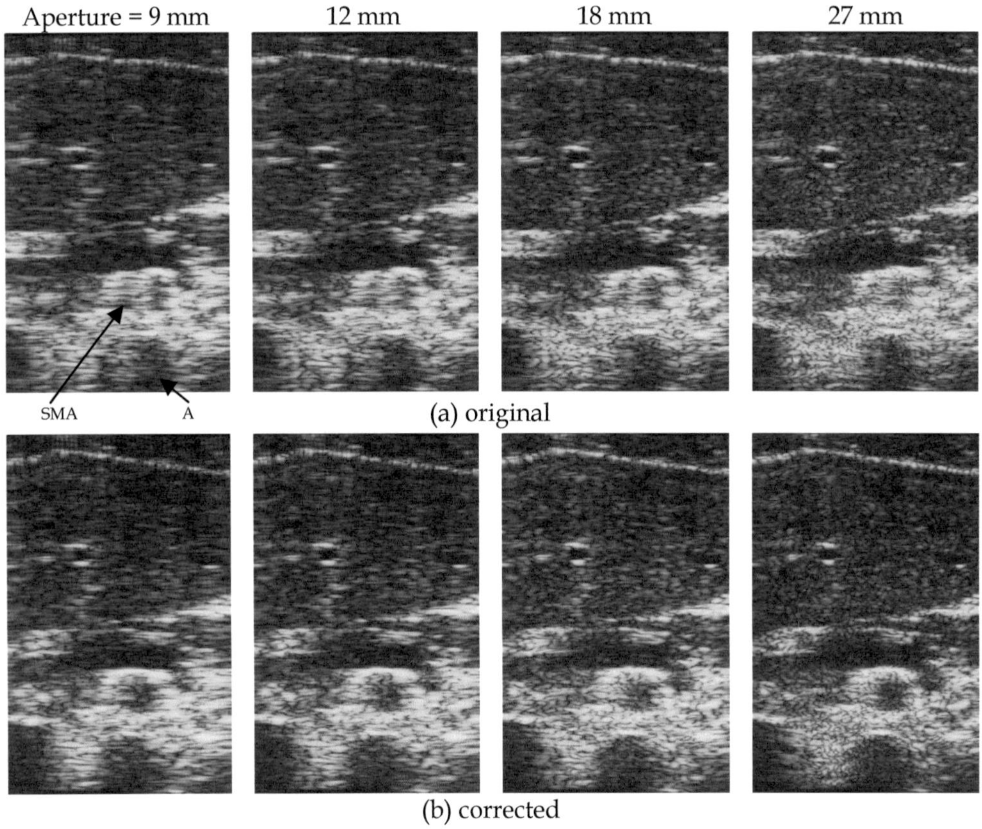

Fig. 1. The resolution of images is only improved with increased aperture size after phase-aberration correction. (a) without phase-aberration correction. (b) with phase-aberration correction.

In astronomical imaging, phase and amplitude aberrations caused by the atmosphere make it difficult to achieve diffraction-limited resolution on the ground. One widely used aberration-correction method is the direct-wave-front-measurement method. This is used when there is a dominant bright star either present or artificially created using laser (Tyson, 2010). A plane wavefront at the aperture should be observed since the dominant point target is in the far field of the imaging aperture. Any departure from a plane wavefront is caused by phase aberration. After measuring the wavefront, the next step is to separate the phase-aberration profile across the aperture from the non-aberrated wavefront. This is not a simple task because the angle of the star is generally unknown. Fortunately, for a target in the far field, such separation is unnecessary since the error of the assumed angle of the star causes a shift of the image position only and has no effect on focusing. Methods using signals received from arbitrary target distributions have also been developed in astronomical imaging. These include maximum-sharpness (Muller & Buffington, 1974; Buffington et al., 1977) and redundant-spacing interferometer methods. (Jennison, 1958; Ishiguro, 1974) Hamaker et al. (Hamaker et al., 1977) pointed out that these methods are all based on the same fundamental principle: signal redundancy. When the target distribution is complex, there is no prior knowledge about the wavefront shape without phase aberrations. Therefore, the aberration profile cannot be separated directly from the unaberrated wavefront in the measured wavefront. In this case, the signal-redundancy principle makes the separation unnecessary. The redundant-spacing interferometer method does not measure the wavefront but the phase difference between redundant signals, and then directly derives the phase-aberration profile across the array. The result also contains an arbitrary steering angle which has no effect on focusing. The maximum-sharpness method uses a trial-and-error method to adjust each antenna's phase. When an indicator is maximized, the system is in focus. This method is also based on the signal-redundancy principle. When the system is in focus, redundant signals are added in phase and the indicators will be maximized.

Phase-aberration correction methods have also been developed for active (pulse-echo) and near-field imaging systems, such as radar, microwave, ultrasonic and seismic imaging systems. Since the number of references is large, they are not listed here and can be found in the references list in (Li, 1997; Li & Robinson, 2008). When there is a dominant point target in the near field, the first step is again to measure the arrival wavefront from the target. Nearest-neighbor-cross-correlation and indicator (maximum sharpness) methods have been used. The next step is to separate the aberration profile from the unaberrated wavefront, which should be spherical. Without knowing the position of the dominant point target, the phase-aberration profile can be obtained only by estimating the target location. The error in the estimated aberration profile because of the wrongly assumed target position will cause de-focusing in the near field case. The image at the dominant point target will still be well focused (at the wrong position) if this inaccurate aberration profile is used to do the correction, since the two errors cancel each other at that position. But, the correction will become increasingly inaccurate away from that point. This correction is therefore only valid in a region around the dominant target. The size of the region depends on the distance from the target to the aperture, the size of the aperture, and the accuracy of the estimated target position. It can be much smaller than the isoplanatic patch, defined as the region where the phase-aberration value is a constant, if the focusing quality is too poor before phase-aberration correction to estimate the dominant point target position with adequate accuracy. Therefore, aberration correction in the near field may have problems even when a dominant point target is available. In some situations, such as forming an image around the dominant target only, estimating the dominant target position accurately is not so important. On the other hand, it is unusual to have a dominant point target in every isoplanatic patch, or even in the entire image, in medical ultrasonic imaging. Techniques have also been developed which use signals from randomly distributed scatterers that generate speckle in an image to measure the wavefront. In the nearest-neighbor-cross-correlation method, a focused beam is transmitted (try to generate an artificial dominant point target) and the phase aberration profile is derived from the cross-correlation measurements between neighboring elements. An iterative method is used to improve the measurement accuracy. The indicator method has also been used in a speckle-generating region. It is an iterative phase-correction procedure in which the timing of acoustic signals transmitted and received from individual elements is adjusted to optimize the quality indicator. In a lens and mirror astronomical imaging system it is the intensity-sensitive recorder that generates the necessary cross-correlation process between signals coming from different locations on the lens aperture to produce redundant signals. Phases of redundant signals are difficult to directly compare at optical frequencies. A trial-and-error method has to be used with a deformable mirror to focus the image by maximizing an indicator; this is time consuming and it may not converge to the right position. On the other hand, in a very large baseline, radio astronomy imaging system, phases of redundant signals can be compared directly. In ultrasonic imaging, radio-frequency (RF) signals can be acquired and their phases can be compared directly. Therefore, direct phase-difference measurement between redundant signals can be used. A comparison of the nearest-neighbor-cross-correlation algorithm, the indicator method, and the near-field-signal-redundancy algorithm discussed in this chapter can be found in (Li & Gill, 1998). In seismic imaging, a phase-aberration correction (surface-consistent residual static correction) method using signals coming from a specular reflecting plane has been developed to correct the phase aberration caused by weathered layers near the ground surface. The specular reflecting plane is a special kind of target. It is similar to a dominant point target in that every receiver element receives a dominant echo from it. The difference is that the position of the reflecting point is different for different transmitter or receiver positions. The non-aberrated arrival wavefront from a specular reflecting plane depends on the angle of the plane and the propagation speed between the plane and the array. Common receiver, common transmitter, and common midpoint signals can be used for the measurement. Common midpoint signals are generally preferred because of several advantages, such as insensitivity to the angle of the reflecting plane. It should be noted that common midpoint signals are not redundant when there is a specular reflecting plane in the near field, because the position of the reflecting point is different for different transmitter or receiver positions. Therefore, the seismic method is not a signal-redundancy method.

A least-mean-squares error-fitting method has been developed in ultrasonic imaging (Hirama & Sato, 1984) to form an image of targets on a plane parallel to the transducer array surface through an inhomogeneous layer. The method uses the complete signal set to build an over-determined equation group which has sufficient equations to estimate the spatial frequency components of the target plane and the aberration profiles across the array. The technique requires the area of the target to be small; when the system is in the Fresnel zone, only an approximated image can be obtained. The method will not apply to targets that extend in range. A least-mean-squares error-fitting method using the far-field signal-redundancy principle to measure the phase aberration profile directly has also been developed (Rachlin, 1990). In this method, first, common midpoint signals are cross correlated directly (without compensating for the near field effect, as shown in (11) in Rachlin, 1990) to find the relative time-shift between them, then an over-determined matrix is used to derive the phase-aberration value for each element. When there is no phase aberration, the relative time-shift between common midpoint signals is zero according to (9) and (10) in (Rachlin, 1990), which is true only in the far field. Therefore, this technique is a far-field signal redundancy technique. The analysis in this chapter shows that for targets in the near field, there is a near-field term in the relative time-shift between common midpoint signals. A dynamic near-field-delay correction is proposed to reduce its effect on the measurement. This is the major difference between the near-field signal-redundancy technique described in this chapter and the technique described in (Rachlin, 1990). In medical ultrasound imaging, dominant point targets, specular reflecting planes, and large areas of uniformly distributed speckle-generating target distributions are unlikely to be found in every isoplanatic patch. The signal redundancy method, which relies very little on target distributions, seems attractive. But, before it can be used in medical ultrasound imaging systems, the near-field effect has to be considered. First, however, the signal redundancy principle for targets in the far field will be reviewed in the next section.

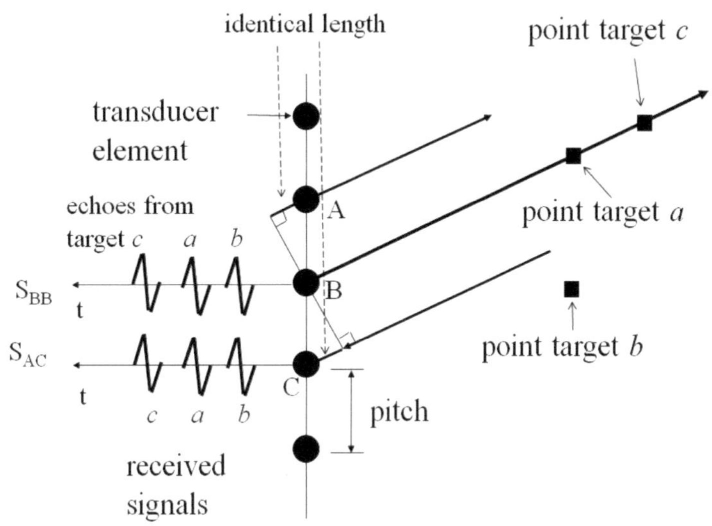

Fig. 2. The signal-redundancy principle for targets in the far field.

2. Signal-redundancy principle in the far field

For an active imaging system, when an array with many small aperture sensors is used to synthesize a larger aperture, it is possible to acquire identical signals using different sensors from arbitrary target distributions in the far field. These signals are termed redundant signals. Common midpoint signals (the middle point position of the transmitter and the receiver is the same) are redundant as shown in Fig. 2. Signal S_{AC} is acquired by transmitting from Element A and receiving at Element C; signal S_{BB} is acquired by transmitting and receiving at Element B. The midpoint of Elements A and C is the center of Element B. Therefore, S_{AC} and S_{BB} are common midpoint signals. When targets are in the far field, *e.g.*, targets *a*, *b* and *c*, S_{AC} and S_{BB} are exactly the same (redundant), because the length of the line segment on the right hand side of Element C and the line segment on the left hand side of Element A in Fig. 2 is the same for targets in all directions. When phase aberrations τ_A, τ_B and τ_C exist at Elements A, B and C, respectively, S_{AC} and S_{BB} will still have the same shape but will have a relative arrival-time difference $2\tau_B$-$(\tau_A+\tau_C)$, and this information can be used to derive the phase-aberration profile across the array.
These results are valid for short as well as long pulsed signals. They are valid generally for arbitrary target distributions provided that targets are in the far field and the propagation speed is homogenous. The effective aperture concept, defined as the convolution of the transmission aperture *T(z)* and the reception aperture *R(z)* for an active imaging system, is based on the assumption that common midpoint signals are identical; the integration of

$R(z')T(z - z')$ over all z' values adds common midpoint signals (midpoint $z/2$) together with the complex weighting of multiplied sensitivities and added phases of $T(z - z')$ and $R(z')$.

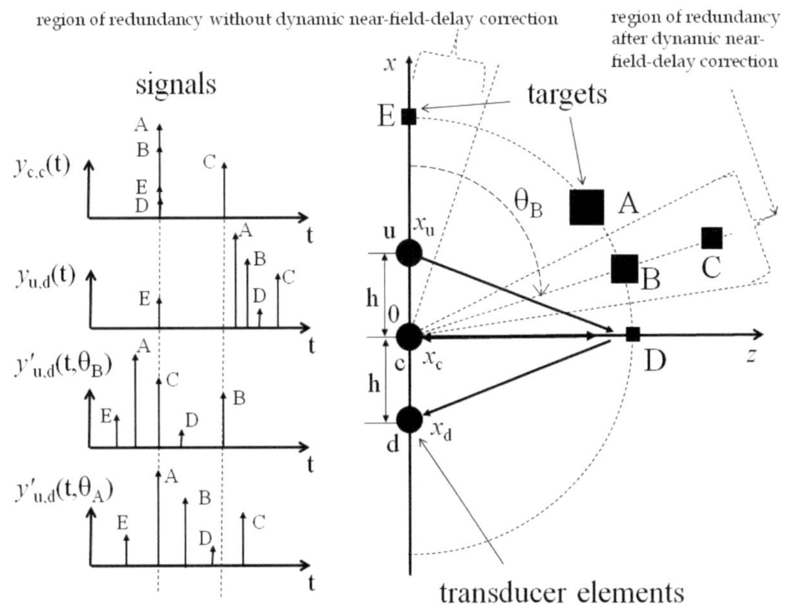

Fig. 3. An active imaging system with targets in the near field and the received and corrected signals when a delta-shaped pulse is transmitted and received.

3. Signal redundancy principle in the near field

For near-field targets, the signal redundancy principle described above is no longer valid. However, although common midpoint signals are not exactly redundant for active near-field imaging, their differences for echoes coming from certain regions can be significantly reduced by a dynamic near-field-delay correction (Li, 1997). Consider a three-element array on the x-axis in Fig. 3. The center element c is located at the origin $x = 0$, and the upper element u and lower element d are located at x_u and x_d respectively. It is assumed that $x_u = - x_d = h$. Let $y_{i,j}(t)$ denotes the received signal at element j when element i is the transmitter; $y_{u,d}(t)$, $y_{d,u}(t)$ and $y_{c,c}(t)$ are common midpoint signals; $y_{u,d}(t)$ and $y_{d,u}(t)$ are reciprocal signals, which are identical even for targets in the near field and inhomogeneous media. Assume that transmitted and received signals are delta-shaped pulses. The received signal $y_{c,c}(t)$ is shown in Fig. 3. Echoes coming from targets A, B, D and E arrive at the same time. The received signal $y_{u,d}(t)$ is also shown in Fig. 3. Even though $y_{u,d}(t)$ and $y_{c,c}(t)$ are common midpoint signals, the difference between them is obvious. The echo from target E, which is located on the x-axis, is the only one at the same location in signals $y_{c,c}(t)$ and $y_{u,d}(t)$.

The echo-location difference is larger for targets at angles nearer to the z-axis and at distances closer to the transducer elements. When the distance between the target and the aperture increases, the echo-location difference in $y_{c,c}(t)$ and $y_{u,d}(t)$ decreases, eventually becoming zero at infinite for the far-field situation. The echo-location difference in $y_{c,c}(t)$ and

$y_{u,d}(t)$ reaches its maximum value $2h/c_0$, where c_0 is the wave-propagation speed in the medium, when the target is at the position of Element c. A dynamic near-field-delay correction can be used to improve the similarity between $y_{c,c}(t)$ and $y_{u,d}(t)$ for echoes from the region around the z-axis of importance for imaging. This correction shifts signals so that envelope peaks of echoes coming from targets in a particular direction line up in the two common midpoint signals. It is the same as the delay process in the "delay-and-sum" dynamic focus image forming algorithm. The signal $y'_{u,d}$ (t, θ_B), which is the corrected version of $y_{u,d}(t)$, with the correction angle in the direction of targets B and C is shown in Fig. 3. The positions of echoes coming from targets B and C in $y'_{u,d}$ (t, θ_B) are the same as those in $y_{c,c}(t)$. That is, for echoes coming from these two targets, $y'_{u,d}$ (t, θ_B) and $y_{c,c}(t)$ are redundant. But the positions of echoes from targets A, D and E in $y'_{u,d}$ (t, θ_B) are different from that in $y_{c,c}(t)$, since these targets are not at the correction angle. The corrected signal $y'_{u,d}$ (t, θ_A) at angle of target A is also shown in Fig. 3.

A pulse with non-zero length will cause problems even for echoes coming from targets at the correction angle. For example, to make the echo from target B identical in $y_{c,c}(t)$ and $y_{u,d}(t)$, the whole pulse has to be moved with the same correction as that for the peak of the pulse envelope. But, since these echoes are overlapping, it is impossible to separate pulses from different depths (and angles) and move them separately. One can only do a dynamic delay correction as for a delta-shaped pulse. This will stretch the echo since the leading part of an echo is always shifted forwards more than its trailing part. Therefore, for a pulse of finite length, the dynamically corrected common midpoint signals are not strictly identical even for echoes coming from targets at the correction angle; the longer the pulse, the larger the difference. Fig. 5 in (Li. 1997) compares echoes coming from targets A, B, and D separately in $y'_{u,d}$ (t, θ_B) and $y_{c,c}(t)$. The echo from target B in $y'_{u,d}$ (t, θ_B) is stretched compared to that in $y_{c,c}(t)$ but their envelope peaks are coincident (Fig. 5(b)). The echo from target A in $y'_{u,d}$ (t, θ_B) is stretched compared with that in $y_{c,c}(t)$, and its envelope peak is shifted forward because of overcorrection. The echo from target D in $y'_{u,d}$ (t, θ_B) is stretched and shifted backward because of undercorrection.

After a dynamic near-field-delay correction, common midpoint signals will not become exactly redundant in the near field. But, they will be more similar for echoes coming from the region of interest. Within a specified error, the echoes coming from the region of interest can be regarded as redundant. The question is, given a pulse length L and an acceptable phase error limit ϕ_0, in what angular range should targets be for their echoes to become redundant in common midpoint signals after a dynamic near-field-delay correction? This question has been answered in (Li, 1997). Before the dynamic near-field-delay correction, the region of redundancy is around the x-axis (Fig. 3), which is not a region of interest. After the dynamic near-field-delay correction, the region of redundancy is around the correction angle. If transducer elements have some degree of directivity, so that their angular response is limited to the region of redundancy around the correction angle, the dynamic near-field-delay correction can increase the similarity between common midpoint signals in the near field. It has been shown in (Li, 1997) that common-midpoint signals are still a special group of signals in the near field because, after the dynamic near-field-delay correction, they are much more similar to one another compared with corrected signals in other signal groups. This is termed the near-field signal-redundancy principle.

For linear arrays, the element size is usually considerably larger than the wavelength. Therefore the beam width of each element is small and most signal energy is from the region of redundancy when the correction angle is around 90°. As a result, common-midpoint signals can be considered as redundant after the dynamic near-field-delay correction.

For phased arrays, the element size is usually smaller than a wave length and the beam of each element is wide. This causes two major problems. One problem is that the similarity between common-midpoint signals is not improved by the dynamic near-field-delay correction. It only shifts the region of redundancy to the area around the correction angle. Another problem is that echoes coming from different angles may experience different aberration values, which makes it impossible to measure the phase aberration profiles using the linear array algorithm. The sub-array method proposed in (Li, 2000a, 2000b; Li & Robinson, 2000b) can be used to solve both problems, if the phase-aberration value for elements in the same sub-array can be considered as the same in all directions. This requirement may limit the maximum size of sub-arrays, and therefore limit the narrowest achievable beamwidth and the maximum spatial frequency of the aberrator that can be successfully measured. In this method, sub-arrays are formed of adjacent groups of elements to narrow the beams used to acquire common-midpoint signals and steer the beam direction, so that the similarity between common-midpoint signals is increased and angle-dependent, phase-aberration profiles can be measured. There are several methods can be used to implement the dynamic near-field-delay correction on common-midpoint signals collected with sub-arrays. These methods have different computation loads and the degree of similarity between common-midpoint signals collected in these methods is also different. The performance of these methods has been analyzed and compared theoretically in (Li, 2000b).

For two-dimensional arrays, besides using elements along a straight line, there is another element configuration that can be used to acquired common-midpoint signals, which does not exist for one-dimensional arrays. Consider four adjacent, point-like transducer elements (Fig. 4) in a two-dimensional array. They are labeled as Element 1, 2, 3 and 4 and located in the x-y plane at $(p_x/2, p_y/2)$, $(-p_x/2, p_y/2)$, $(-p_x/2, -p_y/2)$ and $(p_x/2, -p_y/2)$, respectively, where p_x and p_y are array pitches in the x and y directions respectively. $y_{2,4}(t)$ and $y_{1,3}(t)$ are common midpoint signals, because the midpoints between their transmitters and receivers are located at the same point (the origin in Fig. 4). It has been shown (Li & Robinson, 2008) that without the dynamic near-field-delay correction, the region of redundancy is between two rectangular hyperbolas (Fig. 5), which is in the direction of interest for imaging. This is different from the case of one-dimensional arrays, where, without the dynamic near-field-delay correction, the region of redundancy is in the direction of the axis that goes through the three consecutive transducer elements used to acquire common-midpoint signals (Fig. 3), which is not in the direction of

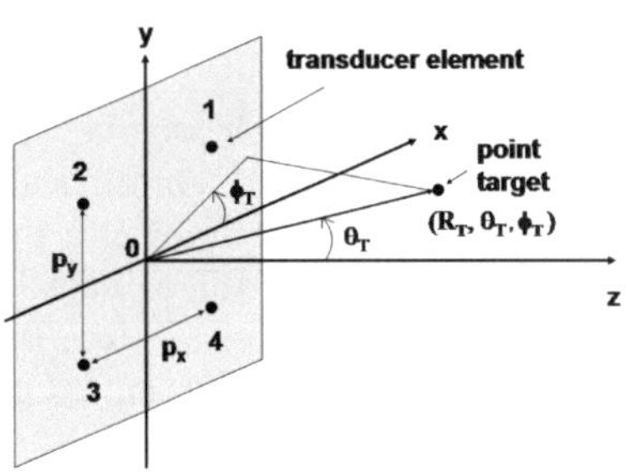

Fig. 4. A four-element sub-aperture in a two-dimensional array.

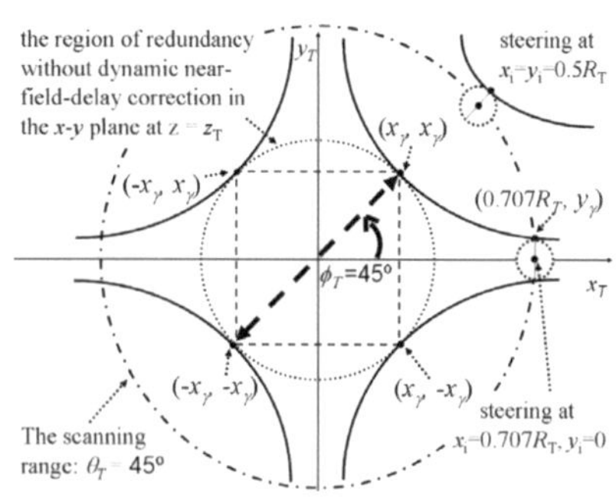

Fig. 5. The region of redundancy (not to scale).

interest for imaging. The region of redundancy is narrowest in the direction of $\phi_T = \pm 45^o$ (Fig. 5). The region of redundancy can be approximately defined as inside the circle within those hyperbolas as shown in Fig. 5. Many properties of the region of redundancy have been theoretically derived in (Li & Robinson, 2008).
As in the case of one-dimensional arrays, the region of redundancy for common-midpoint signals acquired with four adjacent transducer elements can also be shifted to other directions with the dynamic near-field-delay correction. This is a useful property for measuring angle-dependent phase-aberration profiles using sub-arrays and it has been theoretically analyzed in (Li & Robinson, 2008).
In this section, the near-field signal redundancy principles have been discussed for linear, phased and two-dimensional arrays. In the next section, phase-aberration correction algorithms based on these principles are introduced and experimental results are presented.

4. Aberration correction using near field signal redundancy

4.1 Algorithm for linear arrays

Since the array pitch of linear arrays are much larger than the center-frequency wave length of the transmitted pulse, each element has a relatively narrow beam in the z-axis direction. However, the beam cannot be steered. A sub-aperture of the array is used to form an image line and the whole image is formed by sliding the sub-aperture across the array. The linear array algorithm for phase-aberration correction based on the near-field signal-redundancy principle was proposed in (Li, 1997). A few important considerations relating to this algorithm are discussed here.
For each midpoint position, many common midpoint signals can be acquired using a linear array. However, only the closest common midpoint signal pairs (acquired using three adjacent elements) should be used because the near-field effect is smallest for these signals. The received signals are dynamically corrected at the 90° angle. The normalized cross-correlation functions are calculated at a selected depth with a selected window length. The region chosen for correlation should be the region in which one wants to improve the lateral resolution. The length of the correlation window should be chosen so that the signal experiences the same aberration effect, *i.e.* in the same isoplanatic patch. On the other hand, it should be as long as possible to improve the signal-to-noise ratio of cross-correlation functions. The dynamic near-field-delay correction can also be applied at a few angles and the peak position of the cross-correlation function with the maximum cross-correlation coefficient is chosen for deriving the phase-aberration profile.
For an N element array, there are N-2 pairs of common-midpoint signals and measured peak positions. They are related to the phase error at each element by equation (26) in (Li, 1997). The phase aberration profile can be derived assuming that the phase-aberration values for the two elements at the ends of the array are zero. This assumption causes a linear-component error (the ambiguity profile) between the derived phase-aberration profile and the real phase-aberration profile. If the ambiguity profile is small, its effect is approximately a global rotation and range shift of the image. If it is large, it will influence the focusing quality. A detailed analysis of the influence of ambiguity profiles on focusing in the very near field can be found in (Li, 2002a, 2002b).
Errors in peak position measurements of cross-correlation functions will be magnified in the process of deriving the phase aberration profile. Results of theoretical analysis in (Li, 2007) indicate that the accuracy requirement on the peak position measurement is very high for an

array with a large number of elements. For a 64-element array, the bias in the peak-position measurement is magnified by a factor up to 496. Assume that the acceptable largest bias of the derived phase-aberration value is one radian, then the measurement bias needs to be less than 1/496 radians, which is a very strict requirement. Assuming that a constant or linear profile does not influence focusing, the requirement is relaxed to 1/325 radians, and the maximum bias value in the derived phase aberration profile occurs at the ends of the array. The standard deviations of peak position measurements also have to be small in order to measure the phase-aberration profiles accurately. For a 64-element array, the maximum standard deviation in the derived phase-aberration profile is about 72 times the standard deviation of the measured peak position; the *rms* is 52 times, or 25 times if the constant and linear profiles are considered as harmless.

The strict accuracy requirement on peak position measurements creates a new problem. The timing of electronic channels (receiver and transmitter) has to be calibrated accurately. The requirement for channels to be considered as identical is much stricter for phase-aberration measurement than for image formation. Therefore, the system calibration on a commercial machine usually is not accurate enough. The timing errors of channels are part of the phase aberration profile and they make phase aberration profiles for transmission and reception different. When the timing error difference between transmission and reception channels connected to the same element is small enough for the purpose of image formation, the method proposed in (Li, 1997) can be used to solve this problem. The two reciprocal signals $y_{u,d}(t)$ and $y_{d,u}(t)$ (Fig. 3) are dynamically corrected and cross-correlated with $y_{c,c}(t)$ separately. The two peak positions are then averaged and used to derive the phase aberration profile, which can be used for both transmission and reception phase-aberration corrections. There is no need to measure the transmission and reception phase aberration profiles separately. That is, when the difference between transmission and reception phase-aberration profiles is small for image-formation purpose but large for phase-aberration measurement, they have to be treated as different when performing the phase-aberration measurement, but they can be treated as the same in the image-formation process after the measurement. If the difference is large for imaging purpose, they need to be measured separately. In this case, the reciprocal-signal method proposed in (Li, 2008) can be used.

To perform the dynamic near-field-delay correction, the array pitch and the average propagation speed in the medium need to be known. How accurately these parameters need to be known for the near-field signal-redundancy algorithm to perform properly? This has been analyzed in (Li et al., 1996). If the array pitch and propagation speed are not known accurately, the formed image (image formation also uses the two parameters) will also be distorted even if the medium is homogeneous. That is, phase aberrations are introduced by incorrect pitch and speed values and the phase aberration profile across the array is different at different points in the image. It has been shown in (Li et al., 1996) that the near-field signal-redundancy algorithm is capable of correcting phase aberrations generated by pitch and speed errors. Therefore, the array pitch and average propagation speed need not to be known very accurately. However, large errors will reduce the size of the isoplanatic patch and therefore require more phase-aberration profiles to be measured to correct the whole image (Li et al., 1996).

The near-field signal-redundancy algorithm for linear arrays typically includes the following steps:

1. Common midpoint signals are acquired.
2. Dynamic near-field-delay corrections are applied at a proper angle.

3. The dynamically corrected common midpoint signals are cross-correlated at a selected depth with a selected window length.
4. The relative time-shift between common midpoint signals are measured from the peak position of the cross-correlation functions.
5. The relative time-shifts between $y_{u,d}(t)$ and $y_{c,c}(t)$ and between $y_{d,u}(t)$ and $y_{c,c}(t)$ are averaged.
6. The phase-aberration profile across the array is derived.
7. If necessary, the undetermined linear term (ambiguity profile) is adjusted to optimize the performance of the system.

This algorithm has been experimentally tested (Li et al., 1997). The system used to test this algorithm was based on a Toshiba model SAL-32B 8-channel Scanner. This system has 64 transmission channels, 8 reception channels multiplexed across the array. This system is capable of separately transmitting on each individual element, and receiving on eight channels at a time. It can be switched between the normal real-time scan mode and the single-element-transmit/multiple-element-receive data collecting mode. A 64-element linear array was used with a pitch of 1.0 mm and an element width of about 1.0 mm. The element height is 10 mm, and the focus of the lens in the elevation direction is at about 60 mm. The received pulse has a 3.5 MHz centre frequency and 2 MHz bandwidth.

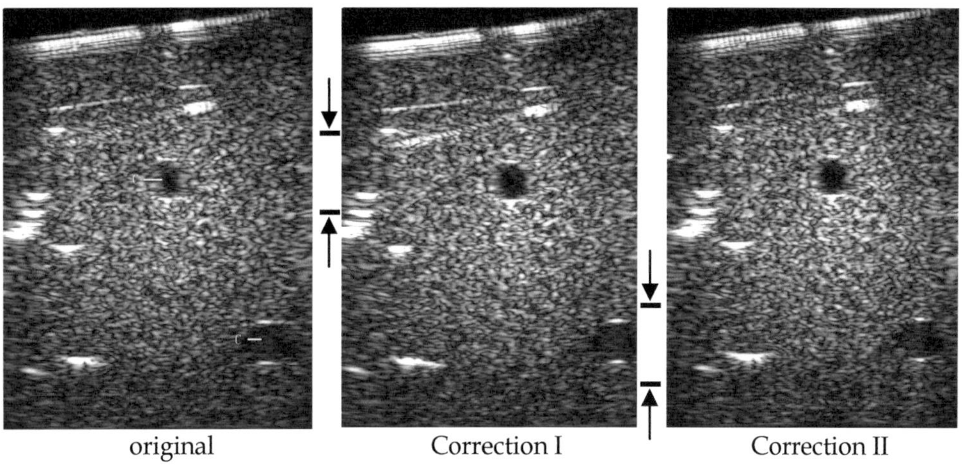

Fig. 6. Correction results of images from a tissue mimicking phantom with an aberrator.

4.1.1 Experimental results from a tissue-mimicking phantom

The data were acquired from a tissue-mimicking phantom overlaid by an aberrator. The aberrator has a speed of 1420 ms^{-1} and an attenuation coefficient 1.2 dB $cm^{-1}MHz^{-1}$. The shape of the aberrator is shown in Fig. 1 in (Li et al., 1997). Two aberrating structures were cut out and put above the two cysts in the phantom. The speed of the aberrator is close to that of fat. Since the array is one-dimensional, the structure of the aberrator is also one-dimensional. The tissue mimicking phantom was RMI-413, but is an earlier version and the cysts are 6 mm, not 7.5 mm, in diameter.

The original aberrated image and two corrected images are shown in Fig. 6. The first correction used signals coming from a depth near the upper cyst (indicated by arrows). The second correction used signals from a depth near the lower cyst. The two cysts are distorted in the original image, and the distortions in the original image are partially corrected in the two corrected images.

For comparison, the results from the same phantom without the aberrator are shown in Fig. 7. The difference between the original and corrected is very small because the measured phase-aberration profile has very small values (Li et al., 1997), which indicates that the noise level and other parameters were reasonable for the successful measurement of phase-aberration profiles.

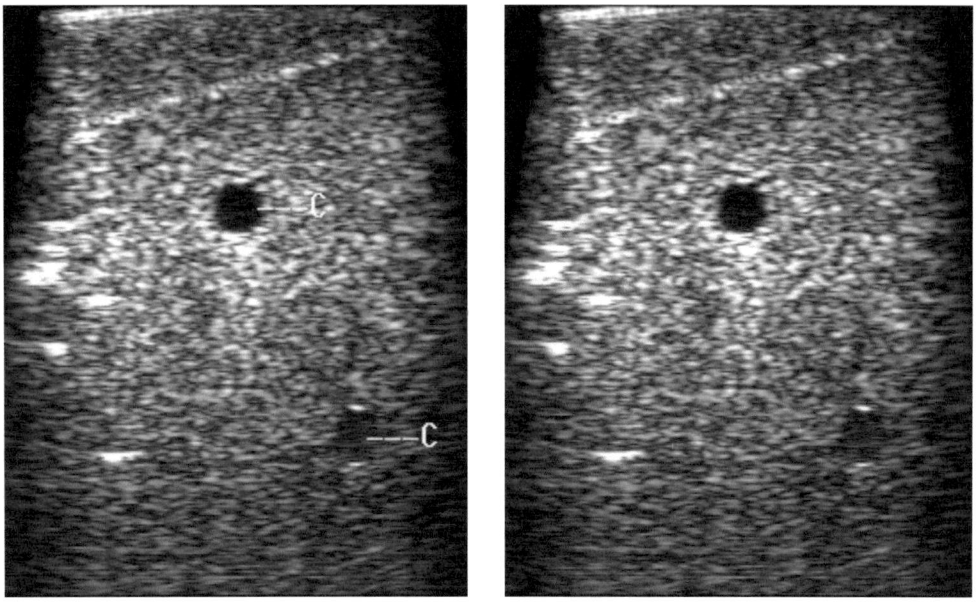

original corrected

Fig. 7. Correction results of images from a tissue mimicking phantom without the aberrator.

4.1.2 Experimental results from volunteers

Data were acquired from a group of volunteer subjects. Since the height of elements in the linear array was large (10 mm) and the algorithm requires that phase aberration values for echoes received at an element can be considered as the same, transverse abdomen scan was used because of the structure of muscles and fat layers in that position. The system was operated in the normal real-time scanning mode to scan for an aberrated image, and then switched to the synthetic-aperture mode to acquire data.

Fig. 8 shows the original and two corrected images from Volunteer 1. The superior-mesenteric-artery (SMA) and the aorta are used as the main objects to evaluate the quality of the images. In the original image the SMA and the aorta are distorted. In the corrected images, their boundaries are much better defined and their shape is more circular. Fig. 9 shows the results from Volunteer 2. The boundaries of the SMA and the aorta are better defined in the corrected image than they are in the original image. Fig. 10 shows the results from Volunteer 3 using data from three different depths. The boundaries of the SMA and the aorta are better defined in the corrected images; the Splenic Vein (SV) is also much clearer in the corrected image. This data set is the same as that used to form images in Fig. 1.

Volunteer 1

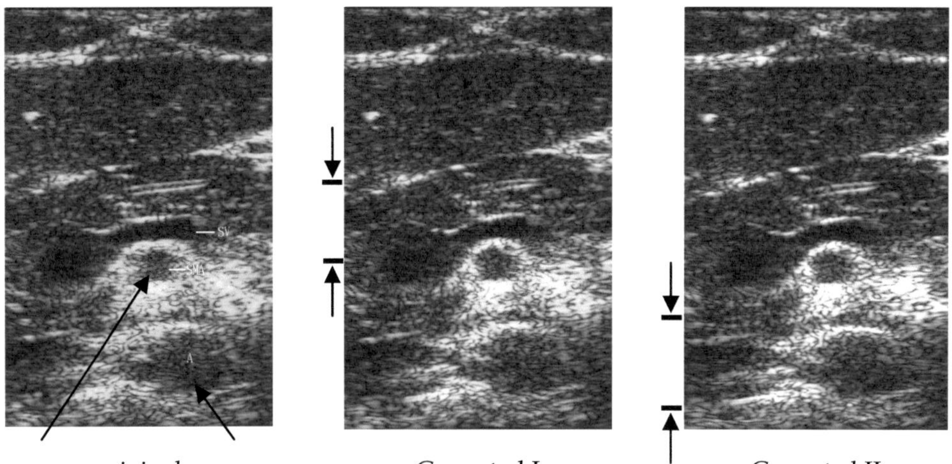

Fig. 8. Correction results of images from Volunteer 1.

Volunteer 2

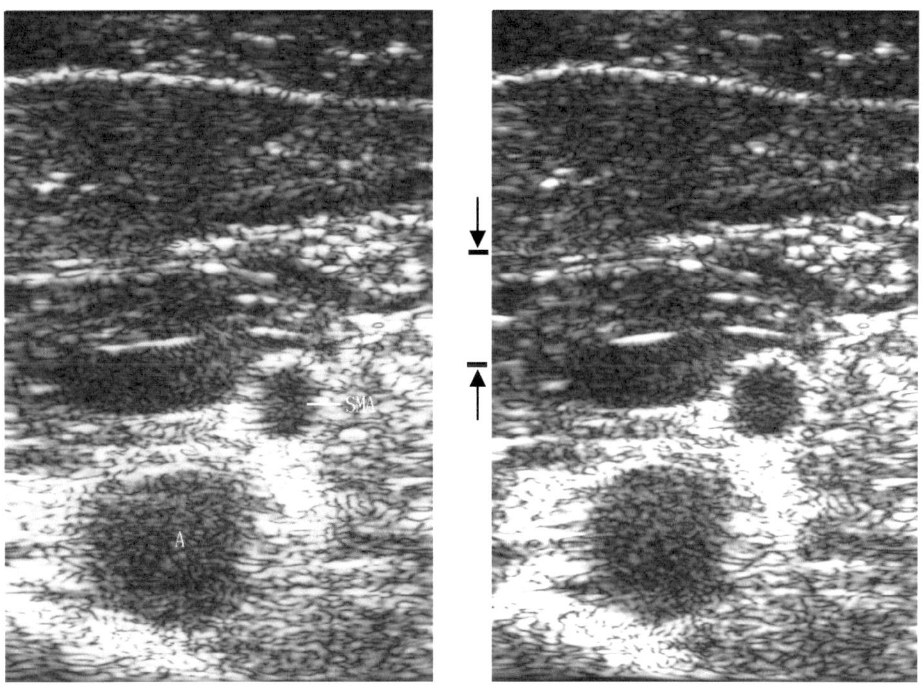

Fig. 9. Correction results of images from Volunteer 2.

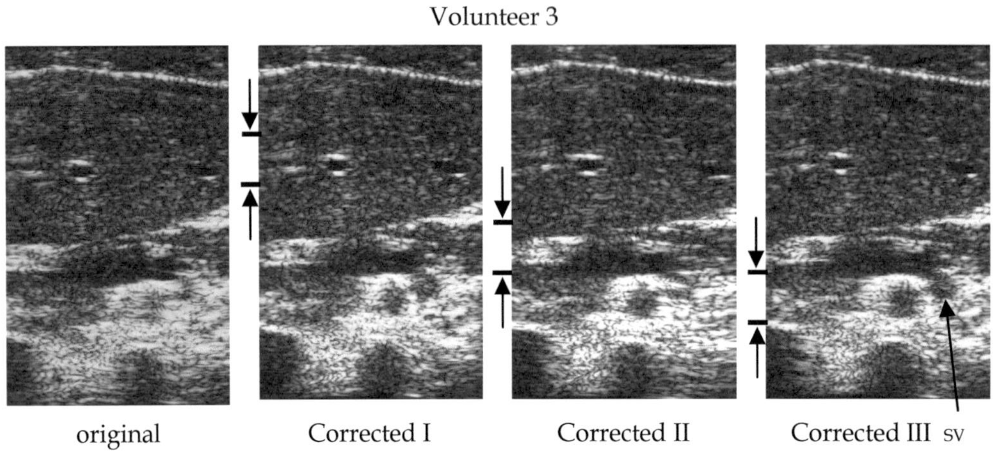

Fig. 10. Correction results of images from Volunteer 3.

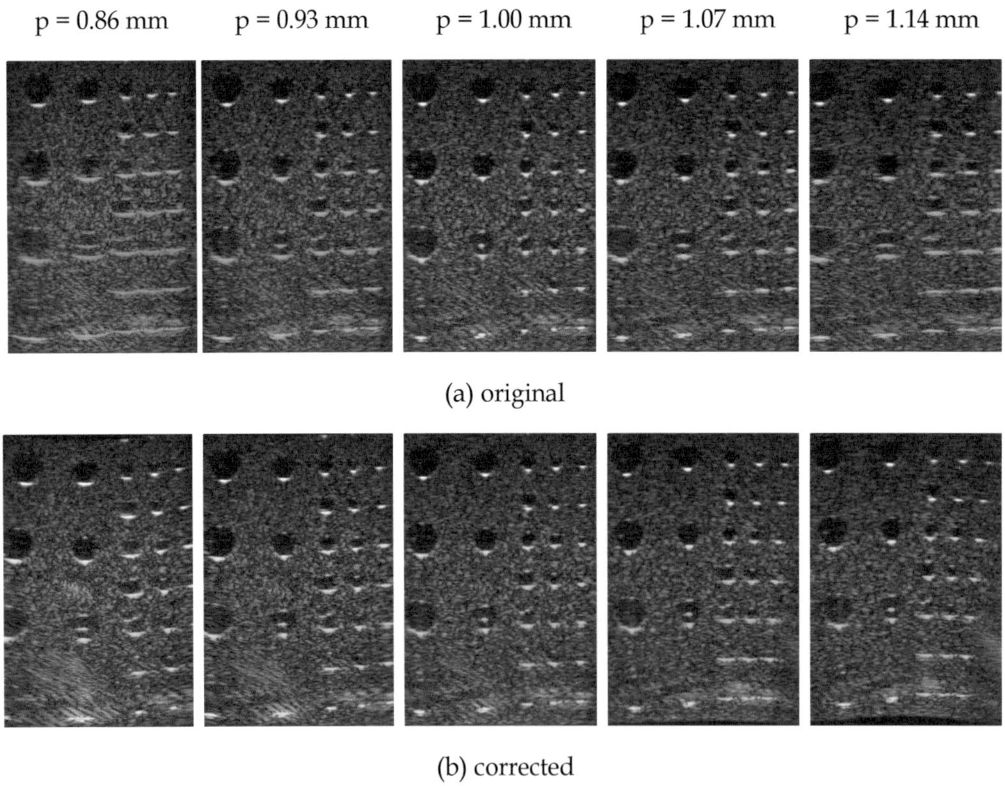

Fig. 11. Results of correcting phase aberrations generated by incorrect pitch values.

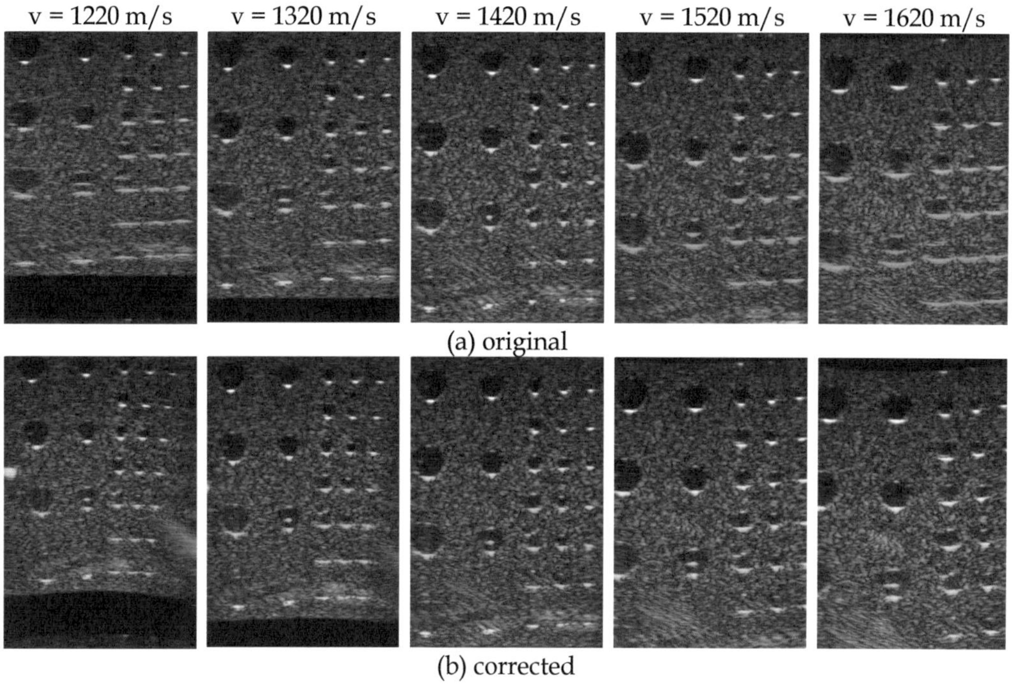

Fig. 12. Results of correcting phase aberrations generated by incorrect speed values.

4.1.3 Experimental results of correcting phase aberrations generated by incorrect pitch and speed values

Data acquired from a tissue-mimicking phantom without any aberrator were used to test the performance of the linear array algorithm on correcting phase aberrations generated by incorrect array pitch and propagation speed values. The phantom had a propagation speed of 1420 m/s. The true array pitch was 1.00 mm. The synthetic aperture image formed using five pitch values and five speed values are shown in Figs. 11(a) and 12(a), respectively, and the image in the middle was formed with the correct value. The size of the images is 45 mm x 55 mm. Images formed with incorrect values are significantly distorted. Phase aberration profiles were measured using the linear array algorithm with the incorrect pitch and speed values. The signal range used in the measurements was around the fourth row of small cysts. The corrected images are shown in Figs. 11(b) and 12(b), respectively. The correction has restored the focus, especially in the region around the fourth row of small cysts. By measuring several phase aberration profiles using signals from different depths, the whole image can be improved, as it is demonstrated later in the chapter with images formed using phased arrays. These corrected images also show distortions (expansion or compression) in both lateral and axial directions caused by ambiguity profiles (Li et al., 1996).

4.2 Algorithm for phased arrays

The sub-array algorithm for small-element arrays has been proposed in (Li & Robinson, 1997; Li, 2000b). It can be used to overcome problems caused by the wide beam and angle-dependent aberration profiles. This sub-array algorithm typically includes the following steps:

1. Choose a sub-array size. The optimal sub-array size depends on the aberrator properties; therefore, it is difficult to determine in advance. A trial-and-error method may have to be used.
2. Acquire individual signals (transmit at one element and receive at one element) by transmitting at one element at a time and receiving at several elements. The number of receiving elements depends on the size of sub-arrays.
3. Form common-midpoint signals acquired with sub-arrays at several steering directions or imaging lines at selected angle intervals.
4. Calculate the normalized cross-correlation function between these common-midpoint signals at a selected depth with a selected window length.
5. Measure relative time-shift between common-midpoint signals from the peak position of these cross-correlation functions.
6. Derive the phase-aberration profiles across the array for each steering angle or image line.
7. Assign the derived phase-aberration value for each sub-array to each element in that sub-array.

4.2.1 Experimental results from a tissue-mimicking phantom

This algorithm has been successfully tested on data acquired from a tissue mimicking phantom with an aberrator (Li & Robinson, 2000b). The imaging system was a modified ATL Ultramark® 8. The transducer used was an ATL 48-element phased-array with 0.28 mm pitch and 3.0 MHz center frequency. The azimuthal cross-section from the center of the transducer is shown in Fig. 13. The aberrator was made from cast RTV, which had a sound

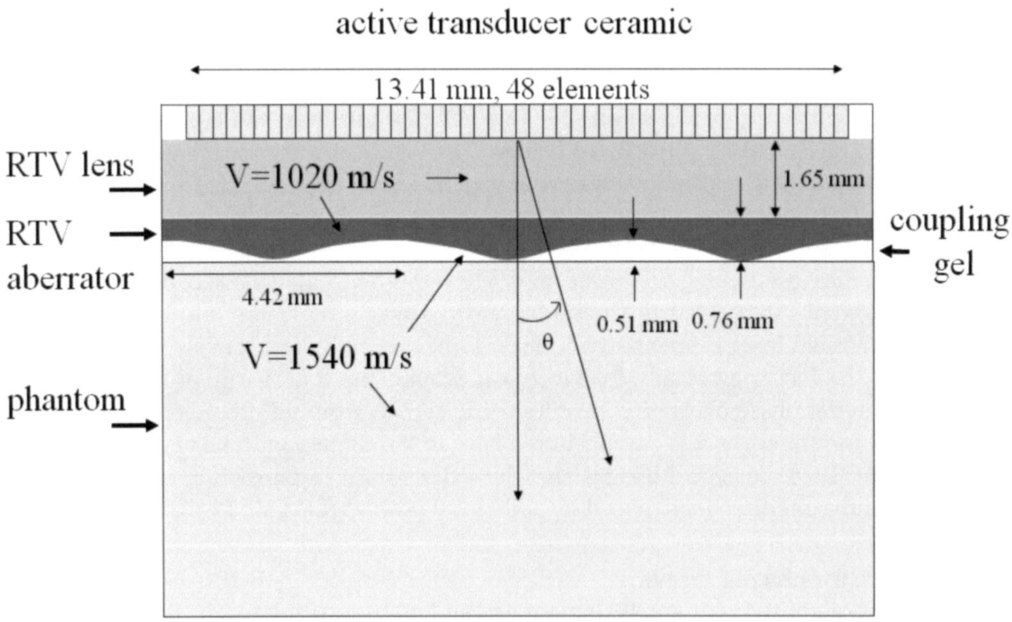

Fig. 13. The azimuthal center cross-section of the ATL transducer with the aberrator attached to its front surface.

velocity of 1020 ms^{-1}, and an attenuation coefficient 1.5 dB mm^{-1} at 3 MHz. The aberrator had a sinusoidal surface, the peak-to-peak range of the sinusoidal wave was 0.51 mm and the period was 4.42 mm. The total active aperture of the array was about 3.03 wavelengths of the sinusoidal wave. The total thickness of the aberrator was about 0.76 mm. The aberrator was cast so that its inner surface conformed to the surface of the elevational focus lens of the array. The potential space between the lens and the aberrator was filled with ultrasound coupling gel, which had a sound speed of 1540 ms^{-1}. Coupling gel also filled the space between the sinusoidal surface of the aberrator and the phantom.

The aberrator introduces a (one-way) phase-error of almost exactly π-radians at 3 MHz. The unaberrated image of the RMI 413 phantom is shown in Fig. 14(a), which was obtained with the same transducer without the aberrator at approximately the same location on the phantom. The image of the phantom from the data set collected with the aberrator attached to the transducer is shown in Fig. 14(b). It is severely aberrated; each point target is tripled with reduced resolution, and the contrast ratio of the anechoic cystic structures is significantly reduced.

To demonstrate the problem related to the wide beam of small elements, we first use the linear-array algorithm to correct the phase aberration. The correction angle for the dynamic near-field-delay correction was at 90° (perpendicular to the array) and the measured profile was used to correct phase aberrations for all image lines (Fig.14(c)). The image quality near the 90° direction has been improved, revealing a column of point targets. The image quality at other directions has not been improved as much. There are no means to measure angle-dependent, phase-aberration profiles without forming sub-arrays. Note that by performing the dynamic near-field-delay correction at different angles in a single-element measurement one does not measure the aberration profiles at different directions. To demonstrate this, phase-aberration profiles were measured with 19 different correction angles, from 45° to 135° at 5° intervals. The measured aberration profiles were very similar for these correction angles (Li & Robinson, 2000b) and the corrected image (Fig. 14(d)) is very similar to that in Fig. 14(c). To measure angle-dependent phase-aberration profiles, sub-arrays need to be formed to narrow and steer the beams. In the sub-array algorithm, each sub-array was formed with three elements (16 sub-arrays in total). The beams of sub-arrays were formed with the synthetic aperture approach and were dynamically focused both on transmission and reception at a correction angle (the beam steering direction). The formed beam had a theoretical -6 dB (two-way) beamwidth of about 20.5° (Li & Robinson, 2000b). It subtended about 0.17 wavelengths of the sinusoidal aberrator. Beams were steered at 19 different angles, from 45° to 135° at 5° intervals, and 19 phase-aberration profiles were derived. The corrected image using the measured phase-aberration profile at the 90° beam steering angle for all images lines is shown in Fig. 15(a) and the focusing quality is only improved around the 90° direction. Similarly, using the phase aberration profile measured at the 105° beam steering angle to correct all images lines only improved the focusing quality around the 105° direction (Fig. 15(b)). The corrected image using all 19 measured profiles is shown in Fig. 15(c) and resolution is improved in all directions. However, the image quality in regions near the left and right boundaries of the image has not improved as much. This is because the strong refraction effect (between RTV and coupling gel) at those angles makes it difficult to measure the aberration profiles accurately in those directions. The aberration values for the two sub-arrays at the two ends of the array are different, and the difference depends on the steering angle. By assuming that they are zeros in the process of deriving the aberration profile, different ambiguity profiles are introduced in the derived aberration profiles at different steering angles. For targets far from the transducer, where the angle from an image pixel to all elements is approximately the same, the changing ambiguity profile will not influence the focusing of the system at each pixel; however, the image may become distorted (change of target shape). For targets near the transducer, where the angle from an image pixel to each element varies, the focusing quality is reduced at that pixel because of the different ambiguity profiles for the derived aberration profiles from different steering angles. The derived aberration profiles were adjusted by adding a proper ambiguity profile and the corrected image is shown in Fig. 15(d). The image quality is further improved.

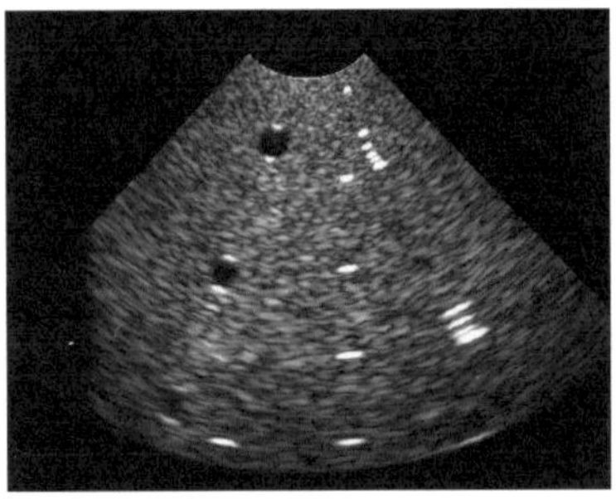

(a) without the aberrator

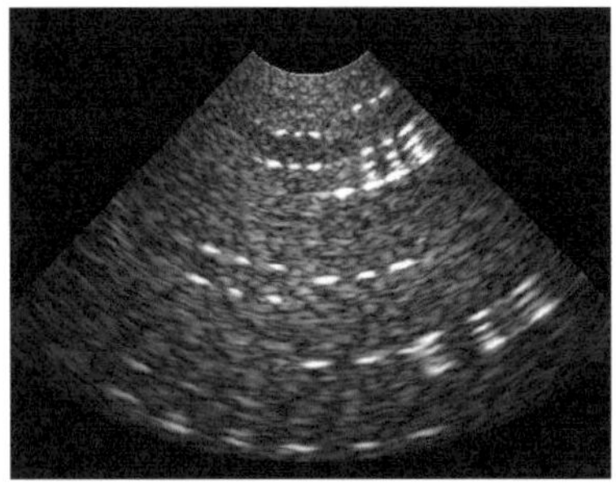

(b) original with the aberrator

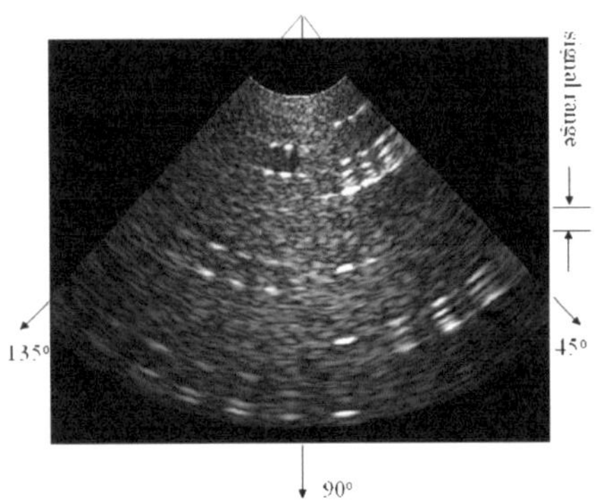

(c) The corrected image using the phase-aberration profile derived without forming sub-arrays at correction angle 90°.

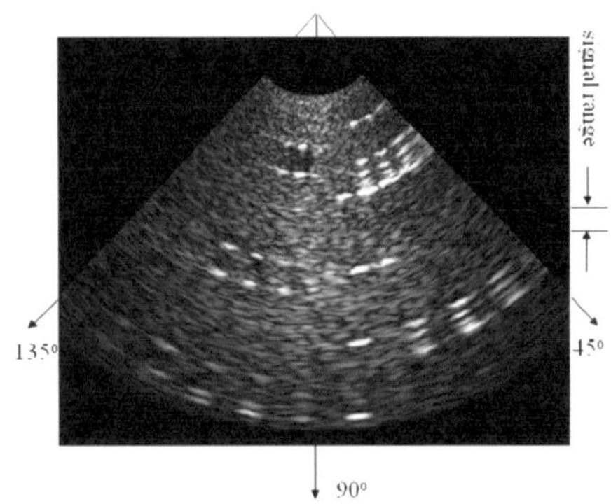

(d) The corrected image using 19 phase-aberration profiles derived without forming sub-arrays and at 19 correction angles between 45° and 135° at 5° intervals.

Fig. 14. (a) Original image without the aberrator. (b) Original image with the aberrator. (c) The corrected image using the phase-aberration profile derived without forming sub-arrays at correction angle 90°. (d) The corrected image using 19 phase-aberration profiles derived without forming sub-arrays and at 19 correction angles between 45° and 135° at 5° intervals.

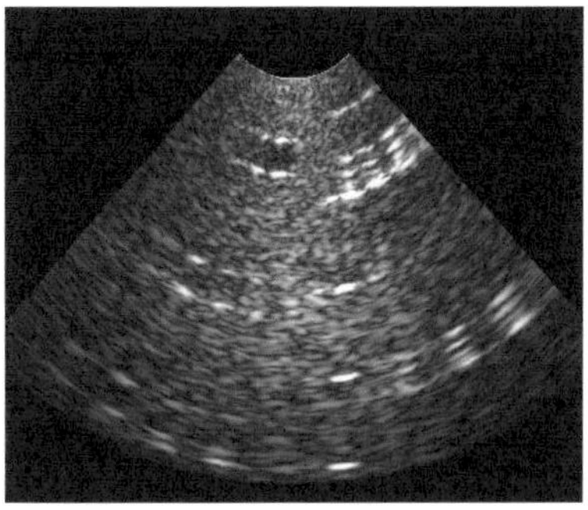

(a) The corrected image using the measured phase-aberration profile at the 90° beam steering angle for all images lines.

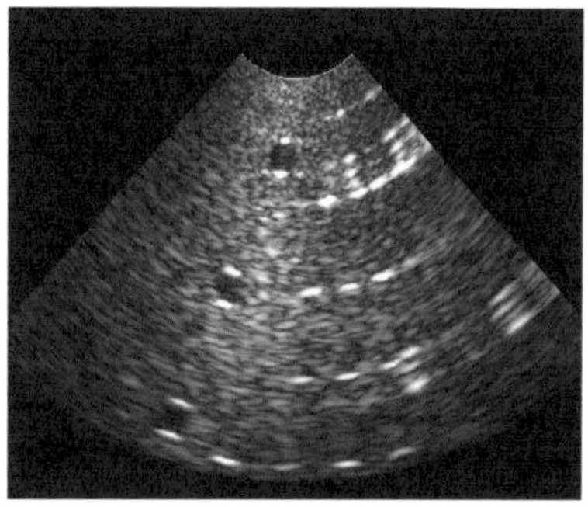

(b) The corrected image using the measured phase-aberration profile at the 105° beam steering angle for all images lines.

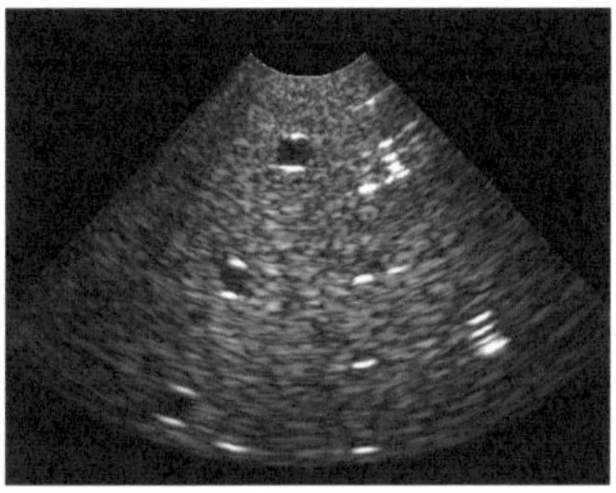

(c) The corrected image using the phase-aberration profile derived with the steering angle-based sub-array method.

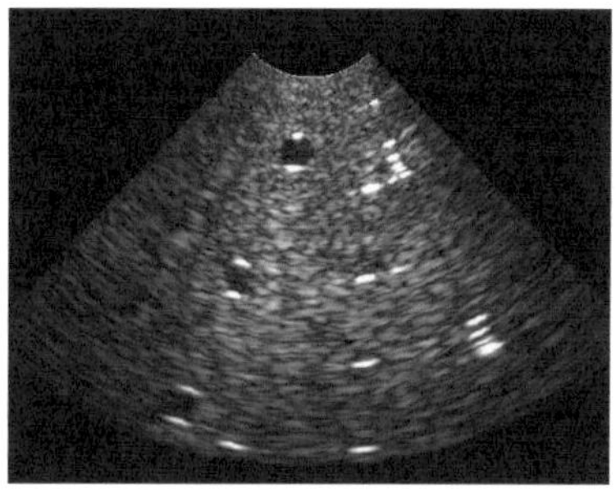

(d) The corrected image using the phase-aberration profiles derived using the steering angle-based sub-array method after manually adjusting ambiguity profiles.

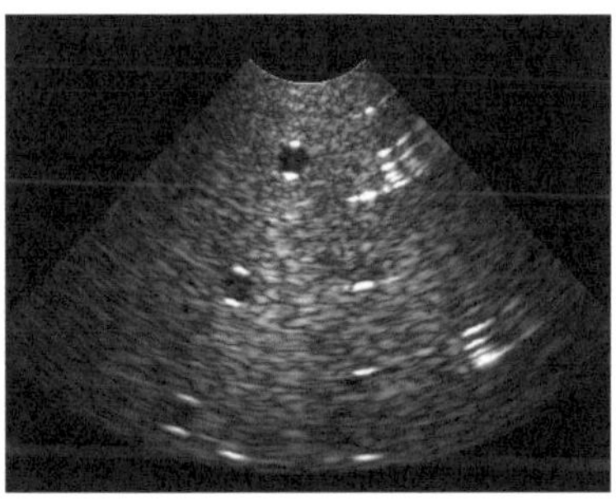

(e) The corrected image using the phase-aberration profiles derived using the image line-based sub-array method without adjusting ambiguity profiles

Fig. 15. Correction results using sub-arrays. (a) The corrected image using the measured phase-aberration profile at the 90° beam steering angle for all images lines. (b) The corrected image using the measured phase-aberration profile at the 105° beam steering angle for all images lines. (c) The corrected image using all 19 measured phase-aberration profiles (d) The corrected image using all 19 measured phase-aberration profiles with manually adjusted ambiguity profiles. (e) The corrected image using 19 measured phase-aberration profiles derived along image lines.

However, this process requires knowledge of the ambiguity profile for all directions, which is usually not available. A better way to measure the phase-aberration profile is to form common-midpoint beams along an image line (Li, 2000b), instead of at a steering angle. The advantage is that the focusing quality of each image pixel will not be influenced by the undetermined linear ambiguity profile; however, the image may still be distorted if the undetermined linear terms are very different for different image lines. The corrected image using this method is shown in Fig. 15(e). Compared with Fig. 15(c), the image quality for pixels near the transducer surface is improved in Fig. 15(e). Note that the derived aberration profiles are not adjusted for the undetermined different steering terms in this case.

4.2.2 Experimental results of correcting phase aberrations generated by incorrect pitch and speed values

The data set acquired from the phantom without the aberrator (Fig. 15(a)) was also used to demonstrate the capability of the sub-array method to correct phase aberrations generated by incorrect array pitch or propagation speed errors (Li et al., 2002). The synthetic aperture image formed using four incorrect pitch values and four incorrect speed values are shown in Figs. 16(a) and 17(a), respectively. The distortions are obvious.

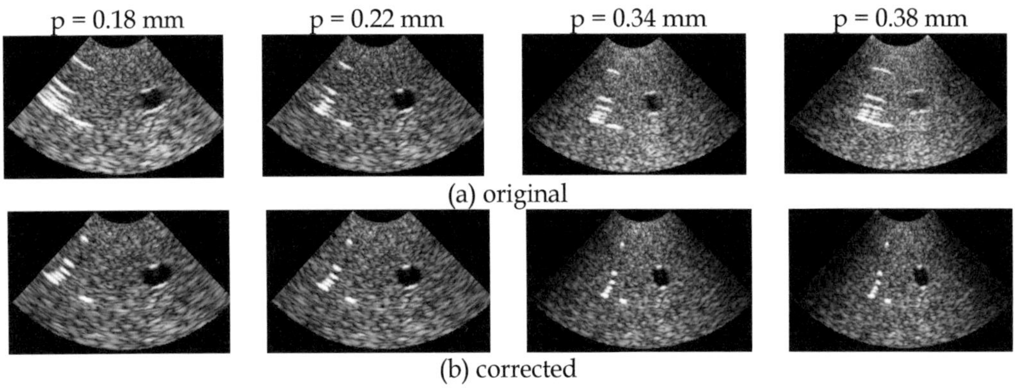

Fig. 16. Correction of phase aberrations generated by incorrect pitch values. (a) original images. (b) corrected images.

Phase aberration profiles were measured using the assumed pitch and speed values. The profile was again derived at 19 steering angles ($45^{o} \leq \theta_{i} \leq 135^{o}$ with 5° interval) and signals around the nearest (to the transducer) point target, the cyst, and the farthest point target vertically below the nearest point target were used to derive three profiles for each direction, resulting in a total of 57 profiles. Figs. 16(b) and 17(b) show images after corrections. These results demonstrated that, after correction, the focusing quality in all the investigated cases is significantly improved in the whole image. These results also show distortions caused by the ambiguity profile (expansion and compression in both lateral and axial directions). The image is compressed (expanded) in the axial direction because the echo from a point target is treated as if it were from a target at a closer (farther) distance from the transducer when the speed is underestimated (overestimated). Different scales were used in Figs. 16 and 17 so that targets of interest occupy a similar image size as that in the un-aberrated image.

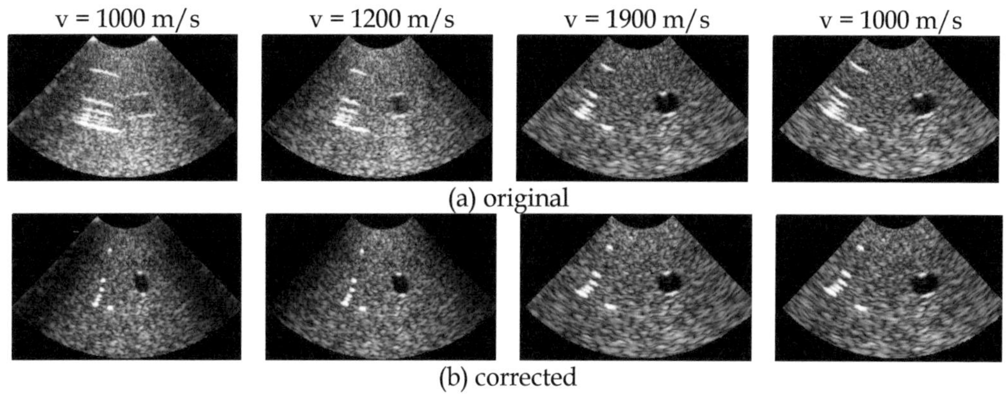

Fig. 17. Correction of phase aberrations generated by incorrect speed values. (a) original images. (b) corrected images.

4.2.3 Experimental results of system-error-difference calibration

The data set acquired using this phased-array system was also used to experimentally test the reciprocal signal algorithm for system-error-difference calibration (Li, 2008). The system has 48 transmission channels and 48 reception channels. Therefore each element has its own transmission and reception channels. Reciprocal signals acquired using each element (the reference element) in the transducer and all other elements were cross correlated. The cross-correlation coefficients between these reciprocal signals are shown in Fig. 18(a). All coefficients are very close to unity, except those that involve Element 12, which indicates that Element 12 was abnormal. Note that the cross-correlation coefficient between reciprocal signals acquired using the reference element and itself is also shown in Fig. 18(a), which is unity because the two reciprocal signals were the same signal. The peak positions of the cross-correlation functions are shown in Fig. 18(b) in grayscale. Each row in Fig. 18(b) is the derived system-error-difference profile using a different reference element. As a consequence, all rows should have identical shape but may have different offsets, if there was no noise (Li, 2008). This can be clearly seen in Fig. 18 (c), where the row profiles are plotted on top of one another. All the rows can be treated as the measurement result using a different element as the reference element. Its advantage is that only a small number of cross-correlation functions needs to be calculated. To improve the measurement accuracy, all row profiles can be averaged and it is shown in Fig. 18(d) together with the one standard deviation (each direction) lines. The profile should have a bias that is the average value of all system-error-difference values (Li, 2008). The peak-to-peak range of system-error-difference values of this system is less than 0.03 microseconds. The period of the transmitted signal at the center frequency (3.5 MHz) is about 0.29 microseconds. Therefore the difference between timing errors in the transmission and reception channels is less than one tenth of a period. Consequently, the transmission and reception phase-aberration profiles can be considered as the same for image formation. There is no need to separately measure transmission and reception channel-timing errors.

4.3 Algorithm for two-dimensional arrays

A few methods have been proposed to implement the near-field signal redundancy algorithm on a two-dimensional array. The all-row-plus-two-column algorithm (Li &

Robinson, 2000a) applies the one-dimensional near-field signal redundancy algorithm on all rows as well as the first and last columns of the transducer array, and then these results are combined to form a two-dimensional phase-aberration profile. However, the ambiguity profile of this method is not linear and a time-consuming iterative method has to be used to linearize the ambiguity profile. To solve this problem, an all-row-plus-two-column-and-a-diagonal algorithm has been proposed (Li & Robinson, 2007). In this algorithm, the one-dimensional algorithm is also applied to elements along a tilted line (the diagonal line if the array is square). The ambiguity profile of this algorithm is linear but it is very sensitive to noise. Another method, the cross algorithm (Li & Robinson, 2008), is based on the two-dimensional near-field signal-redundancy principle discussed in Section 3. In

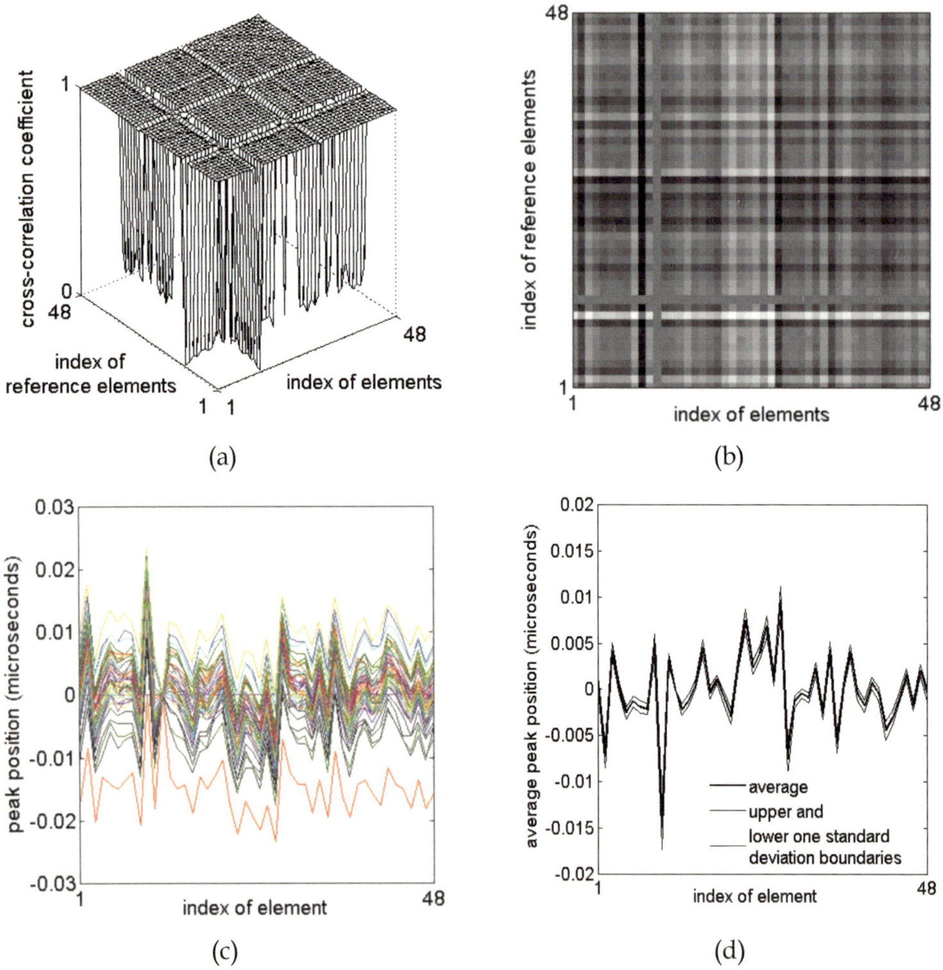

Fig. 18. (a) The cross-correlation coefficient distributions. (b) The peak positions distribution. (c) The peak positions profiles with all reference elements plotted on top of one another. (d) The derived system-error-difference profile by averaging profiles derived with all reference elements. The boundaries of one standard deviation are also plotted.

this algorithm, most common-midpoint signals are acquired using four adjacent transducer elements, which is not available in one-dimensional arrays. An initial two dimensional phase-aberration profile is derived from the peak positions of cross-correlation functions between these common midpoint signals. The boundary conditions needed to drive the final phase-aberration profile are derived by applying the one-dimensional-array algorithm to the first row and the first column of the array. The cross algorithm has a linear ambiguity profile and high signal-to-noise ratio. Due to the lack of experimental data from two-dimensional arrays (still hard to build), the discussed algorithms for two-dimensional arrays have only been tested using simulated data (Li, & Robinson, 2000a, 2007, 2008).

5. Conclusion

Compared with astromical imaging, phase-aberration correction in medical ultrasound imaging is more challenging in the sense that targets are in the near field and aberrators can exist anywhere between the interested targets and the array. Many successful algorithms used in astromical imaging are based on the signal-redundancy principle. However, this principle is invalid in the near field. To use the signal redundancy principle for phase-aberration correction in medical ultrasound images, the near-field effects have to be managed. In this chapter, the near-field signal-redundancy principle has been discussed in depth. Common-midpoint signals are still a special group of signals in the near field because they can be considered as redundant after a dynamic near-field-delay correction. Based on the near-field signal-redundancy principle, phase-aberration-correction algorithms have been developed for linear arrays, phased arrays, and two-dimensional arrays. There are three basic requirements for these algorithms to work properly. One of the requirements is that the phase-aberration effects of aberrators between targets in a region of interest and the transducer array can be approximately modelled as the effects of a phase screen on the transducer surface. The second requirement is that the element size is small enough so that the phase aberration value of the phase screen under each element can be considered as the same. The third requirement is that multi-path echoes are ignorable in common-midpoint signals, because they are not redundant.
The linear array algorithm has been successfully tested on transverse scan of abdomen of volunteers. At this body position, the aberrators are mainly muscle and fat layers under the skin (close to the transducer surface), which makes it easier to model their effect as that of a phase screen on the transducer surface. Another property of the body structure at this location and the transducer orientation is that the thickness of the fat and muscle layers changes very slowly in the direction of element height (10 mm). This property makes it easier to satisfy the second requirement. The high cross-correlation coefficient between common-midpoint signals (Li et al., 1997) also indicated that multi-path echoes were weak in common-midpoint signals and the third requirement was satisfied. Experimental results also show that the measured phase aberration profiles were different for targets from different depths. This could be because the aberration effect of fat and muscle layers near the transducer surface is different for targets at different depths, which is similar to the effect of the aberrator attached to the phased-array transducer surface in phased-array experiments (Section 4.2.1), where the phase screen was different for echoes from targets in different directions. Another possible reason is that the effect of other aberrators between the targets and the transducer surface was included.
For other imaging positions on the body, small element size in both dimensions is usually required to sample the phase screen properly (the second requirement). That is, a two-

dimensional array is needed, but it is still difficult and expensive to build a two-dimensional array. When two-dimensional arrays become available, the near-field signal redundancy algorithm should work at more imaging positions. However, there will be imaging positions where the structure is so complex that the three basic requirements are not satisfied. In this case, the cross-correlation coefficient between common midpoint signals will be low and it can be used as the trigger to abandon the correction.

6. Acknowledgment

The author would like to thank Brent Robinson for many helpful discussions and providing many experimental and simulated data sets.

7. References

Buffington, A.; Crawford, F. S.; Muller, R. A.; Schwemin, A. J. & Smits, R. G. (1997). Correction of atmospheric distortion with an image-sharpening telescope. *J. Opt. Soc. Am.*, Vol. 67, No. 3, (March 1977), pp. 298-303, ISSN: 1084-7529

Goodman, J. W.; Huntley, W. H.; Jackson, Jr., D. W. & Lehmann, M. (1966). Wavefront-reconstruction imaging through random media. *Appl. Phys. Lett.*, Vol. 8, No. 12, (June 1966), pp. 311-312, ISSN: 0003-6951

Hamaker, J. P.; O'Sullivan, J. D. & Noordam, J. E. (1977). Image sharpness, Fourier optics, an redundant-spacing interferometry. *J. Opt. Soc. Am.*, Vol. 67, No. 9, (August 1977), pp. 1122-1123, ISSN: 1084-7529

Hinkelman, L. M.; Mast, T. D., Metlay, L. A., and Waag, R. C. (1998). The effect of abdominal morphology on ultrasonic pulse distortion. Part I. Measurements. *J. Acoust. Soc. Am.* Vol. 104, No. 6, pp. 3635-3649, ISSN: 0001-4966, December 1998.

Hirama M. & Sato, T. (1984). Imaging through an inhomogeneous layer by least-mean-square error fitting. *J. Acoust. Soc. Am.* Vol. 75, No. 4, (April 1984), pp. 1142-1147, ISSN: 0001-4966

Hogg, D. C.; Guirand, F. O & Deckere, M. T. (1981). Measurement of excess radio transmission length on earth-space paths. *Astron. Astrophys.*, Vol. 95, No. 2, (March 1981), pp. 304-307, ISSN: 0004-6361

Ishiguro, M. (1974). Phase error correction in multi-element radio interferometer by data processing. *Astron. Astrophys. Suppl. Ser.*, Vol. 15, (June 1974), pp. 431-443, ISSN: 0004-6361

Jennison, R. C. (1958). A phase sensitive interferometer technique for the measurement of the Fourier transforms of spatial brightness distributions of small angular extent. *Mon. Not. R. Astron. Soc.*, Vol. 118, No. 3, (January 1958), pp. 276-284, ISSN: 1365-2966

Li, Y. & Robinson, B. (2008). The Cross algorithm for phase-aberration correction in medical ultrasound images formed with two-dimensional arrays. *IEEE Trans. Ultrason., Ferroelect., Freq. Cont.*, Vol.55, No.3, (March 2008), pp. 588-601, ISSN 0885-3010

Li, Y. (2008). Timing-error-difference calibration using reciprocal signals. *IEEE Trans. Ultrason., Ferroelect., Freq. Cont.*, Vol.55, No.11, (November 2008), pp. 2405-2417, ISSN 0885-3010

Li, Y. & Robinson, B. (2007). Implementation of the near-field signal redundancy phase-aberration correction algorithm on two-dimensional arrays. *IEEE Trans. Ultrason., Ferroelect., Freq. Cont.*, Vol.54, No.1, (January 2007), pp. 42-51, ISSN 0885-3010

Li, Y. (2002a). The influences of ambiguity phase aberration profiles on focusing quality in the very near field -- part I: single range focusing on transmission. *IEEE Trans. Ultrason., Ferroelect., Freq. Cont.*, Vol.49, No.1, (January 2002), pp. 57-71, ISSN 0885-3010

Li, Y. (2002b). The influences of ambiguity phase aberration profiles on focusing quality in the very near field -- part II: dynamic range focusing on reception. *IEEE Trans. Ultrason., Ferroelect., Freq. Cont.*, Vol.49, No.1, (January 2002), pp. 72-84, ISSN 0885-3010

Li, Y.; Robinson, B.; Drew, P.; Wilson, L.; Price, D. & Gill, R. (2002). Correction of distributed phase aberrations caused by propagation-speed and array-pitch errors. *Proceedings of 2002 IEEE International Ultrasonics Symposium*, pp. 1687-1691, ISBN 0-7803-7583-1, Munich, Germany, October 2002

Li, Y. & Robinson, B (2000a). Phase aberration correction using near-field signal redundancy: two-dimensional array algorithm. *Proceedings of 2000 IEEE International Ultrasonics Symposium*, pp. 1729-1733, ISBN 0-7803-6365-5, *San Juan, Puerto Rico,* October 2000.

Li, Y. & Robinson, B. (2000b). Small-element-array algorithm for correcting phase aberration using near-field signal redundancy-- part II: experimental results. *IEEE Trans. Ultrason., Ferroelect., Freq. Cont.*, Vol.47, No.1, (January 2000), pp. 49-57, ISSN 0885-3010

Li, Y. (2000a). Phase and/or amplitude aberration correction for imaging--continuation. *US Patent Number*: 6,120,450. September 19, 2000

Li, Y. (2000b). Small-element-array algorithm for correcting phase aberration using near-field signal redundancy--part I: principles. *IEEE Trans. Ultrason., Ferroelect., Freq. Cont.*, Vol.47, No.1, (January 2000), pp. 29-48, ISSN 0885-3010

Li, Y. & Gill, R. (1998). A comparison of matched signals used in three different phase-aberration correction algorithms. *Proceedings of 1998 IEEE International Ultrasonics Symposium*, pp. 1707-1712, ISBN 0-7803-4095-7, Sendai, Miyagi, Japan, October 1998.

Li, Y. (1997). Phase-aberration correction using near-field signal redundancy--part I: Principles. *IEEE Trans. Ultrason., Ferroelect., Freq. Cont.*, Vol.44, No.2, (March 1997), pp. 355-371, ISSN 0885-3010

Li, Y.; Robinson, D. & Carpenter D. (1997). Phase-aberration correction using near-field signal redundancy--part II: experimental results. *IEEE Trans. Ultrason., Ferroelect., Freq. Cont.*, Vol.44, No.2, (March 1997), pp. 372-379, ISSN 0885-3010

Li, Y. & Robinson, B. (1997). Phase-aberration-correction algorithm for phased-array transducers using near-field signal redundancy. *Proceedings of 1997 IEEE International Ultrasonics Symposium*, pp. 1729-1732, ISBN 0-7803-4153-8, Ontario, Canada, October 1997.

Li, Y.; Robinson, D.; Carpenter, D. & Kossoff, G. (1996). Phase-aberration correction using near-field signal redundancy: correcting phase aberrations caused by medium-velocity and array-pitch Errors. *Proceedings of 1996 IEEE International Ultrasonics Symposium*, pp. 1367-1370, ISBN 0-7803-3615-1, San Antonio, Texas, November 1996.

Muller, R. A. & Buffington, A. (1974). Real-time correction of atmospherically degraded telescope images through image sharpening. *J. Opt. Soc. Am.*, Vol. 64, No. 9, (September 1974), pp. 1200-1209, ISSN: 1084-7529

O'Donnell M. & Flax, S. W. (1988). Phase aberration measurements in medical ultrasound: human study. *Ultrasonic Imaging*, Vol. 10, No. 1, (January 1988), pp. 1-11, ISSN 0161-7346

Rachlin, D. (1990). Direct estimation of aberration delays in pulse-echo image systems. *J. Acoust. Soc. Am.* Vol. 88, No. 1, (July 1990),pp. 191-198, ISSN: 0001-4966

Robinson, B. S.; Shmulewitz, A. & Burke, T. M. (1994). Waveform aberrations in an animal model. *1994 IEEE Ultrasonics Symposium*, pp. 1619-1624, ISBN: 0-7803-2012-3, Cannes France, November 1994

Shmulewitz, A.; Teefey, S. A. & Robinson, B. S. (1993). Factors affecting image quality and diagnostic efficacy in abdominal sonography: a prospective study of 140 patients," *J. Clinical Ultrasound*, Vol. 21, No. 9, (November 1993), pp. 623-630, ISSN: 1097-0096

Steinberg B. D. & Subbaram, H. M. (1991). Microwave imaging technique. Wiley, ISBN: 047150078X , New York, USA

Tyson, R. K. (2010). *Principle of adaptive optics*. CRC Press, ISBN: 978-1-4398-0859-7, Bota Recon, USA

Yilmaz, O. & Doherty, S. M. (1987). Seismic data processing. *Society of Exploration Geophysicists*, ISBN 10: 0931830400, Tulsa, USA

Zhu, Q. & Steinberg, B. D. (1992). Large transducer measurements of wavefront distortion in the female breast. *Ultrasonic Imaging*, Vol. 14, No. 3, (July 1992), pp. 276-299, 1992. , ISSN 0161-7346

5

The Role of 3D Ultrasound in Assessment of Endometrial Receptivity and Follicular Vascularity to Predict the Quality Oocyte

T. Žáčková[1,2], I.Y. Järvelä[1] and T. Marděšič
[1]*Department of Obstetrics and Gynecology, Oulu University Hospital, Oulu*
[2]*Institute for the Care of Mother and Child (UPMD), Department of IVF*
Charles University, Prague
[3]*Sanatorium Pronatal, Praha*
[1]*Finland*
[2,3]*Czech Republic*

1. Introduction

The success of human and embryo implantation depends on maternal and embryonic factors and their interactions. To asses uterine receptivity one must take various factors into account. Current advances in transvaginal 3D ultrasonography have allowed us to examine in detail and visualize pelvic organ structures to analyse their volumes with great accuracy (Alcazar et al., 2006),(Raga et al., 1999). It is reasonable to believe that an analysis of power Doppler signals in a volume better reflects the overall vascularization in an organ than analysis of a two-dimensional (2D) ultrasound image or measurement of blood flow velocity in a single or a few vessels. Using 3D Power Doppler Angiography we can assess both arterial and venous circulation also the whole architecture of the vascular net into a volumetric image with the posibility of an overall evaluation of blood flows , and computer analysis makes this assessment objective (Jokubkiene et al., 2006). The VOCAL (Virtual Organ Computer - aided Analysis) and volume calculation is semi-authomatic type of calculating volumes starting from the rotation of the organ target of study. Allows to calculate partial volumes and at the same time the of vascular system and flows into the region of interest. Two dimensional Doppler sonography provides a subjective estimation of uterine and ovarian vascularity. Is it limited, however, by providing flow depiction in a single plane as opposed to the sample volume as obtained by free dimensional imaging. Therefore, three dimensional ultrasound and power Doppler angiography (3D US-PDA) have advantage of assessing simultaneously both the endometrial blood flow and endometrial volume (EV) (Merce et al., 2008) and improves better traditional ultrasound scanning imaging with the posibility of storing information for further analysis or share datasets through telemedicine.
The follicular blood flow seems to play a major role during the growth and development of the follicle containing the oocyte (Chui et al. ,1997),(Coulam et al.,1999). The surge in perifolicullar angiogenesis during selection of dominant follicles and following the LH surge or HCG can be detected by measurment of perifolicular flow/velocities. This allows identification of those follicles likely to produce high quality eggs and embryos. 3D surface

rendering at 4xmagnification can show the blood vessels in the follicular wall and can identify features incompatible with successfull oocyte retrieval (Cambell,2010).

2. Evaluation of endometrial receptivity

Failure of implantation remains the main reason why most IVF treatment fails to result in pregnancy. Angiogenesis plays a critical role in various female reproductive processes such as development of dominant follicle, formation of a corpus luteum, growth of endometrium and implantation. A good blood supply towards the endometrium is usually considered as an essentials requirement for implantation. The ability to identify a receptive uterus prospectively by a noninvasive method would have an invaluable clinical impact on treatment efficiency and succes rates. This chapter explores the role of transvaginal three dimensional ultrasound (3d US) and 3D power -Doppler ultrasound (3D-PDA) in evaluation of endometrial receptivity.

2.1 Technical aspects and three dimensional data analysis

3D US images can be obtained by two methods: freehand and automated. The freehand method requires manual movement of the transducer through the ROI. The automated method acquires the images using dedicated 3D transducers. When these probes are activated, the transducer elements automatically sweep through the ROI selected by the operator (the so-called "volume box") while the probe is held stationary. This provides more accuracy to this method as compared with the freehand systems, in which speed of sweep is more difficult to maintain constant manually by the operator. The digitally stored volume data can be manipulated and presented in various displays: multiplanar display, "niche" mode or surface rendering mode. Probably, the most used and useful display is multiplanar display, which simultaneously shows three perpendicular planes (axial, sagital and coronal), allowing navigation through these three planes with the possibility of switch over any desired plane (Alcazar et al, 2006). There are two basic methods employed to calculate volume from a three dimensional dataset :the convencional „full planar„ or „contour„ method and the more recently introduced ‚rotational„ method possible through the VOCAL -imaging program (Virtuala Organ Computer aided analysis).This rotational method based on rotations in given steps (6°, 9°, 15°, 30°) on a given orthogonal plane (A, B or C).Vascularization of tissues within the ROI can be also assessed using 3D Power -Doppler ultrasound (3D PDA) and the VOCAL program. Three Indices of vascularity are calculated: the Vascularization Index (VI) reflects the ratio of power Dopler information within the total dataset relative to both colour and grey information, the Flow Index (FI) represents the mean power Doppler signal intensity and the Vascularisation Flow index represents a combination of the two (Pairleitner et al., 1999). Using the „shell„ function it is possible to calculate a volume at different thickness around the predetermined endometrium and estimate the vascularization in this „shell„.This allows the assessment of the so-called „subendometrial region„ (Alcazar et al, 2006).

2.2 Results and authors studies

The pregnancy outcome of frozen embryo transfer is known to be dependent on multiple clinical and embryological factors, including the age of the woman at IVF/ICSI treatment; (Salumets et.al, 2006),(Wang et. al, 2001), the method of oocyte fertilization used (Van Steirteghem et. Al , 1994),(Salumets et al., 2006), the developmental stage of embryos at freezing (Salumets et al., 2003), the embryo quality before freezing (Schalkoff et al., 1993), the extent of embryo damage after thawing (Edgar et al., 2000) and the resumption of post-thaw blastomere divisions (Van der Elst et al., 1997). On the other hand the risk of pregnancy loss is similar after cryopreservation and fresh IVF or ICSI (Aytoz et al., 1999) and embryo morphology is not related to the miscarriage rates in any of the treatment modalities studied (Veleva et al., 2008). Several ultrasound parameters of the endometrium and the evaluation of uterine and endometrial blood flow have been proposed for assessing endometrial receptivity, including endometrial thickness, endometrial pattern and endometrial and subendometrial blood floow and considered as implantation markers in vitro fertilization (IVF) and embryo transfer cycles. These parameters may identify patients with low implantation potential. However, their positive predictive value is low. No differences were find in endometrial thickness, endometrial volume, endometrial pattern, uterine PI, uterine RI, endometrial and subendometrial 3D power Doppler flow indeces between the nonpregnant and pregnant groups on LH+1(1 day after the LH surge) during frozen -thawed embryo transfer cycles (Ng et al., 2006). Nevertheless another studies suggested any corelations between the thickness of endometrium and pregnancy rate during the treatment with assisted reproductive technology. There was the endometrial thickness decreases as function of the patients age on the day of HCG administration during an IVF cycle. (Amir et.al., 2007). In our study at the time of embryo transfer only the structure of endometrium seems to be of significance and 3D power Doppler ultrasound and steroids levels does not provide us any additional information at this point . The 3D transvaginal ultrasound measurements (Voluson Expert 730, Kretz, Zipf, Austria) were performed on the day of the FET and repeated about one week later, at the time of the expected implantation. The 3D ultrasound technique enabled the determination of endometrial, subendometrial, and ovarian volume, including possible changes in the vascular network. Identical preinstalled instrument settings (frequency, mid; dynamic set, 2; balance, G>170; smooth, 5/5; ensemble, 16; line density, 7; power Doppler map, 5; and the setting conditions for the power Doppler mode were gain, -5.6; quality, normal; wall motion filter, low 1; peak repetitive frequency PRF, 0.9 kHz) were applied for all patients. At the second visit, the power Doppler mode was not used to examine the uterus. During the ultrasound examination, the uterus was first visualized in two-dimensional (2D) B-mode after the patient had emptied her bladder. The power Doppler mode was switched on, and the power Doppler box was positioned to cover the whole uterus. The 3D facility was engaged by switching to 'volume mode. The volume sector angle was preset to 80°, and the fast volume acquisition (low-resolution) setting was selected to avoid artifacts. Thereafter, the ovaries were examined similarly. The ultrasonographic volume data were saved on the hard drive and analyzed later using the built-in virtual organ computer-aided analysis imaging program (VOCAL, GE Healthcare, Zipf, Austria) for 3D power Doppler histogram analysis. The manual mode of the VOCAL Contour Editor was used to cover the whole 3D volume of the region of interest (ROI), with 15° rotation steps. Hence, 12 contour planes were analyzed for each ROI to cover 360°. After obtaining the total volume of the ROI, the program calculated the ratio of color voxels to all the voxels; this ratio (%) was expressed as the vascularization index (VI). The vascularized volume (unit mL) in the endometrium or in the ovary was calculated by multiplying the total volume of the ROI by its VI. The VOCAL program automatically calculated the index for mean grayness (MG) in the ROI, which presents the average grayness in the gray-scale voxels. We have reported only vascularization index and vascularized volume(VI x volume),since only the last one has been shown to reflex corpus luteal function in several studies(Järvelä et al., 2007; Järvelä et al.,2008; Niinimäki et al 2009).We have not analysed any data concerning VI or VFI , neither do we have any intention to analyse them,because we are unaware what kind of physiological phenomena they reflect (Zackova et al., 2009).

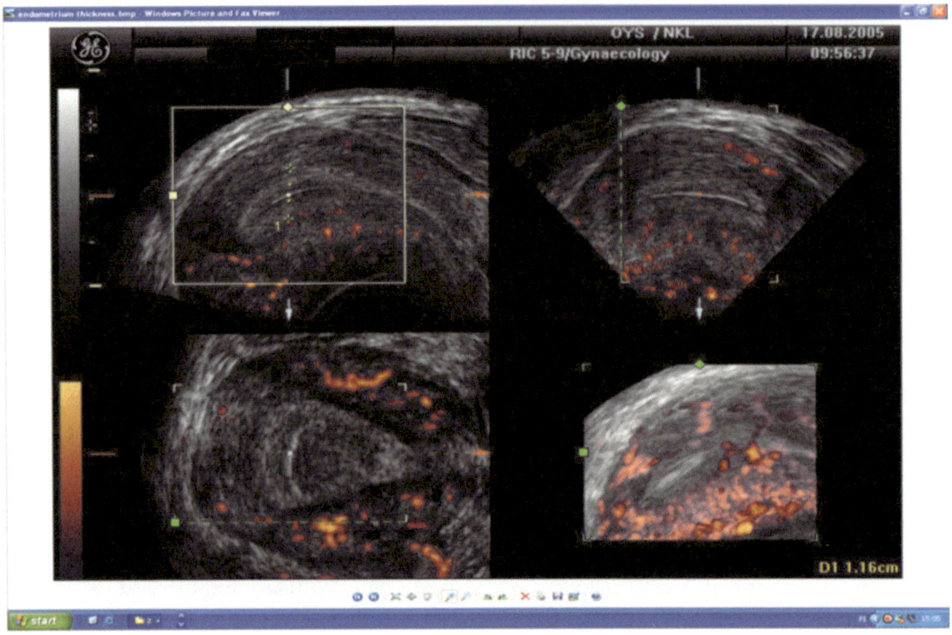

Fig. 1. Three dimensional multiplanar depicting multiplanar display of the uterus. All three ortogonal planes can be displayed using this technique. Endometrium thickness meassurment.

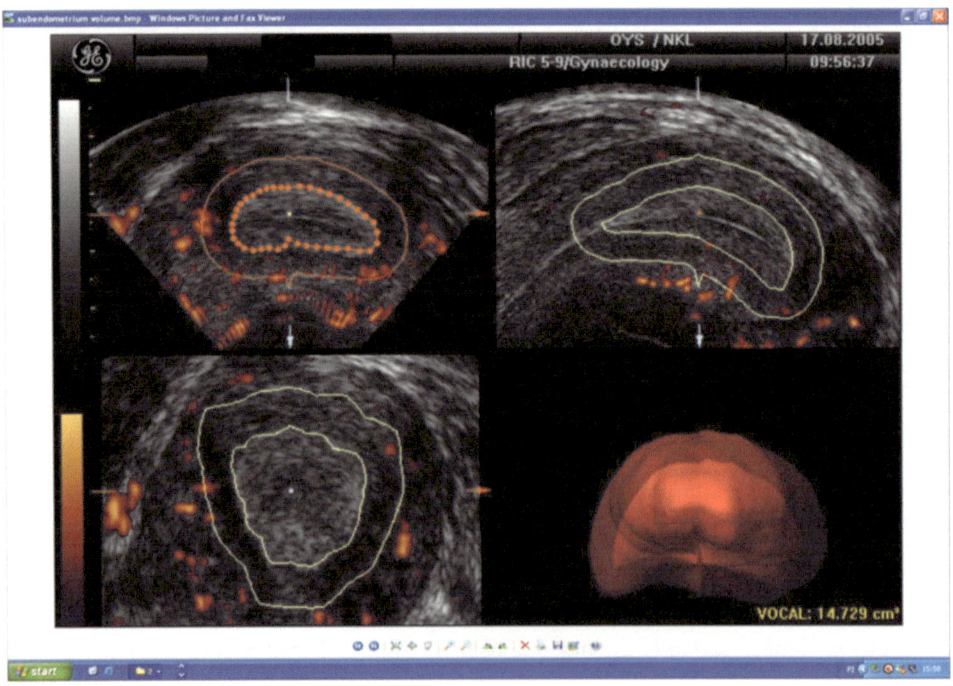

Fig. 2. Endometrial volume calculation by using VOCAL software after three dimensional ultrasound . Determination of the subendometrial area volume by using the „shell „ facility. In this case 5 mm has been chosen.

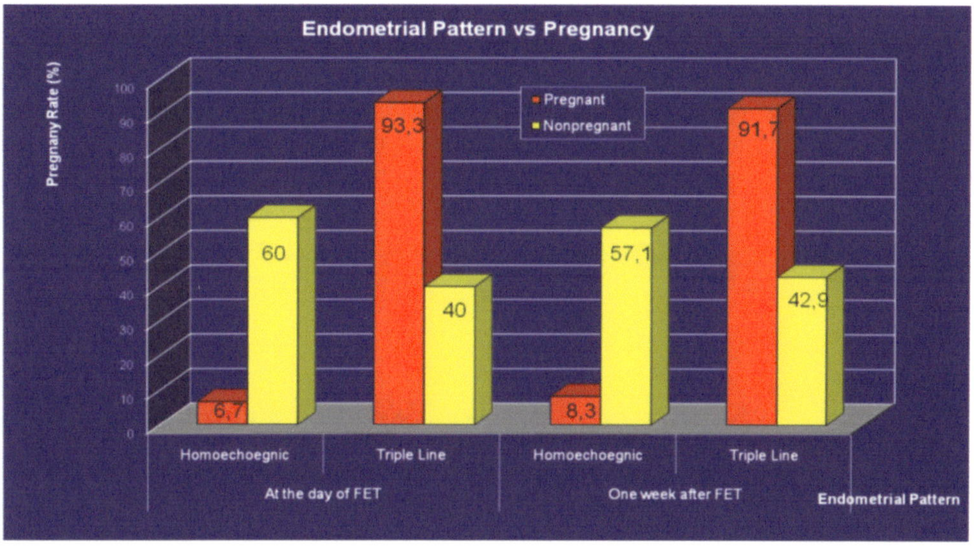

Fig. 3. The endometrial echo patterns in the pregnant group (93.3% *vs.* 40.0%, 95% CI 25.5-81.2%) on the day of FET and one week after (91.7% *vs.* 42.9%, 95% CI 18.5-79.1%) .No differences were observed in the dominant ovarian vasculature.

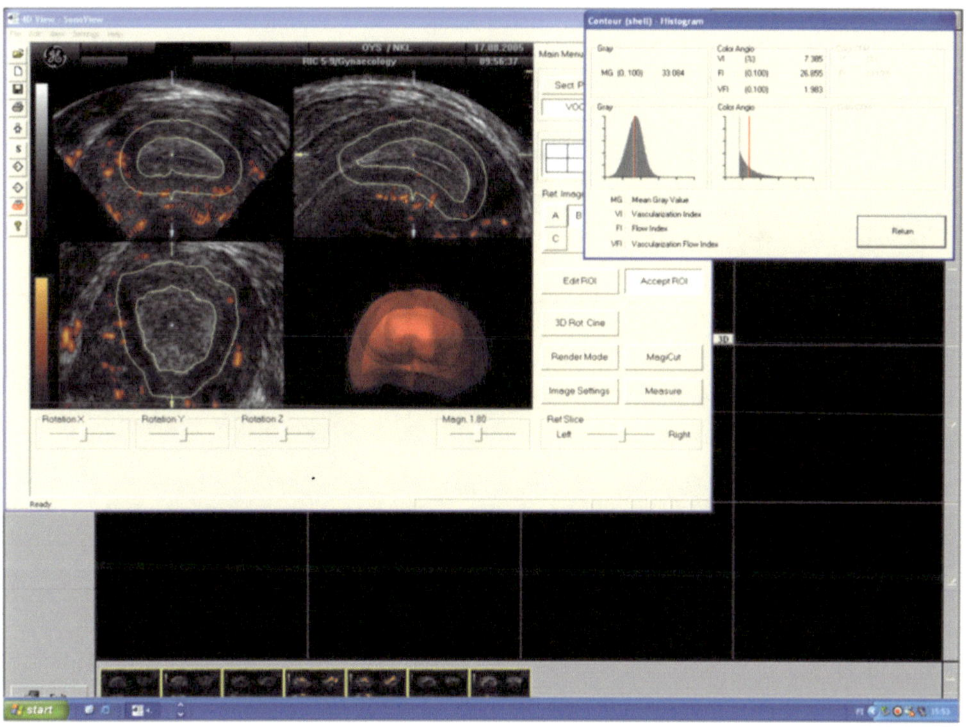

Fig. 4. Vascularization of the subendometrial area by 3D -Power Doppler . 3D power doppler indexes VI,FI, and VFI refers to the shell area- subendometrium. Determination of the subendometrial area volume by using the „shell „ facility. I n this case 5 mm has been chosen

2.3 Assessment of endometrial echogenicity

In the recent literature there has been interest in the possible relationship between the degree of endometrial echogenicity an IVF-ET outcome and the cycles sorted into six groups according to the extent of the upward hyperechogenic transformation of the endometrium. In contrast to the similiraty in individual , control ovarian hyperstimulation /COH / and embryology data among groups, they observed a dramatic decrease in clinical and ongoing pregnancy as well as in implantation rates from the lowest to the highest endometrial

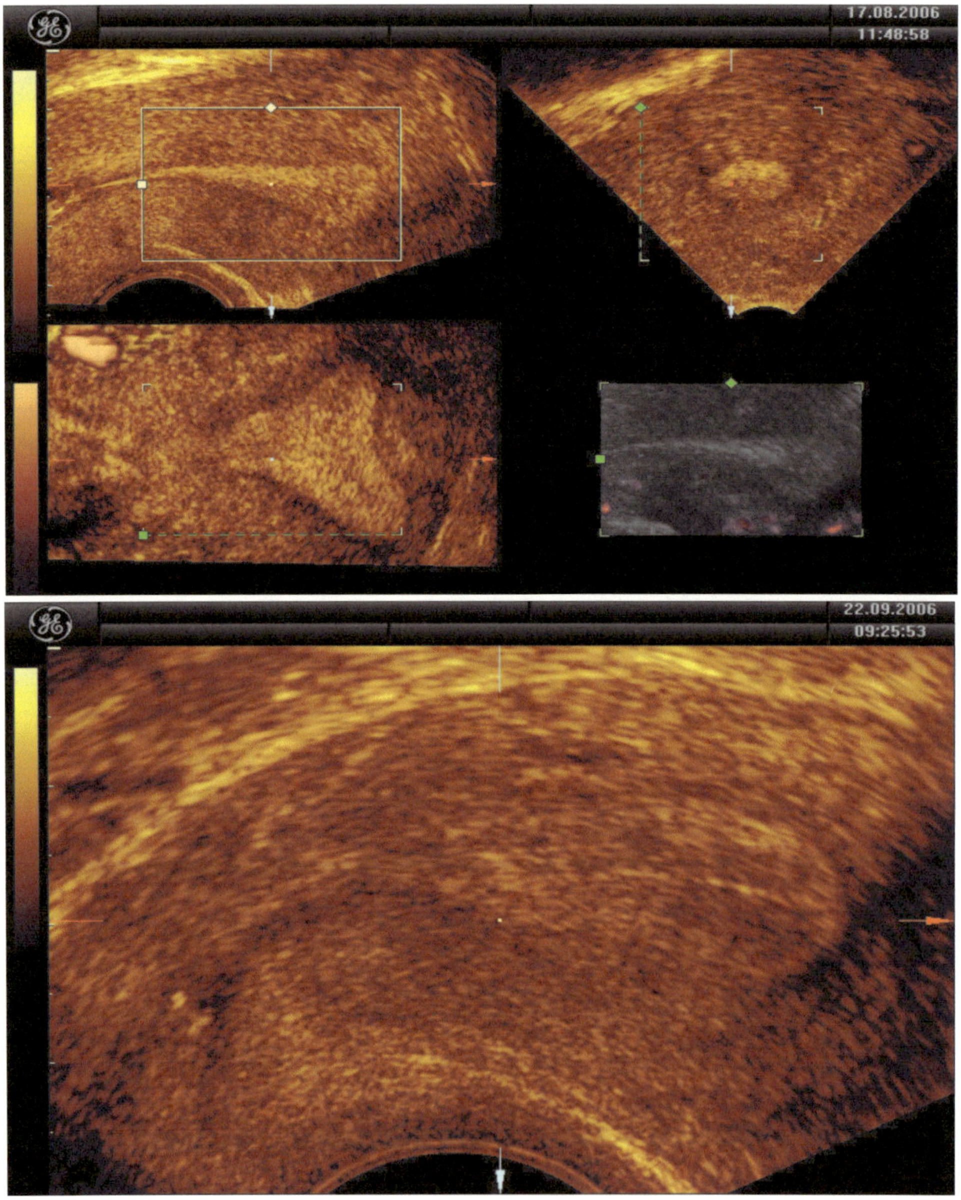

Fig. 5. The endometrial pattern ,which was assessed in the longitudinal section and described as triple -line or homoechogenic.

echogenicity groups. Conversely, no relationship between endometrial thickness on the day of hCG administration and IVF-ET outcome was observed (Fanchin et al., 2001). This ultrasonographic aspect may be reflection of glandular straightness, reduced glandular secretion, and reduced stromal edema that characterize the proliferative endometrium, with a decreased number of interfaces to ultrasound. Since the echogenity of the secretory endometrium is usually higher than in the surrounding myometrium, we assessed the echogenity in these two areas subjectively and used software to provide the MG values. A strong correlation between these two methods was observed. Future studies will show whether this index has clinical value (Zackova et al., 2009).

3. Color Doppler sonography for the the optimization of follicular vascularity

The 2D color Doppler studies have show that perifolicular blood flow of individual follicles during IVF treatment correlates with oocyte recovery (Nargund et al., 1996) ,oocyte developmental potential (Van Blerkom et al., 1997), embryo quality (Nargund et al., 1996), (Chui et al., 1997) and pregnancy rate (Coulam et al.,1999). We analysed relationship between kind of stimulated protokol and cause of sterility to determine ovarian and dominant follicle blood flow characteristics using three dimensional power Doppler ultrasound , grading system of perifollicular vascularity (Chui et al, ,1997) and power doppler index PI and RI of dominant follicle artery in the prospective pilot study of 17 women in IVF/ICSI stimulation.

Materials and methods. 17 the patients were stimulated in a long protocol (GnRh agonist-Zoladex, Decapeptyl) on 22-th day of their period and subsequently with rekombinant FSH (puregon /gonal pen) 15 days after downregulation / no follicles more than 10 mm, endometrium thickness less than 5 mm and level of Estradiol /E2/ less than 50 pg/ml. We exluded the women, who didn ' t agree with the examination on the day of ovum pick up futher such as women , whose stimulation was stopped for the risk of OHSS, women with the operation of right or left ovary, women with ovarectomy , women with uterine malformation , women with FSH level more than 10 mIU/l in early follicular period or women with ovarian cysts. On the basis of male factor infertility exclusion we provided always ICSI Method. The 3D ultrasound examinations and power doppler sonography of the ovary and dominant follicle we provided on the day HCG (pregnyl) before ovum pick up. All the 3D ultrasound and PDA examinations were carried out by a single observer (T.Z) and all the patients were explored in a gynaecological position using Voluson Expert 760, Kretz, Zipf, Austria equipped with vaginal multifrequency (from 3 to 9 mHz) volume transducer, which has a 146 ° field of view. The volume of the ovary and dominant follicle, vascularization index /VI/, flow index /FI/, vascularization flow index / VFI / , mean grayness , perifolicular vascularity and PI a RI of the dominant follicle was determined for each ovary separately. The dominant follicle is presented by maximal mean diameter (MD). Follicular volume (FV) was etermined for each follicle according to the sphere formula : FV (ml) = 4,1888 x $(MD/2\ (cm))^3$. The power dopler Windows was placed on the maximum longitudinal plane of both ovaries,including the whole ovarian surface. The following Doppler predetermined characteristics were applied in every patient (colour gain from -3 to -7 ,normal colour quality, wall motion filter,low 1, peak repetitive frequency PRF ,0.9 KHz). When an adequate power Doppler signal was achieved, we placed the 3D box to aquire the volume from the region of interest (ROI). The VOCAL imaging program was used tu calculate the ovarian volume and 3D power Dopler indices . Using the manual mode, the contour of the different ovarain slices was traced by taking 15° rotational steps by using the longitudinal plane as the work plane. 3D power Dopller indices were calculated using the histogram facility. Vascularization Index (VI) is the number of colour voxels in the volume studied, symbolizing in this way the number of vessels arriving to the organ, expressed as a percentage.The Flow Index (FI) is the metan colour value of the colour voxels,thus representing the average blood flow intensity, expressed as a whole number rating from 0 to 100. VFI integrates both vascularization and blood flow (tisues perfusion). It si also expressed as a whole number rating from 0 to 100, and represents color value of grey and colour voxels in the studied ROI (Pairleitner et al., 1999). The Grading system (Chui, et al. 1997) was used to assess perifollicular vascularity. (a) shows 25% circumferential flow (Grade1); (b) 26–50% flow (Grade 2); (c) 51–75% flow (Grade 3) and (d)75% flow (Grade 4), where follicles of high grade follicular vascularity are associated with grade 3 and 4. The oocyte of the dominant follicle from both ovaries was fertilized by ICSI and observed his embryogeny. The embryos were classified into four morphological grades in accordance with our conventional criteria (Kondo *et al.*, 1996) consisting of blastomere size and the amount of anucleate fragmentation (conventional method): grade 1 (g1), blastomere uniform in size and shape and little or no fragmentation; grade 2 (g2), blastomeres uneven in size and shape and/or fragmentation <10% of the embryonic surface; grade 3 (g3), fragmentation of 10–30% of the embryonic surface; and grade 4 (g4), fragments >30% of the embryonic surface. On the day of ovum pick up we have collected the samples of follicular fluid of dominanat follicle without of blood contamination. After the collecting of samples of follicular fluid of dominant follicle and serum we provided their centrifugate and stored at -40 C until their planned biochemical analysis after the completed collection of the samples at all intended 80 patients.

Results .The IVF/ICSI cycle was evaluated in 17 women, among which 5 were pregnant (29.4 %) and 12 non-pregnant (70.6 %). The median age of the women was 32 (range 26-36). The causes of the infertility were male in 12 cases (70.6 %), tubal in 2 cases (11.8 %) and mixed in 3 cases (17.6 %). There were 11 cases (64.7 %) of primary and 6 cases (35.3 %) of secondary infertility.Statistical analysis of the data was performed with R programming language (http://cran.r-project.org), version 2.4.1. We have computed descriptive statistics and p-values of hypothesis tests for comparing the group of pregnant and non-pregnant patients. For continuous data the normality is not assumed because of small sample sizes and asymmetry of the data distribution. The following tables give the median and range (minimum and maximum) of each continuous variable together with the p-value of the two-sample Wilcoxon test. For categorical data we list the tables of counts with percentages of cases. To compare the two groups, the p-value of Fisher's exact test is computed (also for tables larger 2 by 2). Ultrasonography and Doppler angiography parameters measured on both ovaries are analyzed for each ovary separately.There is no significant difference between groups in the age of patients, type and causes of infertility and other general and clinical characteristics. In the group of pregnant women, there is a significantly larger number of grade 1 embryos on transfer day, a significantly larger flow index dx and there is a significant difference in the degree of morphological preimplantation quality of the 1. and 2. transferred embryos and in the degree of perifollicular vascularity of the right follicle dx. Other variables yield a non-significant difference between the pregnant and non-pregnant group because of small sizes of the data samples; however the p-values are near the 5%-level for the vascularization index and vascularization flow index, for which the observed values have the tendency to be larger for pregnant women and a future research with a larger number of patients is intended to attain significant results.

Implications. The follicular vascularity assesment with 3D ultrasonography and PDA of ovaries may represent a possible predictors of the the outcome of assisted conception therapy. Future research with a larger number of patients is intended to attain significant results ant to confirm these findings .

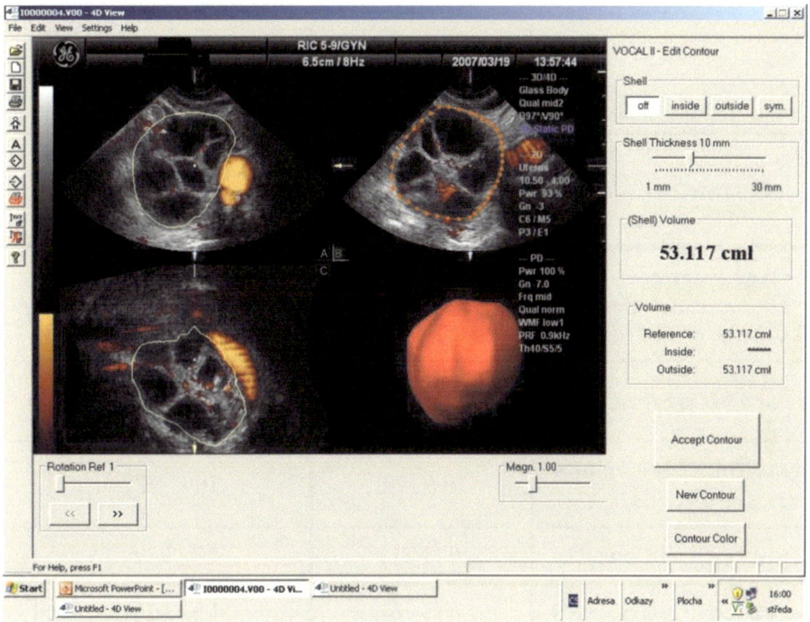

Fig. 6. Assessment of the ovarian volume by the virtual organ computer-aided analysis (VOCAL). Using the manual mode, the contour of different ovarian slices was traced by rotational steps every 15 ° taking the longitudinal plane as the work pattern.

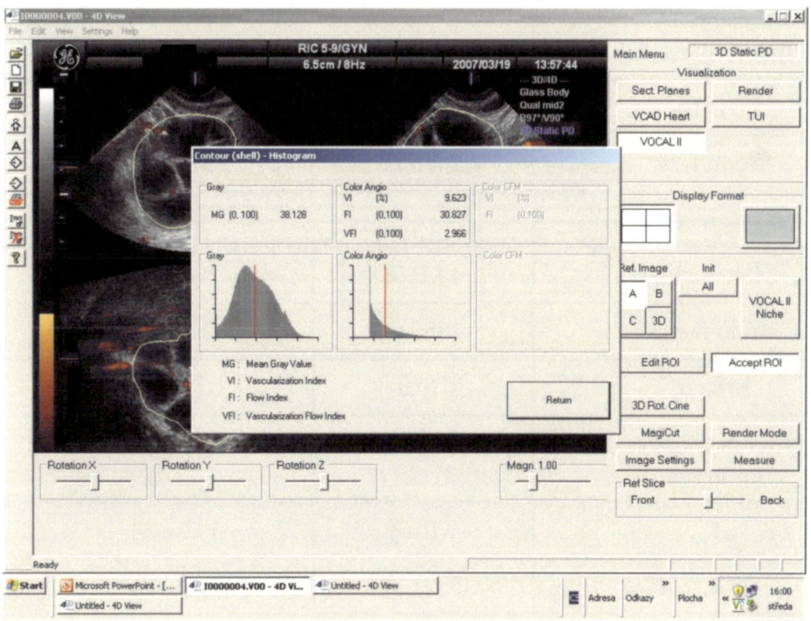

Fig. 7. Evaluation of the ovarian vascularity by three-dimensional power Doppler indices: vascualrization index (VI), flow index (FI) and vascularization flow index (VFI).These indices were calculated using the histogram facility provided by the virtual organ computer - aided analysis (VOCAL) program.

Parametrs	Pregnant (n=5)	Non pregnant (n=12)	P-value
Age (years)	32 (26-34)	32 (29-36)	0.488
Total dosage of FSH (IU)	2250 (1500-2825)	2250 (1 800-3 750)	0.560
Days of FSH treatment	14 (10-15)	13 (10-19)	0.873
Number of follicles > 16 mm on day of OPU	10 (6-28)	10 (5-17)	1.000
Number of retrieved oocytes	6 (4-21)	7.5 (3-14)	0.792
Number of fertilized oocytes	6 (3-16)	4.5 (3-10)	0.486
Number of grade 1 embryos on transfer day	3 (2-4)	0 (0-2)	0.001
Day of embryo transfer	3 (2-5)	3 (0-5)	0.914
Type of infertility			0.600
Primary	4 (36.3)	7 (63.6)	
Secondary	1 (16.7)	5 (83.3)	
Cause of infertility			0.547
Male factor	4 (33.3)	8 (66.7)	
Tubal factor	1 (50.0)	1 (50.0)	
Mixed	0 (0.0)	3 (100.0)	
Number of transferred embryos			1.000
1	0 (0.0)	1 (100.0)	
2	5 (31.2)	11 (68.8)	

Table 1. General and clinical parameters in relation to IVF/ICSI outcome

Parameters	Pregnant (n=5)	Non pregnant (n=12)	P-value
Degree of morphological preimplantation quality of transferred embryos 1.			0.029
1	5 (55.6)	4 (44.4)	
2	0 (0.0)	8 (100.0)	
3	0	0	
4	0	0	
Degree of morphological preimplantation quality of transferred embryos 2.			0.020
1	4 (80.0)	1 (20.0)	
2	1(14.3)	6 (85.7)	
3	0 (0.0)	4 (100.0)	
4	0	0	
Not obtained	0 (0.0)	1 (100.0)	
Grade of morphological reimplantationquality of selected oocytes from 3D measures dominant follicles dx			0.080
1	2 (100.0)	0 (0.0)	
2	3 (33.3)	6 (66.7)	
3	0 (0.0)	4 (100.0)	
4	0 (0.0)	1 (100.0)	
Not obtained	0 (0.0)	1 (100.0)	
Grade of morphological preimplantation quality of selected oocytes from 3D measuresdominant follicles sin			0.755
1	2 (66.7)	1 (33.3)	
2	1 (33.3)	2 (66.7)	
3	2 (28.6)	5 (71.4)	
4	0	0	
Not obtained	0 (0.0)	4 (100.0)	

Table 2. Embryological parameters in relation to IVF/ICSI outcome

Parameters	Pregnant(n=5)	Nonpregnant (n=12)	p-value
Total ovarian volume OV (ml) dx	43.96 (41.69-138.13)	42.55 (19.52-108.60)	0.279
Total ovarian volume OV (ml) sin	45.06 (43.86-116.96)	42.06 (11.32-102.38)	0.316
Volume of the dominant follicle FV (ml) l.dx	6.08 (5.28-6.43)	5.38 (2.36-7.05)	0.154
Volume of the dominant follicle FV (ml) l.sin	5.09 (4.08-5.65)	4.98 (3.26-9.63)	0.570
Vascularization index VI l.dx	12.47 (8.66-20.06)	8.22 (2.61-19.06)	0.066
Vascularization index VI l.sin	10.38 (5.02-25.43)	8.54 (6.20-11.72)	0.107
Flow index FI l.dx	47.85 (42.78-52.25)	40.46 (32.31-57.66)	0.044
Flow index FI l.sin	46.90 (35.23-48.90)	41.91 (28.83-51.47)	0.099
Vascularization flow index VFI l.dx	4.95 (2.85-8.46)	4.00 (0.90-10.05)	0.065
Vascularization flow index VFI l.sin	4.84 (2.30-10.05)	3.91 (2.82-4.62)	0.087
Resistence index Doppler of the dominant follicle l.dx	0.56 (0.55-0.62)	0.53 (0.42-0.67)	0.081
Resistence index Doppler of the dominant follicle l.sin	0.58 (0.50-0.62)	0.55 (0.38-0.71)	0.691
Pulsatility index Doppler of the dominant follicle l.dx	0.89 (0.83-1.00)	0.82 (0.65-1.24)	0.224

Table 3. Three - dimensional ultrasonography , Power doppler angiography parametrs on the HCG day in relation to IVF/ICSI outcome . Date are presented as mean +/- standart deviation.

Parameters	Pregnant(n=5)	Nonpregnant (n=12)	p-value
Degree of perifollicular vascularity of the dominant follicle l.dx			0.029
1.	1 (11.1)	8 (88.9)	
2.	1 (20.0)	4 (80.0)	
3.	3 (100.0)	0 (0.0)	
Degree of perifollicular vascularity of the dominant follicle l.sin			0.093
1.	1 (12.5)	7 (87.5)	
2.	2 (33.3)	4 (66.7)	
3.	2 (100.0)	0 (0.0)	

Table 4. Perifollicular vascularity grading score on the HCG day in relation to IVF/ICSI outcome. Date are presented as mean +/- standart deviation. Grading system (Chui, et al. 1997) used to assess perifollicular vascularity.

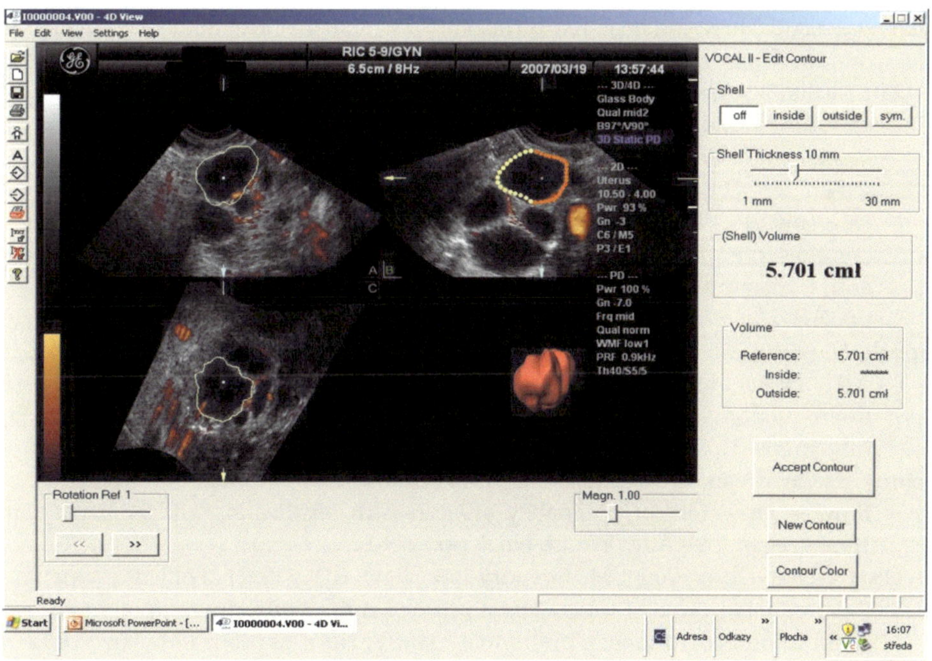

Fig. 8. Dominant follicle volume calculation by using the VOCAL software after three-dimensional ultrasound. The dominant follicle is presented by maximal mean diameter (MD). Follicular volume (FV) was determined for each follicle according to the sphere formula : FV (ml) = 4,1888 x (MD/2 (cm))3.

4. Conclusions

Developments in infertility treatment assisted reproduction methods are directed to transfer a single high quality embryo, while maintaining a high standard of treatment success. In this context, in recent years recede into the background, the standard "stimulation protocols using higher doses of FSH, often with a higher number of oocytes. The importance of more and more become "soft stimulation protocols aimed at, although a smaller number of growing follicles, which are a source of high-quality oocytes. The Natural / Mild IVF managment / ISMAAR / requires greater understanding of medical physiology, follicular growth and endometrial receptivity, which can be investigated using high-quality 2D and 3D ultrasound Dopler ultrasound and ultrasound, as evidenced by the results of our work. In this context, early identification of high-quality follicles might serve as one means of enabling a timely selection of oocytes and embryos with high developmental competence and the hope of a successful implantation. The follicular vascularity assessment with 3D ultrasonography and PDA of ovaries may represent a possible predictors of the the ooutcome of assisted conception therapy. Future research with a larger number of patients is intended to attain significant results and to confirm these findings . Definition of new applications of 3D ultrasound in the diagnosis of women enrolled in the program of assisted reproduction and the definition of predictive factors in the evaluation of the oocyte quality would have a significant contribution to our everyday clinical practice.

5. References

Alcazar ,JL.(2006). Three-dimensional ultrasound assessment of endometrial receptivity: a review. *Reprod Biol Endocrinol. Vo.4* , November 9,pp.56, ISSN1477-7827

Amir ,W.; Micha, B.; Ariel ,H.; Liat, LG.; Jehoshua ,D. &Adrian, S. (2007) Predicting factors for endometrial thickness during treatment with assisted reproductive technology. *Fertil Steril. 2007* Apr; Vol. 87, No. 4, pp.799-804. Epub 2007 Jan 4.

Aytoz, A.; Van den Abbeel, E.; Bonduelle. M.; Camus, M.; Joris, H.; Van Steirteghem, A. & Devroey, P.(1999).Obstetric outcome of pregnancies after the transfer of cryopreserved and fresh embryos obtained by conventional in-vitro fertilization and intracytoplasmic sperm injection. *Hum Reprod.* 1999 Oct;Vol. 14, No. 10, pp.2619-24.

Campbell, S. (2010)The role of advanced ultrasound in the managment of natural/mild ART, Proceedings of The Third Word congress on Mild Approaches in assisted Reproduction -embracing Mild IVF and IVM, venue: Pacifik Yokohama, Japan, July 30 and 31, 2010.

Coulam, CB.; Goodman, C. & Rinehart JS.(1999) Colour Doppler indices of follicular blood flow as predictors of pregnancy after in-vitro fertilization and embryo transfer. *Hum Reprod.* 1999 Aug; Vol.14, No.8, pp.1979-82.

Chui, DK.; Pugh ,ND.; Walker ,SM.; Gregory L.& Shaw, RW. (1997) . Follicular vascularity--the predictive value of transvaginal power Doppler ultrasonography in an in-vitro fertilization programme: a preliminary study. Hum Reprod. 1997 Jan; vol.12 No.1, pp :191-6.

Edgar ,DH.; Bourne, H.; Jericho, H. & McBain, JC.(2000). The developmental potential of cryopreserved human embryos. *Mol Cell Endocrinol. 2000* Nov 27; Vol. 169, No.1-2), pp.69-72.

Fanchin R. (2001).Assessing uterine receptivity in 2001: ultrasonographic glances at the new millennium. *Ann N Y Acad Sci.* 2001 Sep; Vol.943, pp.185-202.

Järvelä ,IY.; Niinimäki, M.; Martikainen, H.; Ruokonen, A. & Tapanainen ,JS.(2007). Ovarian response to the human chorionic gonadotrophin stimulation test in normal ovulatory women: the impact of regressing corpus luteum. *Fertil Steril.* 2007 May; Vol. 87, No.5 , pp.1122-30. Epub 2007 Jan 22.

Järvelä, IY.; Ruokonen ,A. & Tekay, A.(2008). Effect of rising hCG levels on the human corpus luteum during early pregnancy. *Hum Reprod.* 2008 Dec;Vol. 23,No.12, pp.2775-81. Epub 2008,Aug 10

Jokubkiene L.; Sladkevicius ,P.; Rovas, L. &Valentin L.(2006). Assessment of changes in endometrial and subendometrial volume and vascularity during the normal menstrual cycle using three-dimensional power Doppler ultrasound. *Ultrasound Obstet Gynecol.* 2006 Jun; Vol 27 No. 6, pp.672-9.

Kondo, I.; Suganuma, N.; Ando, T.; Asada,Y.; Furuhashi ,M. & Tomoda, Y.(1996). Clinical factors for successful cryopreserved-thawed embryo transfer. *J Assist Reprod Genet.* 1996 Mar;Vol.13, No. 3, pp.201-6.

Mercé, LT.; Barco ,MJ.; Bau ,S. &Troyano, J. Are endometrial parameters by three-dimensional ultrasound and power Doppler angiography related to in vitro fertilization/embryo transfer outcome?*Fertil Steril. 2008 Jan;89(1)* pp.111-7. Epub 2007 Jun 6.

Nargund, G.; Bourne, T.; Doyle, P.; Parsons, J.; Cheng, W.; Campbell , S & Collins, W.(1996).Associations between ultrasound indices of follicular blood flow, oocyte recovery and preimplantation embryo quality. *Hum Reprod.* 1996 Jan; Vol. 11,No.1, pp.109-13.

Ng , EH.; Chan ,CC.; Tang ,OS.; Yeung, WS. & Ho ,PC.(2006). The role of endometrial and subendometrial vascularity measured by three- dimensional power Doppler ultrasound in the prediction of pregnancy during frozen-thawed embryo transfer cycles. *Hum Reprod.* 2006 Jun; Vol.21, No.6, pp .1612-7. Epub 2006 Jan 31.

Niinimäki, M.; Ruokonen, A.; Tapanainen, JS & Järvelä ,IY.(2009). Effect of mifepristone on the corpus luteum in early pregnancy. *Ultrasound Obstet Gynecol.* 2009 Oct; Vol.34 , no.4,pp.448-53.

Pairleitner, H.; Steiner, H.; Hasenoehrl ,G. & Staudach A.(1999). Three-dimensional power Doppler sonography: imaging and quantifying blood flow and vascularization.*Ultrasound Obstet Gynecol. 1999* Aug; vol. 14, No.2, pp.139-43.

Raga, F.; Bonilla-Musoles, F.;Casan, E. M.;Klein, O. &Bonilla, F.(1999). Assessment of endometrial volume by three-dimensional ultrasound prior to embryo transfer: clues to endometrial receptivity. *Hum Reprod.Vol 14 ,No11, pp.2851-4,*

Salumets, A. ;Suikkari ,AM.; Mäkinen, S.; Karro, H.; Roos, A. & Tuuri ,T.(2006). Frozen embryo transfers: implications of clinical and embryological factors on the pregnancy outcome. *Hum Reprod. 2006* Sep; Vol.21, no. 9, pp. 2368-74. Epub 2006 May 9.

Salumets , A.; Tuuri ,T.; Mäkinen, S.; Vilska, S.; Husu ,L.; Tainio ,R. & Suikarri Am (2003). Effect of developmental stage of embryo at freezing on pregnancy outcome of frozen-thawed embryo transfer.*Hum Reprod.* 2003 Sep; Vol. 18, No. 9, pp.1890-5.

Schalkoff , ME. ; Oskowitz ,SP . & Powers ,RD.(1993). A multifactorial analysis of the pregnancy outcome in a successful embryo cryopreservation program. *Fertil Steril.* 1993 May; Vol. 59, No. 5, pp :1070-4.

Van Blerkom, J.; Antczak, M. & Schrader, R.(1997). The developmental potential of the human oocyte is related to the dissolved oxygen content of follicular fluid: association with vascular endothelial growth factor levels and perifollicular blood flow characteristics. *Hum Reprod.* 1997 May; Vol. 12, No. 5, pp .1047-55.

Van Steirteghem, AC .; Van der Elst , J.; Van den Abbeel, E.; Joris, H.;Camus ,M.& Devroey P(1994). Cryopreservation of supernumerary multicellular human embryos obtained after intracytoplasmic sperm injection. *Fertil Steril.* 1994 Oct;Vol. 62, No. 4, pp .775-80.

Van der Elst, J.; Van den Abbeel ,E.; Vitrier, S.; Camus, M.; Devroey, P. & Van Steirteghem ,AC.(1997) Selective transfer of cryopreserved human embryos with further cleavage after thawing increases delivery and implantation rates. *Hum Reprod.* 1997 Jul;Vol. 12, No. 7, pp. 1513-21.

Veleva, Z. ;Tiitinen, A.; Vilska ,S.; Hydén-Granskog, C.; Tomás, C.; Martikainen, H & Tapanainen, JS. (2005) High and low BMI increase the risk of miscarriage after IVF/ICSI and FET. *Hum Reprod.* 2008 Apr;Vol.23, No.4,pp. 878-84. Epub 2008 Feb 15.

Wang, JX.; Yap ,YY. & Matthews ,CD.(2001). Frozen-thawed embryo transfer: influence of clinical factors on implantation rate and risk of multiple conception. *Hum Reprod. 2001* Nov; Vol. 16, No. 11, pp .2316-9.

Zackova, T.; Järvelä ,IY.; Tapanainen, JS. . & Feyereisl, J. (2009).Assessment of endometrial and ovarian characteristics using three dimensional power Doppler ultrasound to predict response in frozen embryo transfer cycles. *Reprod Biol Endocrinol.* 2009 Dec 25; Vol. 7, pp.151.

6

Atherosclerotic Plaque Regression and Arterial Reverse Remodelling in Carotid and Femoral Arteries by Statin Use in Primary Prevention Setting: Ultrasound Findings

Cesare Rusconi, Riccardo Raddino,
Eleftheria Trichaki and Livio Dei Cas
Department of Cardiology, Faculty of Medicine University of Brescia
Study & Research Center - Gino Giribardi Gymnasium -
Science and Prevention of Cardiovascular Aging, Brescia
Italy

1. Introduction

Atherosclerosis is a generalized process which begins early in childhood (first decade of life) and develops silently and more or less rapidly during adolescence and young adulthood (Stary et al., 1994). Recent investigation using whole body multislice computed tomography in 52 ancient Egyptians mummies (mean age 45.1 ± 9.2 years) from the Middle Kingdom to the Greco-Roman period, a time span of more than 2,000 years, Allam et al. (Allam et al., 2011) showed that atherosclerosis (as in contemporary humans) was more evident and extensive with advancig age, and as common and devastating disease as at present time.

Atherosclerotic cardiovascular (CV) disease, which includes coronary artery disease, stroke and peripheral arterial disease, is the most common cause of premature death in the industrialized world thereby constituting an immense public health problem. This disease was formerly considered an inevitable consequence of aging. The Framingham Heart Study, the most important and influential investigation in CV diseases which laid the foundation for preventive medicine and for CV disorders in particular (Greenberg, 2010), enrolled its first patient in 1948. In the following 40 years a large body of scientific evidence from the Framingham cohort and other major epidemiological studies definitely established that multiple CV risks were responsible of the growing CV disease burden, mainly in high-income countries (Mendis 2010). The scientific Framingham Community gave foundation to the risk factor concept providing insights into their prevalence, incidence and prognostic value. Due to variation in prevalence of individual risk factors in different geographic regions specific approaches to CV disease prevention have been implemented in various countries. Accordingly, a WHO survey on CV risk factors in 2002 showed that more than three quarters of the global CV disease burden was attributable to the following 3: tobacco, blood pressure and cholesterol. And the INTERHART case-control study (Yusuf et al., 2004), involving 27,000 subjects from 52 countries representing all inhabited continents, provided evidence that approximately 80% of the population attributable risk of acute myocardial infarction was predicted by smoking, lipids, hypertension, diabetes and obesity.

As demonstrated in the Karelia Community (Puska, 2010), despite recent attempts to include new CV events predictors, it appears that targeting the already known major risk factors, identified 50 years ago in the Framingham community, remains a priority for the present time and the future. In addition to tobacco the most important modifiable risk factors are hypertension and hypercholesterolemia: due to distinct pathways of atherosclerosis in intracranial versus extracranial disease in patients with hypertension this risk factor has been thought to have major responsibility in the pathogenesis of cerebrovascular diseses whereas the second in coronary artery disese (Napoli et al., 2006). Increasing evidence suggests that atherosclerosis is a diffuse disease with first clinical manifestation in one territory often followed by symptoms coming from other vascular districts. Accordingly, a very high burden of preclinical (silent) coronary artery disease has been recently documented in patients with cerebral infarction (Amarenco, et al., 2010) In recent years, despite the wishful statement by the nobel prize winners Brown and Gldstein "heart attacks: gone with the century? (Brown & Godstein, 1996) CV diseases still remain the undisputed number one killer in most countries and will remain in the next future with an increasing contribution from eastern countries. The well known different gender susceptibility to advanced atherosclerotic lesions observed some 20 years before the occurence of clinical events, supports the pediatrician's view that early preventive measures in young male people can significantly postpone the onset of clinical manifestations (Mc-Gill & McMahan, 2006). Some optimism comes from the percentage decrease (44% to 76%) in death due to coronary artery disease (CAD) during 1980 through 2000 attributed to risk-factor changes in 10 studies in different populations across the globe (Ford et al., 2007). According to Jeremia Stamler (Stamler et al., 2006) an important goal is to increase the population at low risk until it will be the overwhelming majority. He also mentioned the importance of improving life style from the time of preconception to birth and through school age to young adult: a statement in line with studies pioneered by DJP Barker (Barker 1992) on the association between measures of fetal growth and increased risk of CV diseses later in life. Somehow in line with these observations, it has been reported that maternal hypercholesterolemia is associated with enhanced lipid deposition in human fetal arteries (Napoli et al., 2006).

As far as the lipid story is concerned, after early pathological investigations demonstrating that younger hypercholesterolemic people manifest atheroscerotic plaques in their first or second decade of life, it became clear that serum cholesterol was responsible of the intimal atherosclerotic plaque formation laiding the foundation of the science of atherosclerosis as a major research target for the present time and years to come. It has been consistently shown in studies that on average each 1% raise in cholesterolemia is associated with an approximate 3% increase in risk for CV events, and that on the contrary, the HDL cholesterol level is inversely associated with CV diseases in both sexes at all ages ((Barker 1992). At present a great number of experimental, genetic, and epidemiologic papers support the notion that LDL cholesterol is the most important risk factor for atherosclerosis and responsible for clinical events both in men and women (Freeman et al., 2006; Napoli et al.,2006). Moreover, as a relevant finding from the ARIC study it has been shown that a lifelong history of reduced LDL cholesterol levels (by a nonsense mutations in PCSK9) over a 15-year period was associated with 47% reduction of coronary artery disease risk even in presence of multiple risk factors (Cohen et al., 2006), a larger result compared to that predicted from other LDL-lowering trials. These findings strongly support the view that benefits from cholesterol lowering treatments with statins are expected in relation with the effective duration of treatment along years. According to William Robert (Roberts, 2002) substantial evidence exists that keeping serum total cholesterol <150 mg/dl, LDL-cholesterol <100 mg/dl, and HDL cholesterol at least >20 mg/dl, the chances of forming atherosclerotic plaques are slim. Statins have been available since late-eighties and yet, more than 20 years later, most patients who have had atherosclerotic events or who are at high risk for atherosclerotic events unfortunately are not on statin therapy despite its proven benefit in decreasing first and repeated atherosclerotic events.

2. The atherosclerotic plaque

Atherosclerotic plaques develop over many years. Initiating event is focal subendothelial retention of apoB lipoproteins on extracellular matrix molecules particularly proteoglycans (Tabas et al., 2007). These retained molecules become aggregated and oxidized and induce a series of biological modifications producing a maladaptive inflammatory response by which monocytes enter the subendothelium and become cholesterol enriched foam cells after incorporating the modified lipoproteins. The fibrous cap of such a plaque may become thin and rupture as a result of the depletion of matrix components through the activation of proteolytic enzymes such as matrix-degrading proteinases. It has been shown that lipoprotein retention is amplified and retention continues to accelerate once lesions become established. This implies that lesions are more dangerous when formed early in life and suggests the great gain young subjects can have if don't leave untreated their high blood cholesterol level and other risk factors. Endothelial dysfunction is the first step in atherosclerosis and the combined association of a decreased NO production with an increase of NO inactivation appears to be a marker of this condition. Major responsibility in the formation and progression of atherosclerotic is attributed to reduced adiponectin plasma levels. Adiponectin is thought to be also involved in the regulating of necrotic core development (see 3.4 section of this chapter).
Of note, arterial wall reverse (outward) remodelling is usually associated with vulnerable plaques with higher risk of rupture. Their vulnerability is defined as a relatively large necrotic lipid core, intraplaque haemorrhage, abundant vasa vasorum and/or calcification. They are also covered by a thin, inflamed, fibrous cap that may fissure (Naghavi et al., 2003; Virmani et al., 2005). Collagenous fibrous cap represents a form of scar-like response promoted by smooth muscle cells migration into the intima. Of note, plaque progression (Fig.1) is associated with dying macrophages giving rise to areas of necrosis with cholesterol crystals, extracellular debris, proteases and prothrombotic agents (Tabas et al., 2007). These advanced plaques (Fig. 2) are characterized by fibrous cap thinning, plaque erosion and rupture as a result of the depletion of matrix components through the activation of proteolytic enzymes such as matrix-degrading proteinases (MMPs) that are highly concentrated in atherosclerotic plaques by inflammatory cells (macrophages, foam cells), smooth muscle cells and endothelial cells, ultimately being responsible of clinical thrombotic events such as acute myocardial infarction or stroke. A number of research lines have been identified and a therapeutic window of opportunity appears to exist to selectively block proretentive subendothelial matrix-lipoprotein interaction with a potential for regression of advanced plaques
Great advancement of the knowledge in coronary plaque structure has been obtained in recent years by intravascular imaging modalities which can characterize the plaque

according to the presence of thin fibrous cap and other findings such as active inflammation, lipid core disruption and severe stenosis, with high sensitivity specificity and predictive accuracy (Valgimigli et al., 2006; Hong et al., 2009). Much interest has been recently focused on the role of calcium which is incorporated into the plaque with an active process resembling bone formation preceded by apoptosis of smooth muscle cells and generation of apoptotic bodies acting as calcification sites with further steps ultimately leading to hydroxyapatite deposition (Mamm et al., 2011).

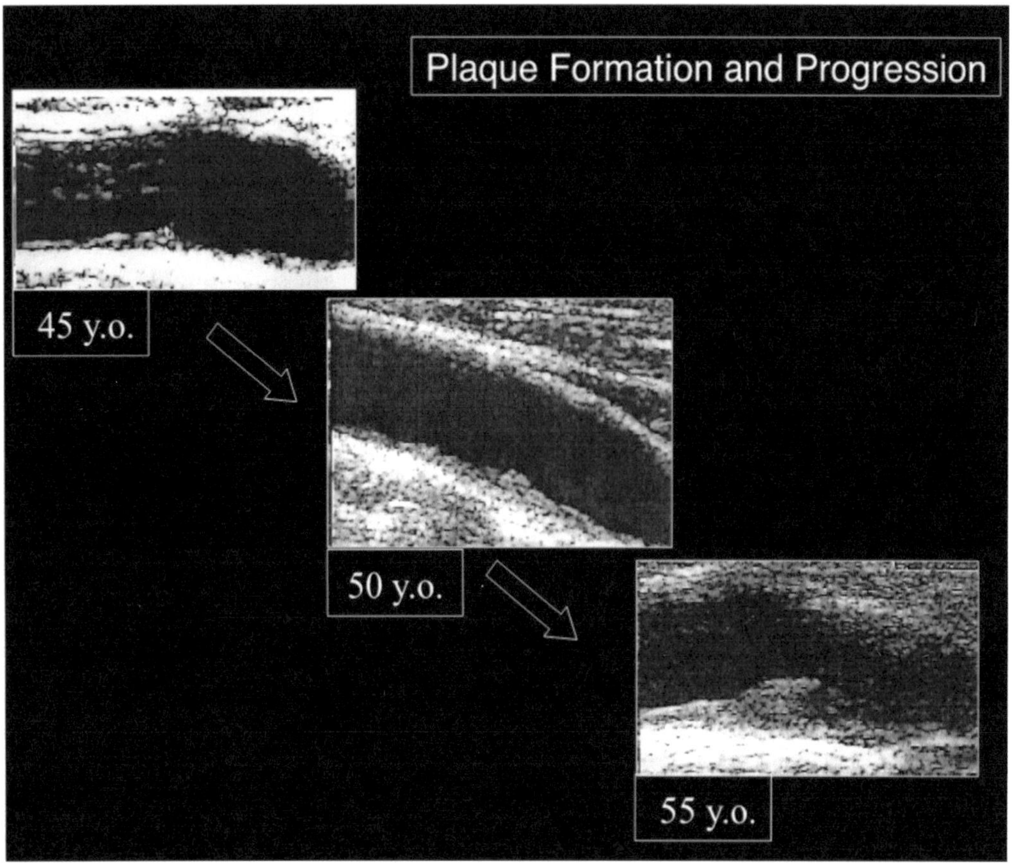

Fig. 1. Plaque formation and progression in the carotid artery. B-mode ultrasound imaging of the left carotid artery in a long-axis during a 10 years period follow-up (1998-2008) in a healthy man from 45 to 55 years of age. Of note, this subject was normotensive and had surprisingly normal blood lipids level (total chol. 165 mg/dl, HDL chol. 71 mg/dl and tryglicerides 64 mg/dl). In 1998, at age 45 y.o., a small plaque was present (maximum short axis diameter: 1.3 mm). In the following ten years a progressive increase in plaque dimension occurred associated with a mild expansive arterial wall remodelling [Glagov phenomenon (Glagov et al., 1987)] in the far field in the year 2003, with a marked step-up increase of the outward arterial remodelling in 2008. The large echo-lucent (black) area within the plaque in 2008 is associated with a thin fibrous cap indicating a high risk of plaque rupture in this subject.

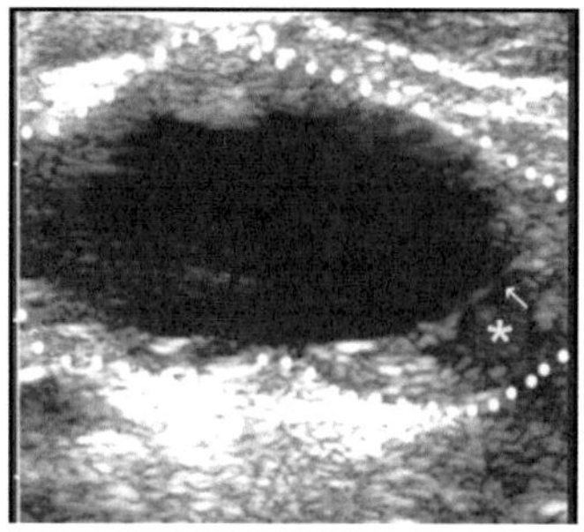

Fig. 2. Vulnerable plaque of the carotid artery bifurcation referring to type VI lesion of the AHA plaque nomenclature. The asterisk indicates the area of the lipid necrotic core covered by a very thin fibrous cap (small arrow) with high risk of rupture. The plaque is associated with a marked outward vessel remodelling keeping intact the lumen of the artery.

Moreover, a recent non invasive ultrasound study of femoral arteries in animals opened a door for clinical application of quantification of adventitial vasa vasorum proliferation, a feature of plaque progression (Moguillansky et al., 2011). But evidence exists that despite core in vivo imaging strategies are promising, their invasive nature and limited spatial resolution, as well as ionizing radiation and poor penetration, limit their possible application in human beings. A future however most exists for hybrid technologies and advanced reconstruction and post-processing techniques.

Summarizing, atherosclerosis has top responsibility in total and CV mortality, either industrialized and in the developing countries, it is a cholesterol dependent disease, progressive in nature and characterized by a very long preclinical period. Total cholesterol plasma level > 130 mg/dl is the necessary causing factor. This process starts in the early decade of life and is accelerated by other major risk factors like hypertension, smoking, diabetes, obesity and male gender. It can be easily identified by B-Mode ultrasound of carotid and femoral arteries during the asymptomatic (preclinical) period long before clinical manifestations do occur, opening a window for early diagnosis and lipid-lowering interventions.

2.1 Plaque regression and stabilization

An ischemic event is usually associated with an advanced atherosclerotic lesion. Early studies in animals showed that removal of atherogenic factors reduced the prevalence of atherosclerotic lesions. As far as the regression studies of atherosclerosis in human beings is concerned, we must first acknowledge those studies pioneered at the University of California in 1978 by David Blankenhorn and his group (Blankenhorn et al., 1978; Blankenohorn 1978). These authors used advanced computer techniques for image processing derived from space-fly technology with a digital array depicting up to 256 shades of gray. This group first demonstrated the regression by treatment of atherosclerotic lesions with serial femoral artery angiograms (two exams at 13 months interval) performed in 25 hyperlipidemic subjects. During the following 15 years nine arteriographic human studies have been conducted by different groups with a total of 2.101 patients and a mean follow-up of 3,3 (1 to 10) years. These studies have been reviewed by Brown et al. (Brown et al., 1993). Despite several diversities among these studies the analysis showed a benefit from treatment: whether by diet, diet plus life style changes, by hypolipidemic drugs niacin and lovastatin, or plus ileal by-pass associated with resins (cholestipol or cholestiramine). The mean numbers of angiographic outcomes were the following: 53% progression and 8% regression in the control group, versus 26% progression and 26% regression in the treated groups. The authors concluded that this analysis has confirmed the hypothesis that lipid lowering therapy selectively depletes the atherosclerotic plaques lipid content and prevents plaque disruption and the associated clinical events. For what the plaque instability is concerned many factors concur to the phenomenon. The mechanical strength of the cap appears to be one of these and depends on the amount and structure of collagen and other tissue protein determinants of plaque rupture.

Mechanisms by which lipid lowering may stabilize vulnerable plaques in humans have been extensively investigated in recent years. Specific cellular and molecular alterations consequent to lipid lowering have been identified: matrix metalloproteinase (MMP) activity reduction with associated increase of collagen content in plaques appears to have major importance. Smooth muscle cells have a central role in the formation and stabilisation of the fibrous cap because they produce connective tissue matrix proteins. It has been suggested that the combination of lipid lowering and antioxidant agents has a rationale for preserving fibrous cap stabilization (Davies, 1998). On this line it has been shown (Aikawa et al., 1998; Crisby et al., 2001) that pravastatin not only decreases lipid content, oxydized LDL and inflammation, but also MMPs-2 and cell death, whereas it increases collagen content providing the first strong evidence of plaque stabilizing effect by statins in humans.

In 2001 Corti et al. (Corti et al., 2001) using serial black-blood MRI of the aorta and carotid arteries at baseline, 6 and 12 months after lipid-lowering therapy with simvastatin in hypercholesterolemic patients with aortic and/or carotid atherosclerotic plaques, demonstrated that persistent reduction in total and LDL cholesterol levels was associated with a significant inverse remodeling and lumen preservation of both aorta and carotid arteries at 12 months. In the REVERSAL study, published in 2004 by Nissen et al. (Nissen et al., 2005) intravascular ultrasound have been used in 502 patients divided into equal sized groups receiving either pravastatin 40 mg or atorvastatin 80 mg daily dose for 18 months: a complete halting of coronary disease progression was observed in the atorvastatin-treated patients but a continued disease progression occurred in the pravastatin-treated group, thereby suggesting that a very low levels of LDL cholesterol are needed to arrest and stabilize the ongoing atherosclerotic process and that 40 mg pravastatin is inadequate to this end. A step up progression of the results from lipid reducing drugs has been demonstrated by Corti et al. (Corti et al., 2005) in a further study in which a significant regression of atherosclerotic plaques has been obtained by effective and protracted lipid-lowering therapy: moreover and of major importance, the study suggested that the degree of LDL-cholesterol reduction rather than the statin dose was associated with plaque regression. Differently from previous intravascular studies in which statins administration was accompanied only by slowing or halting of the atherosclerotic process, Nissen et al. (Nissen et al., 2006) first demonstrated in 2006 a significant regression of coronary atherosclerosis with serial intravascular ultrasound examinations in the ASTEROID trial: the study was conducted during 24 months period in 349 patients submitted to high-intensity statin therapy with rosuvastatin 40 mg. Of interest, a 10-12 months period appears to be the appropriate time interval for initial appreciation of plaque regression in carotid and femoral arteries during statin treatment also in our experience in the last ten years period (Rusconi C, 2008; Rusconi et al., 2011). Thus, evidence exists allowing us to conclude that with appropriate statin use plaque regression and stabilization do occur. The phenomenon can be assessed non-invasively in patients using ultrasound imaging of carotid and femoral arteries and is further examined and described in details in the last part of this chapter.

3. The 4S trial and the statins story

As far as the story of secondary CV events prevention is concerned, it is worthy to mention the pioneering Scandinavian Simvastatin Survival Study (4S) trial (The Lancet, 1994) and its promoter Prof. Terjie Pedersen who opened the door to evidence based secondary CAD prevention by statin use. In this study it has been shown for the first time that simvastatin reduced mortality in patients with a high cardiovascular risk. Many large outcome trials of statins have been performed during the following years confirming the results of the 4S trial. Further recent confirmation that statin use continues to be useful comes from a double-blind randomised trial (SEARCH Study, 2007) comparing 80 versus 20 mg simvastatin administration in 12,064 men and women 18–80 years old with a history of myocardial infarction. In this study the higher simvastatin dosage has reduced from 25,7% to 24,5% (with 6% proportional reduction) the major vascular events. Consistent with previous trials, this result has been obtained by an average 0·35 mmol/L greater reduction in LDL cholesterol. In this study the risk of statin-related myopathy was low with the 20–40 mg simvastatin dosage (about one per 10,000 patients per year) but increased about ten times (to about one per 1000 patients per year) with 80 mg simvastatin daily. Of importance, the excess risk mainly occurred during the first year and has been largely confined to those people carrying *SLCO1B1* genetic variants which can be otherwise detected before starting treatment and may be useful for tailoring the statin dose in the first year of treatment, especially when certain other drugs are simultaneously used (The Search Collaborative Group, 2008). In this study clear evidence has come out that lowering LDL cholesterol concentrations lowers the risk of major vascular events and that intensive LDL cholesterol lowering reduces the risk even more. Based on these results the authors suggested that "for patients deemed to be at sufficient risk of major cardiovascular events a more appropriate strategy - by contrast with current guidance - could be to consider regimens which involve newer, more potent, statins (80 mg atorvastatin or 20–40 mg rosuvastatin daily) or the combination of standard doses of generic statins (40 mg simvastatin daily) with other agents that can lower LDL cholesterol substantially, without producing such increases in the risk of myopathy". On the subject of the recent statins introduction in the armamentarium of cardiovascular therapy Scott Grundy (Grundy, 2004) wrote the following statement: "lowering low-density lipoproteins by statin therapy to reduce the risk for major clinical events in patients with clinical atherosclerotic CV disease represents a therapeutic triumph of modern medicine". After a seven years period from this statement a surprising sequence of successes has so far characterized the statins story, also extending the positive results to apparently healthy people with preclinical atherosclerosis. According to the extraordinary evidence on the issue and in agreement with the SHAPE Group strategy in USA-Texas State, (Naghavi, M., Libby, P., & Falk, E. 2003) we think that the time has come to go by far beyond such evidence by applying effective preventive measures also to the great group of individuals with preclinical atherosclerosis.

There are now available multiple noninvasive imaging modalities that can identify subclinical atherosclerosis in different vascular beds. They include ultrasonography, coronary CCS assessment by CT, noninvasive CT angiography and MRI. All these methods have advantages and draw backs, but only CCS and ultrasonography have been mostly used. The CCS has provided powerful prognostic information in both sexes of multiple ethnic populations and a systematic review of both symptomatic and asymptomatic populations led investigators to conclude that who have a negative CCS are highly unlikely to have CAD (Sewer et al. 2009). But discordant results have been also reported. In our view, due to the associated radiation exposure and the need of repeated examination in the course of years also to establish the right moment for an interventional procedure, the coronary CCS should be used to this end only after careful evaluation of risk/benefit ratio. The issue will be later thoroughly treated in this chapter.

3.1 Statins-induced event reduction in primary prevention setting

Patients with established CHD or other clinical manifestation of atherosclerosis, or diabetes, have by definition a substantial risk for future cardiovascular events and premature death. These people should have intensive lipid-lowering therapy because the benefit from these drugs is estimated to largely overweight the risk associated with such a treatment, even if low baseline LDL concentration is present (Cheung & Lam, 2010). On the other side, according to the results of several studies statin treatment appears appropriate in primary prevention setting only in presence of specific risk factors.

The first clinical trial to study the effect of statins in primary prevention setting in patients with a relatively low risk was the WOSCOPS trial (Shepherd et al., 1995) performed in 6.595 hypercholesterolemic patients using 40 mg pravastatin, obtaining a 32% risk reduction in major CV events during a 4.9 years period of follow-up. The following AFCAPS trial (Downs et al., 2001) studied the effects of lovastatin in healthy men and women and was associated with 39% reduction in major coronary events definitely confirming the benefits of statin treatment in healthy individuals. The results of the subsequent PROSPER trial (Shepherd et al., 2002) in 1,585 subjects taking pravastatin raised the question of the potential cancers risk and the problem of side effects with statins. The concern has been subsequently negated by the following studies: ASCOT (Sever et al., 2003) in 5,168 hypertensive patients, HPS (Heart Protection Study Collaborative Group, 2002) in 20,536 patients, CARDS (Colhoun et al. 2004.) in 1.428 diabetic patients, ASPEN (Knoop et al., 2006) in 959 diabetic patients. All the aforementioned studies have demonstrated mostly positive results on the incidence of coronary and cerebrovascular disease without increasing cancer risk.

Recently, in primary prevention setting the MEGA trial (Nakamura et al., 2006) in 3.966 hypercholesterolemic Japanese women during a mean follow-up of 5.3 years, randomly assigned to diet or diet plus 10-20 mg pravastatin, it has been shown that pravastatin reduced coronary events by 23% without any difference in the incidence of cancer or other adverse events between the two groups, suggesting that treatment with a low dose of pravastatin reduces the risk of coronary heart disease in Japan by much the same amount as higher doses have shown in Europe and the USA. In the year 2004 a meta-analysis (Grundy et al., 2004) from the National Cholesterol Education Program Adult Treatment Panel III Guidelines, including 26 randomized trial, 5 of them planned *more vs less statins* and 21 planned *statins vs control* (also including the eight studies just mentioned in previous lines) with a total of 170.000 participants, the authors conclude that further reductions in LDL-cholesterol safely produce definite further reductions in the incidence of heart attack, revascularisation and ischemic stroke, reducing the annual rate of these major vascular events by just over a fifth with each 1.0 mmol/L of LDL-cholesterol reduction. Furthermore, no evidence of any threshold within the cholesterol range studied was found suggesting that by 2-3 mmol/L plasma lowering of LDL-cholesterol would reduce risk by about 40-50% respectively. Of importance, further reduction of LDL-cholesterol did not produce any adverse effects even in those subjects with baseline LDL- cholesterol lower than 2.0 mmol/L. A meta-analyses of more versus less intensive therapy, and of statins versus control, did not discovered any adverse effects on cancer incidence (CTT Trialists, 2005). A number of other important conclusions for clinical practice have been drawn in this meta-analysis: 1) the primary goal for patients at high CV risk should be to achieve the largest LDL-cholesterol reduction possible, without materially increasing myopathy risk, 2) lowering of LDL-cholesterol further below the limit established by NECP in 2004 (Grundy et al., 2004) of 70 mg/dL (1.8 mmol/L) to achieve additional benefits, without an increased risk of cancer or non-vascular mortality, 3) to achieve these benefits, with newer more potent statins such as 80 mg atorvastatin or 20 mg rosuvastatin daily, 4) to use combination of standard doses of generic statins (40 mg simvastatin or pravastatin daily) with other LDL-cholesterol lowering therapies.

In primary prevention setting (asymptomatic and apparently healthy subjects) statins are used in presence of risk factors and hypercholesterolemia in particular. Prototypic condition in which aggressive LDL-cholesterol reduction is mandatory is familial hypercholesterolemia. General agreement exists that in these patients should be used the highest tolerated statin dosage. In a study on this subset of patients it has been shown that atorvastatin 80 mg treatment was accompanied by regression of carotid intima media thickness whereas conventional LDL-cholesterol lowering was not (Smilde et al., 2001). Similarly, the great number of apparently healthy subjects with documented atherosclerosis, either by 2D-echo of carotid/femoral arteries or by CT scan of coronary calcium, in addition to life style modifications and other risk factors control, statin treatment appears appropriate according to the severity of the atherosclerotic process and the number and weight of risk factors.

Of note, for what the dietary alcohol is concerned, it has been shown that comparing alcohol consumers and abstainers for a 3 years period follow-up after femoral or carotid artery surgery, alcohol consumers had less cardiovascular event rate as well as more stable plaque cores and less macrophage infiltration (Gisbertz et al., 2011) confirming that mild-to moderate alcohol consumption may help to reduce atherosclerosis progression.

3.2 HDL-cholesterol and statins

Clinical, experimental and epidemiological evidence consistently demonstrated the inverse association and causal relationship between low HDL levels and the risk of coronary artery disease (Gordon & Rifkind, 1989). Statin treatment of cardiovascular patients reduces clinical events by 25 to 45%. High-density lipoprotein (HDL) has been proposed as a therapeutic target to further reduce this residual cardiovascular risk. The primary role of HDL and reverse cholesterol transport in the reduction of CHD risk is supported by a considerable amount of experimental data. The mechanism by which HDL can mediate protection from atherosclerosis is complex and multifactorial and evolving concepts of the role of HDL in protection from atherosclerosis have been recently pointed out (Farmer & Liao, 2011).

The HDL particles exert a strong antiatherosclerotic action through several mechanisms. These include a facilitating cholesterol efflux from cholesterol-loaded foam cells, an antiinflammatory action, a positive effect on nitric oxide synthesis, serving as a plasma transport lipoprotein for biologically important proteins and as an antithrombotic agent by improving thrombolytic balance. In addition to their beneficial effects on the coagulation system the HDL molecules have a favorable complex interaction with the protein C and protein S system and have a significant natural antioxidant effect which improves endothelial function and inhibits the oxidative step required for LDL uptake by the macrophage. These properties of HDL have been demonstrated to decreased apoptosis and promote endothelial repair. Clinical trials with new HDL-raising drugs are currently under way to provide definitive evidence that increasing HDL will reduce cardiovascular events (Brewer, 2011).

Low HDL levels are present in about 10% of the general population and represent the most frequent form of dyslipidemia in patients with CAD. Reduced HDL concentrations seem to be unable to eliminate efficiently the cholesterol excess at vascular wall level, contributing to the onset of the inflammatory response that typically occurs in the pathogenesis of atherosclerosis from its earliest stages. In keeping with this evidence the results of numerous studies quite convincingly suggest that HDL is capable of exerting anti-inflammatory activity either directly or by modulating the expression of a number of acute phase reactants. Endothelial repair and reduced apoptosis are other mechanism by which HDLs preserve vascular function (Kera et al., 2011).

In a recent careful examination of 20 randomized control trials (completed in the period from 1991 to 2009) in which statins have been used, for the first time clear evidence emerged that despite statin treatment a low HDL-cholesterol plasma level remains an independent predictor of higher cardiac events (Jafri et al., 2010) A post-hoc analysis of one of these studies, the TNT trial (Waters et al., 2004), showed that low levels of HDL-cholesterol was predictive of high rate of major CV events even at very low level of LDL-cholesterol thus suggesting that low levels of HDL and high levels of LDL cholesterol are indipendently important predictors of cardiovascular disease. Similarly, in another meta-analysis of 23 trials of various lipid-modifying drugs the sum of LDL-cholesterol percentage reduction and the HDL-cholesterol increase better predicted the benefit than the individual lipoprotein changes: it has been calculated that each 0.26 mmol/L (10 mg/dL) decrease in HDL-cholesterol level was associated with 7 additional myocardial infarction and 4 additional CV events/1000 person-years (Brown et al., 2004). It has been also underlined that despite the aforementioned undisputable evidence of the benefit associated with higher HDL-lipoprotein plasma levels, certain drugs (fibrates) do not appear to be associated with clear benefit (Joy et al., 2008).

In a recent and important study Kera et al. (Kera et al. 2011), measured the cholesterol efflux capacity from macrophages (a metric of HDL function) in 203 healthy volunteers who underwent carotid artery IMT assessment and in 442 angiographycally confirmed coronary patients, as well as in 351 patients without angiographic confirmed disease: in this study the authors demonstrated the followings: 1) HDL-cholesterol levels and apolipoprotein A-1 (the major protein component of HDL) were significant determinants of cholesterol efflux capacity accounting for less than 40% of the observed variation, 2) the efflux capacity was inversely related to IMT and was a strong inverse predictor of coronary artery disease status. The authors concluded that this capacity "is not explained simply by circulating levels of HDL-cholesterol or apoliprotein A-I and is independently related to both the presence and extent of atherosclerosis".

Therapeutic options for raising HDL-cholesterol plasma levels still appear inconsistent either in experimental or in preclinical setting and, up to now, in clinical studies the cholesterol efflux capacity has not been enhanced in statins treated patients. Due to inability of statins to further reduce the risk associated with low HDL-cholesterol, a treatment has been suggested (Cziraky et al., 2008) to promote optimal lipid values in several at risk patients-populations based on the association of a statin with extended-release niacin, the most effective agent for raising HDL-cholesterol levels. This approach appears most justified in type 2 diabetes which is characterized by two to three times higher prevalence of hypertrigliceridemia usually associated with decreased HDL-cholesterol levels and increased small dense LDL-cholesterol particles, forming the powerful risk factor of the lipid triad (Temelkova- Kurktschiev & Hanefeld, 2004). As far as the antioxidant potential of HDL particles is concerned it has been shown that distribution of HDL subpopulations according to their particle mean size has important implication for their antioxidant potential and that HDL3 particles are more resistant to oxidation (Shuhei, 2010).

3.3 Inflammation, C-reactive protein and lipoprotein (a)

Inflammation and inflammatory pathways appear to have a fundamental role in the pathogenesis of atherosclerosis and coronary artery disease in particular (Hansson, 2005). Accelerated atherosclerosis has been described in patients with chronic inflammatory diseases such as rheumatoid arthritis, psoriasis and systemic lupus erythematosus. High sensitivity C-reactive protein (hsCRP), an acute phase reactant produced by the liver is the most studied, although nonspecific, marker of inflammation. In 1997 Ridker et al. (Ridker et al., 1997) gave first demonstration of hsCRP ability to predict future myocardial infarction and stroke in apparently healthy asymptomatic subjects, and several papers have been published in recent years on the subject supporting Ridker's conclusions that hsCRP is a strong predictor of future major cardiovascular events. Moreover, evidence +has been published that the magnitude of this effect is similar to that of cholesterol and blood pressure and that also people with elevated hsCRP levels but without hyperlipidemia might benefit from statin treatment (Ridker et al., 2008).

However, in a recent report of the Heart Protection Study (HPS Collaborative Group, 2002) with 20.536 high risk patients randomly assigned to simvastatin 40 mg versus placebo for 5 years, it has been observed a 29% reduction of major vascular events without any significant difference between the four subgroup (defined by the combination of low or high baseline LDL-cholesterol and CRP) with clear evidence of benefits mainly in those with both low LDL-cholesterol and low CRP. These findings suggested that LDL-cholesterol reduction is the necessary condition to reduce the risk of cardiovascular events, independently of CRP changes. According to the authors, this conclusion appears to be mainly supported by the finding that LDL-cholesterol reduction by simvastatin reduced the event risk to a similar extent irrespective of baseline CRP levels. At present, it appears uncertain whether hsCRP should be considered only a clinically useful disease marker or whether it also may play a causal role in the atherothrombotic process. Of interest, in a recent study in the TNT study population (Arsenault et al., 2011) investigating the effects of atorvastatin 80 mg versus 10 mg in patients with stable coronary artery disease, it has been shown that in contrast to the blood lipid levels almost none among several non-lipid biomarkers predicted recurrent CV events after 1 year of treatment. According to the authors' suggestion the cardiovascular benefits were primarily due to the effects of statins on lipids biomarkers rather than on non-lipid ones. According to 2009 Canadian Lipid Guidelines (Jenest et al., 2009) hsCRP should not performed on everyone but only in selected subjects and in patients with metabolic syndrome for better risk stratification.

More recent data from Molenkampf et al. (Molenkampf et al., 2011) suggest that in primary prevention setting hsCRP may help selecting in the general population those people with highest risk of coronary events but with low coronary calcium score (CCS). In particular they demonstrated that CCS was superior to hsCRP in the discrimination and reclassification of coronary risk and that further improvement in coronary risk assessment was obtained when CCS was added to Framingham risk variables and hsCRP, whereas adding hsCRP to Framingham risk variables and CCS did not increase risk prediction. In any case, and in complete agreement with the authors, in asymptomatic subjects and for all individuals, the first-line recommendation remains a healthy lifestyle including quit smoking, regular physical activity, healthy diet, blood pressure and weight control. The efforts that are necessary to implement effective lifestyle modification in larger cohorts must be weighed against the costs of extended risk assessment and, for what CCS is concerned, the risk attributable to radiation exposure (see later). Being hsCRP a nonspecific marker of inflammation, it has been suggested that among the other inflammatory markers interleukine-6 may provide valuable additional prognostic information. In conclusion, at present time it appears that hsCRP should not be considered neither a major player in the atherosclerotic process nor a major predictor for future events, but may be thought to better stratify the risk and to support clinical decision in the individual patient.

Finally, as far as the lipoprotein-(a) [Lp(a)] is concerned, the results from the recently published Young Finnish Study [a prospective population-based cohort study of 939 men and 1,141 women followed-up from the mean age of 17 and 38 years with repeated Lp(a) and both carotid IMT and flow-mediated dilation tests] do not provide any support for an early atherogenic effect of increased Lp (a) plasma levels (Kivimaki et al., 2010).

3.4 Adiponectin

Adiponectin is the most abundant adipokine released by adipocytes in response to extracellular stimuli and metabolic changes (Berseghian, 2011). It is predominately, but not exclusively, produced by adipose tissue and recent studies suggest that it is also synthesized and secreted by human cardiomyocytes (Pineiro et al., 2005). It is reduced in obesity and type 2 diabetes and low plasma concentration has been associated with an increased risk of CAD and acute coronary syndrome in several though not all studies. Low plasma levels of adiponectin are also associated with increased NO inactivation combined with decreased NO production, both of which contribute to endothelial dysfunction, the first step in atherosclerosis. Adiponectin is thought to be also involved in the regulation of necrotic core development. In patients with stable CAD and in acute coronary syndrome, a decrease in plasma adiponectin values has been found to be associated with an increase in necrotic core in both culprit and non-culprit lesions assessed by intravascular ultrasounds, suggesting that in this clinical setting lower adiponectin levels reflect plaque vulnerability (Otake et al., 2008). Accordingly, the association of decreased plasma adiponectin level and increased necrotic core ratio has not been demonstrated in patients with stable CAD (Sawada et al., 2010). Although produced by adipocytes, adiponectin exhibits plasma levels inversely proportional to body mass index and visceral adiposity (Bajaj & Ben-Yehuda, 2006). Adiponectin is thought to decrease atherosclerosis progression through inhibition of both neointimal thickening and SMC proliferation and migration into the intima. As recently suggested by Barseghian et al. (Barseghian et al., 2011) direct adiponectin administration in humans is premature and warrants further investigation but indirect methods such as lifestyle modifications and pharmacological interventions may be used to increase adiponectin plasma levels at present time (Hermann et al., 2006). On this line, a meta-analysis of 19 studies confirmed an increase of endogenous adiponectin levels with thiazolidinediones use. Accordingly, pioglitazone exhibited the potential of coronary plaque stabilization in patients with type 2 diabetes by increasing adiponectin levels and reducing the necrotic-core component (Ogasawara et al., 2009; Riera-Guardia & Rothenbacher, 2008).

3.5 Lipids and stroke prevention

The stroke represents the second leading cause of death and is a major contributor to health-care cost. As recently reviewed by Endres et al (Endres et al., 2011) variations have been found between the main risk factors for haemorrhagic vs ischemic stroke and overwhelming evidence suggests that hypertension is a major cause of brain damage and that brain benefits more from high blood pressure treatment. Moreover, it has been indicated (Pischon et al., 2007) that the main modifiable risk factors such as diabetes, smoking, hypertension, and hypercholesterolemia, explain only 55% of variance for stroke events compared to 88% variance for myocardial infarction. In that review (Endres et al., 2011) it has been underlined that actually no randomized clinical trial exists providing a blood pressure target for effective prevention of first strokes. In several studies a close relationship between cholesterol plasma levels and stroke has not been found and hypercholesterolemia is thought to have major responsibility in atherothrombotic stroke only Endres et al., 2011). Although it is still unsettled whether statin use is useful in primary prevention of atherothrombotic stroke in subjects with mild hypercholesterolemia, evidence exists on the other side (Naghavi et al,. 2003) that even mild carotid atherosclerosis in apparently healthy subjects, and independently of lipid plasma values, identifies those subjects with more or less generalized subclinical disease which should be appropriately treated with statins.

3.6 LDL-cholesterol and cancer

Several cancer subtypes (gastrointestinal, hematological, female-specific, urologic and lung cancer) have been observed to be associated with low LDL-cholesterol levels and the mechanisms by which preclinical cancer might induce low LDL-cholesterol plasma levels are largely unknown. The issue of a potential increased risk of cancer in patients treated with hypolipidemic drugs has been already faced in previous pages (see section 3.1) where substantial evidence has been provided on the safety of statin use. The problem of an increased risk of cancer by hypolipidemic drugs has been raised since the late seventhies by the Clofibrate trial, a WHO Cooperative Trial on primary prevention of ischemic heart disease using clofibrate (Oliver et al., 1978). In this study a 47% excess mortality occurred in the treated group during the study period but it has not continued in the follow-up period with only 5% excess mortality after treatment has ended. Recent meta-analyses (Benn et al., 2011) from more than 90,000 patients have lessened the concern, raised in the previous three decades, on risk of cancer using LDL-cholesterol lowering drugs (Rose et al. 1974). However, the pendulum of the potential damage from cholesterol lowering thearpy has been again a little bit forced forward by the results from two studies in Denmark - the Copenhagen City Heart Study (CCHS) and the Copenhagen General Population Study (CGPS) on 59,566 and 6,816 subjects respectively- which have shown that, indipendently of statin use, participants with low plasma cholesterol level (<87 mg/dL) were associated with a 47% increased risk of cancer, a finding not observed in those patients with innate low plasma LDL-cholesterol level identified by genetic study of single-nucleotide polymorphisms in PCSK9, ABACG8 and APOE (Benn et al., 2011). This study has left unsettled the issue of the potential cause-effect relationship between LDL-cholesterol lowering by statin use and cancer. However, a recent metaanalysis of data on cancer from 166,000 paricipants in 25 randomized trials, it has been concluded that, at least in the five years treatment period no evidence emerged of any effect of statin therapy on cancer incidence or mortality at any particular site (Emerson et al., 2010). Has the story come to an end?

4. Imaging of atherosclerosis

Atherosclerosis has been generally viewed as a chronic and inevitably progressive disease characterized by continuous accumulation of atheromatous plaque within the arterial wall. In the last 25 years an important step-up progression occurred with the introduction of a variety of anti-atherosclerotic therapies, the most important of which are the so called statins, which rank among the most extensively studied therapies in contemporary medicine, opening the door to an effective anti-atherosclerotic treatment in addition to standard non pharmacologic measures. Almost simultaneously, invasive and non-invasive imaging techniques of atherosclerosis have been attempted in the course of years and an extraordinary development in non-invasive assessment has been realized during the last two decades. X-ray angiography is still considered the gold standard imaging technique for vessel patency studies but it does not usually allow obtaining information on plaque structure as well as differentiating stable from unstable plaques and the risk of rupture. This technique typically suffers from these limitations and even to day many cardiologists unfortunately still behave as if the absence of angiographic abnormalities indicates the normality of coronary artery anatomy and absence of atherosclerosis (Davis et al., 2004) In a decreasing degree of complexity the new imaging modalities are represented by the following: 1) magnetic resonance imaging (MRI), 2) CT angiography, 3) CCS ,4) B-mode ultrasonography of carotid and femoral arteries as well as abdominal aorta. All these methods are used in clinical setting and the type of investigation closely dependent on the clinical problem the individual patient has and on which techniques are locally available. As it has already been discussed in previous pages high-quality studies have demonstrated that a correlation exits between the severity of atherosclerosis in one arterial territory and involvement of other arteries and that these tests can predict the risk of future CAD events (Fowkes et al., 2008). Accordingly, noninvasive atherosclerosis imaging has evolved into a central method in clinical cardiology and both CCS and B-mode ultrasonography have recently become the most used techniques as first line approach for atherosclerosis detection in primary prevention setting (Greenland et al., 2003). Expert recommendations have endorsed the use of these imaging modalities in primary prevention (Stein et al., 2008) allowing a step-up progression towards an individualised CAD prevention through more effective use of drugs. According to 2009 Canadian Lipid Guidelines (Genest et al., 2009) the screening for high risk subjects should include the following as Class I Recommendation Grade, Level of Evidence C:

- All men over 40 and postmenopausal women
- Anyone with atherosclerosis or diabetes regardless of age
- Anyone with family history of premature (< 60 yrs) cardiovascular event
- All patients with hypertension or dyslipidemia
- All patients with inflammatory diseases such as lupus, rheumatoid arthritis and psoriasis
- Children of patients with severe dyslipidemia
- Subjects with xanthomas, xanthelasma or premature arcus corneus
- Erectile dysfunction
- Chronic renal disease.

Moreover, the following test for atherosclerosis are suggested as Class IIa Recommendation Grade, Level of Evidence C :

- Ankle brachial index
- Exercise stress test

- Carotid B mode ultrasonography
- Cardiac Computed Tomography

These guidelines (Genest et al., 2009) indicate that the presence of atherosclerosis in one of these tests places the individual in the high risk category. In the following pages in addition to a brief review on the usefulness of noninvasive techniques the attention will be focused on noninvasive plaque imaging by ultrasound (which is available in every clinical setting) enabling first line study of plaque burden and structure with assessment of potential regression during statin treatment.

4.1 Magnetic resonance and CT imaging

Due to inability of surface ultrasound to imaging coronary artery circulation, attention has focused on other techniques such as CT and MRI (Kim et al., 2001). As far as MRI is concerned , appropriate sequences are needed for plaque imaging and the contrast-enhanced MRI used for clinical purposes is inadequate to this end (Fig. 3).

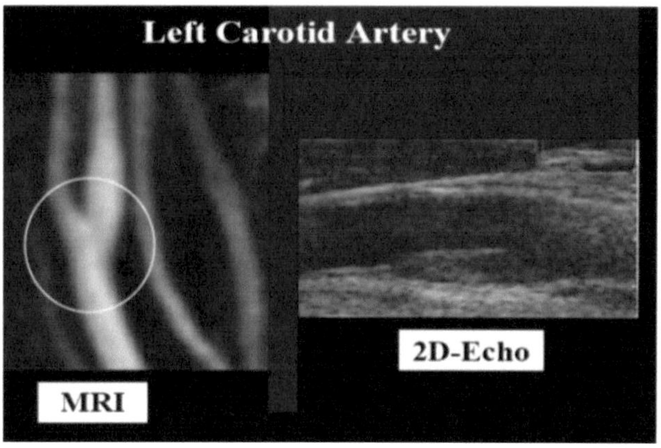

Fig. 3. Contrast-Enhanced MRI (left panel) and B-mode ultrasonography (right panel) of the left crotid artery in a patient with carotid atherosclerosis. In this case the MRI exam has been perfomed for the clinical purpose of a better assessment of vessel stenosis. Plaque imaging would have required a different exam with T1-T2 weighted sequences.

Due to its non-invasiveness carotid MRI has been recently proposed as tool for monitoring individual response to cardiovascular therapy (Yuan, 2008). High-resolution MRI has been recently used for the noninvasive evaluation of carotid plaques showing that is possible to analyze the structure and molecules inside the plaque and to distinguish symptomatic from asymptomatic plaques and patients with low versus high risk through identification of iron deposition (Raman et al., 2008). Moreover, discrimination between lipid core, fibrous cap, intraplaque haemorrhage and calcification as well as distinguishing macrophage-rich from macrophage-poor lesions is possible (Kooi et al., 2003). From these studies emerged the finding that patients with a lipid-rich necrotic core with or without intraplaque haemorrhage represent the desired phenotype for monitoring treatment effects. It has been recently also suggested (Underhill et al., 20011) that throughout advanced tissue specific sequences, acquisition resolution and scan time, in association with techniques allowing monitoring of inflammation and mechanical forces, this technique will enable early assessment of response to therapy.

As far as CT is concerned, significant advances in the last ten years helped this technology to evolve as a real non-invasive alternative to conventional catheter based coronary angiography with the additional great advantage of the possibility of establishing the atherosclerotic burden and plaque characteristics with a radiation exposure less than 1mSv (when a heart rate is kept <60 bpm) which is less than the radiation dose of current CCS imaging. But new evidence that even low-dose ionizing radiation from cardiac imaging and therapeutic procedures is associated with an increased risk of cancer (Eisenberg et al., 2011), suggests that a new word of caution is worthy on the issue and that if the benefits to patients of a single cardiac imaging test probably outweigh any small excess risk of cancer, repeated examinations can induce more harm than good.

4.2 B-mode ultrasound and CCS

During the last 25 years, after the seminal papers by Pignoli and his coworkers (Pignoli, 1984; Poli et al., 1984) in mid eighties, on the feasibility of direct measurement of arterial wall thickness with B-mode imaging in vitro of specimens of human aortic and common carotid arteries, the use of this noninvasive approach through the measurement of the carotid intima-media thickness (CIMT) has become the standard reference method in assessing the presence and the amount of clinical atherosclerosis. Since early studies (Salonen & Salonen, 1991) it has been demonstrated that the presence of different degrees of carotid atherosclerosis (normal, thickening, plaque, stenosis) was associated with a progressive increase of coronary events incidence during a 4-years follow-up period. But at present, after dozens of published studies, the evidence to quantitatively support the use of a CIMT measurement to help in risk stratification on top of a risk function is limited (Platinga et al., 2009). As it will be reported later on, plaque detection by B-Mode ultrasound has become the method of choice for early detection and follow-up treatment in patients deemed to be at higher risk because of preclincal atherosclerosis by carotid and/or femoral plaques, a more reliable manifestation of atherosclerosis as well as stronger prognosticator for future events. Carotid artery plaque are defined as the presence of focal thickening 50% greater than that of the surrounding vessel wall, with a minimal thickness of 1.2 mm (Hurst et al., 2010)Cardiac CT began with electron-beam CT in the early 1980s and continues with multidetector CT. In early studies with electron-beam CT high risk subjects have been identified by a score greater than 80-160 (O'Rourke et al., 2000). The advent of modern CT and high resolution MRI, ranked these techniques at the first approach in the assessment of preclinical atherosclerosis by the American Heart Association guidelines (Greenland et al., 2007). Quantification of coronary artery calcium, the so called coronary calcium score (CCS), as an estimate of atherosclerotic plaque burden has become the current major application of non-contrast CT. Plaque burden is quantified by the Agatston score: according to different tertiles of CCS values (Tertile I = CCS 0-99, Tertile II = CCS 100-309, Tertile III = CCS ≥ 400) the estimated annual risk of CAD death or myocardial infarction rate appears to be 0,4%, 1,3% and 2.4% respectively (Greenland et al., 2007). It has been generally suggested that a zero CCS might exclude the need for coronary angiography among asymptomatic patients. However, it has been also shown in studies that increasing the cut-point for calcification markedly improved the specificity but decreased the sensitivity. For patients with CCS >100 the sensitivity to predict significant coronary artery stenosis on angiography was 87% and the specifity 79% (Haberl et al., 2001). Of note, in a meta-analysis a CCS grater than 400 was associated with an increased risk of CAD (Third Report of NCEP, 2002). But a number of recent studies challenged this statement. The first study (Lester et al., 2009) in a young to middle-aged population with a low Framingham risk score where CCS was less sensitive than CIMT in the identification of preclinical atherosclerosis. The second from Mohlenkamp et al. (Mohlenkamp et al., 2011) in a group of 1934 healthy participants in whom, despite an improved discrimination was possible by adding CCS to traditional risk factors, the reclassification and the overall event rates appeared to low to justify CCS testing in all subjects. Moreover, and in contrast with the published recommendations on the subject, a third new study from Gottlieb et al. (Gottlieb et al., 2011) showed that even total coronary occlusion frequently occurs in the absence of any detectable calcification, definitely suggesting that a zero CCS value does not exclude obstructive stenosis or even the need for revascularization among patients with high enough clinical suspicion of coronary artery disease to be referred for coronary angiography. The finding of very low or even absent coronary calcium by CT in patients with documented carotid and femoral atherosclerosis has been found in a preliminary study from our group (Fig. 3) suggesting that B-Mode ultrasound imaging of carotid and femoral arteries probably overcomes the CCS approach for preclinical screening of atherosclerosis. As far as the effect on CCS by statin treatment is concerned, initial retrospective studies and observational data suggested that statin treatment resulted in reduction of coronary calcium but a recent exam of five randomized controlled trials proved that statin treatment does not reduce CCS values, with similar progression in either the treated and placebo group (Gill Jr, 2010).

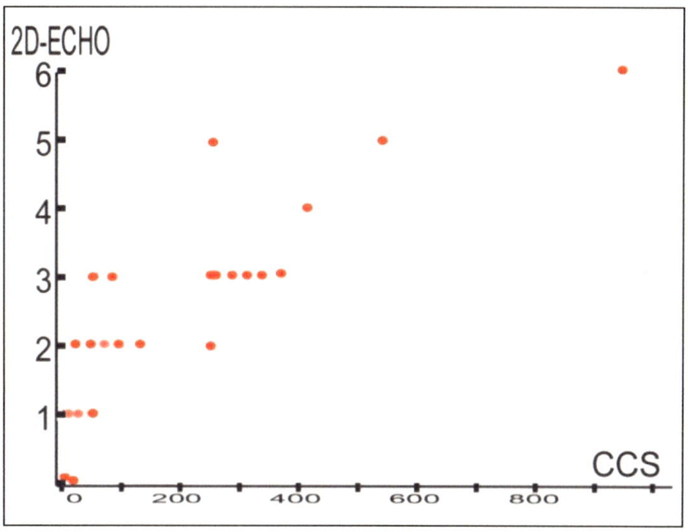

Fig. 4. Relationship between carotid and/or femoral atherosclerosis as assessed by B-Mode ultrasound (2D-ECHO) and CCS by compute tomography in 23 men, 35 to 65 y.o. The amount of carotid atherosclerosis has been arbitrarily graded into 6 grades from low to severe according to the amount of plaques in both arteries (IMT value has not been taken into account). CCS has been graded according to Agatstone score units. Close relationship exists on the presence and the amount of atherosclerosis between the two methods, with ultrasound findings being more sensitive than CCS in identifying subjects with atherosclerosis. These findings have been confirmed in studies and support the view that ultrasounds should be considered the first line approach in the screening for atherosclerosis in apparently healthy people with CV risk factors.

Of note, other clinical circumstances have been suggested to take advantage from use of CCS measurement, these include: 1) distinguishing ischemic from non-ischemic etiology of dilated cardiomyopathy, 2) identifying patients in emergency department with chest pain and nonspecific ECG, 3) predicting very low subsequent event rates in patients with acute MI and negative CCS test. However, and differently from asymptomatic patients setting, prognostic studies in symptomatic patients are lacking probably because a very large number of patients is needed in this setting to obtain the evidence. In any case, according to 2007 guidelines (Greenland et al., 2007) clinical monitoring of CCS progression is not recommended.

Finally, as far as the role of the race is concerned, despite a generally higher prevalence of cardiovascular risk factors also included a broad trait of endothelial dysfunction in this population group (Friedewald et al., 2008) a lower prevalence and extent of coronary calcification has been demonstrated in blacks. Accordingly, the Prospective Army Coronary Calcium (PACC) Project has found a higher prevalence of CCS in white (19.2%) than in black (10.3 %) military personnel with a mean age of 42 years (Mohlenkamp et al., 2011). Higher CCS scores have been also found in whites compared with blacks in the Cardiovascular Health Study (Raman et al., 2008) and lower prevalence of coronary calcium has been observed in Japanese (13%) than in the American men (47%). Overall, as reported in recent guidelines, despite a higher prevalence of cardiovascular risk factors in blacks, the majority of studies demonstrated a lower prevalence and amount of coronary calcification compared to whites. The recently published MESA study (Multi-Ethnic Study of Atherosclerosis) showed that traditional CV-risk-factor-based prediction models, such as the Framingham score, are improved by the addition of CCS especially in patients at intermediate risk for future coronary artery disease, ultimately suggesting the superiority of CCS and CIMT vs the Framingham risk score for risk prediction. In line with these conclusions are the results from the recent Heinz Nixdorf Recall study of 4,129 subjects (age 45 to 75 years, 53% female) without overt coronary artery disease at baseline in whom traditional risk factors and CCS scores were measured. The CCS resulted in a high reclassification rate in the intermediate-risk cohort, demonstrating the benefit of imaging of subclinical coronary atherosclerosis in carefully selected individuals with intermediate risk (Erbel R, et al. 2008)In any case, in the recently published ESNIER (Early Identification of Subclinical Atherosclerosis by Noninvasive Imaging Research) prospective randomized trial, it has been shown that compared with no scanning, the simple randomization to CAC scanning appears to improve patients' lifestyle health behaviours (Rozanski et al. 2011).

As far as the CIMT is concerned, a recent reclassification analysis of the ten-year follow-up of the Carotid Atherosclerosis Progression Study (CAPS) has challenged its value as a marker of future CV events rate and did not support its clinical usefulness for risk stratification in primary prevention setting (Lorentz et al, 2010). But evidence has been provided that when associated with risk factor assessment the CIMT may still be a valid tool in risk prediction in dyslipidemic patients (Baldassarre et al, 2007). The bottom line was that we have clear evidence that these two noninvasive methods of risk assessment are superior to Framingham risk score alone, and we think that the time has come to incorporate into new guidelines the cheaper, and completely safe, B-Mode ultrasound technique in primary prevention setting mainly focused on plaque detection.

The new high-resolution imaging technologies have enhanced our understanding of the atherosclerotic disease process and recently a new modified American Heart Association

classification scheme system based on morphological plaque features and the propensity of plaque for thrombosis has been suggested for use (Donnelly et al., 2010). Based on lipid deposition, fibrous cap thickening, lipid pool transition into necrotic core, calcium deposition, plaque disruption, haemorrhage and thrombosis, a number of categories of coronary atherosclerotic lesions have been identified and reported in Table 1 (Stary et al. 1994; Virmani et al. 1999; Virmani et al 2000; Donnelly et al, 2010).
Present status of CT technology clearly indicate that its diagnostic accuracy for the detection of the presence of atherosclerosis is superior over the detection of significant stenosis ultimately suggesting a progressive shift of this technique in the future towards the study of the atherosclerotic process per se rather than to simply assess the stenosis severity (Van Velzen et al., 2011).

AHA Plaque Nomenclature

Type	Finding
Early lesions (Type I-II)	Intimal thickening - Intimal xantoma
Progressive lesions (type III)	Pathological intimal thickening or preatheroma
Progressive lesions (type IV)	Fibrous cap atheroma
Progressive lesions (type Va,Vb,Vc)	Healed cap rupture (with or without Ca++)
Progressive lesions (Type VI)	Thin fibrous cap atheroma
Progressive lesion (Type VI)	Plaque hemorrhage and/or plaque rupture

Table 1.

Although primarily established for coronary lesions, in accordance with the recently emerged clinically relevant idea that carotid and femoral arteries can be considered the "sentinel vessels" of the coronary artery status (Heinecke, 2011., Joy & Hegel, 2008) we think that this classification can be usefully applied to the analysis of these vessels. As atherosclerosis begins early in life and then remains clinically silent for decades, a distinct opportunity for early intervention comes from the identification of subclinical stages of the disease. Accordingly, the concept that atherosclerosis must be viewed as a preventable disease, which should be approached not only in terms of risk-factor control but also in terms of early disease detection, plaque prevention and plaque stabilization, has rapidly gained acceptance (Naghavi et al., 2003). But even plaque regression (the holy grail for therapeutic interventions) appears possible and has become a new target in our clinical practice during the last ten years. Together with a proposal for a strategy for primary CV disease prevention this evidence will be accordingly presented in the following pages.

4.3 Preclinical atherosclerosis and risk prediction

Coronary atherosclerosis starts early in the life and it is progressive in nature and when angiograficallly identified as minimal vessel stenosis its burden is already diffuse. By the time a patient has developed minor obstructive disease on angiography, an extensive systemic atheroma is already present. This finding underscores the importance of an aggressive risk factor modification (and statin use) since early stages of atherosclerosis in asymptomatic subjects (Lavoie et al., 2010). In recent years several studies addressed the prognostic implications of detecting asymptomatic atherosclerosis in the general apparently healthy population. Pathological, epidemiological and clinical studies indicate tha atherosclerosis is a systemic disease which develops with a variable extension and severity in all conduit arteries. In particular, an almost constant association exists between carotid, femoral, and coronary artery disease, with first clinical manifestation usually due to a CAD. Ten years ago in the CAFES-CAVE study (Belcaro et al., 2001), subclinical carotid and femoral artery plaques have been found strongly and independently associated with future adverse cardiovascular events rate in low risk subjects by Framingham criteria. Similarly, the presence of peripheral (occlusive or sub-occlusive) artery disease independently predicted myocardial infarction and death in 1,325 individuals with either carotid or femoral plaques by ultrasound (Lamina et al., 2006). And early atherosclerosis (increased IMT) in femoral arteries predicted single-vessel CAD whereas advanced atherosclerotic (plaques) was usually associated with more severe CAD (Sosnowski et al., 2007). Evidence of the systemic nature of the atherosclerotic process comes also fromseveral studies of prevalence of occult CAD in patients with peripheral artery disease or stroke. In a recent study in patients with cerebral infarction without history of CAD (Amarenco et al., 2011) it has been shown that a silent CAD was present in 62% of patients and that 31% and 26% had a 3 vessel disease and vessel stenosis > 50% respectively, and similar findings have been reported in another recent study in which the atherosclerotic process was quite advanced in coronary as well as in peripheral arteries of patients at their first presentation for acute coronary artery disease (Kranjec, 2011). Evidence of high prevalence of subclinical atherosclerosis in the general population comes also from another recent study on a randomly selected sample of 292 subjects (mean age 59.5 years, 50% women) from the offspring cohort of the Framingham Heart Study free of clinically apparent cardiovascular disease, who exhibited high levels of subclinical atherosclerosis on more than 2 imaging tests including MRI of abdominal and thoracic aorta, coronary artery calcification by EBCT, and CIMT by ultrasonography (Kathiresan et al., 2007). Also on this line are the results from the mass screening recently introduced in United Kingdom where an ultrasound scan of the abdomen is offered to all men over 64 years for the screening of abdominal aorta aneurysm by ultrasonography. In a large randomized trial in 67,770 men, age 65 to 74 years, it has been shown that in the group invited for screening the mortality was halved (because of elective surgery): an approach that additionally proved to be highly cost-effective (Kim et al., 2007).

As far as the role of carotid IMT as a predictor of future events is concerned, in a recent meta-anlaysis of 41 randomized trials it has been shown (Costanzo et al., 2010) that regression or slowed progression of carotid IMT by cardiovascular drugs is not accompanied by reduction in cardiovascular events, definitely suggesting that this parameter has a very limited role in cardiovascular risk prediction. Similarly, a recent review including 13.145 patients (Masson et al., 2011) has shown that presence of carotid plaques predicted future risk better than IMT value, supporting the view that when detecting plaque we are not just evaluating a surrogate objective but a process that in itself indicates the presence of the atherosclerotic disease.

The American Society of Echocardiography consensus document (Stein et al., 2008) and the recently published Canadian guidelines (Genest et al., 2009) which formally classify patients with subclinical atherosclerosis as high risk and recommend preventive measures as intensive as those to be used in patients with clinically established atherosclerotic disease, are both in line with this suggestion. Neither those persons with a past history of intensive professional sport activity appear protected by the atherosclerotic assault of modern life as demonstrated by a recent paper in which former professional football players, despite their elite athletic histories, have a similar prevalence of advanced subclinical atherosclerosis as a clinically referred population of overweight and obese men (Hurst et al., 2010). In response to the wall lipid infiltration and plaque formation the arterial wall changes its structure according to two types of anatomical remodelling, positive and negative. Positive remodelling is characterized by outward expansion and negative remodelling by vessel shrinkage. Paradoxically the apparent beneficial and more frequent phenomenon of outward wall expansion is associated with the feature of unstable lesions (fig. 1) i.e. with histological characteristics of plaque vulnerability such as a large lipid core and high plaque macrophage content (Pasternak et al., 1998). These important morphological features have been studied in coronary vessels by intravascular ultrasound (IVUS) and angioscopy, but optical coherence tomography with its unique ability of identifying lipid content, fibrous cap thickness and its macrophage density, is the method of choice (Yabushita et al., 2002; Raffel et al., 2008). Recently, a first report on virtual histology-IVUS assessment of natural history (1 year follow-up with repeated examinations) of coronary artery lesions morphology has been published (Kubo et al., 2010). In this study it has been demonstrated that most thin capped fibroatheroma had plaque progression (most stabilized or healed but new developed) whereas fibrotic and fibrocalcific plaque did not demonstrate any geometric changes during the follow-up and no spontaneous plaque regression has been observed, as usual.

AS highlighted in previous pages an ischemic event is usually associated with an advanced atherosclerotic lesion. And since early regression studies (Blankenhorn et al., 1978; Corti et al., 2001), the evidence clearly emerged that persistent and marked reduction of total and LDL cholesterol plasma levels (with LDL-cholesterol in the range of 50 mg /dl) is the key element for obtaining atherosclerosis regression and significant inverse remodelling with lumen preservation of both aorta and carotid arteries at 12 months, and that the degree of LDL-cholesterol reduction rather than the statin dose was associated with plaque regression. According to this line of conduct we have had evidence in the last 10 years on the possibility to induce plaque regression even up to complete disappearance: moreover we have realized how B-mode ultrasound imaging can help us and motivate patients in many ways in primary prevention setting. As it will be suggested in the next pages, our experience has confirmed the hypothesis that lipid lowering therapy selectively depletes the atherosclerotic plaques lipid content and prevents plaque disruption.

5. Plaque monitoring by ultrasound imaging and plaque regression by statin use

Notwithstanding large-scale clinical trials have proved that both primary and secondary prevention reduce myocardial infarction, stroke and overall mortality, the optimal level of plasma lipids to achieve these goals remains unresolved. Recent trend suggests "the lower the better" for all risk factors, but recent data suggest that lipid lowering appears to have larger impact than blood pressure lowering on plaque progression (Chhatriwalla et al., 2009) and hence also supporting the view that only intensive plasma lipid reduction can induced plaque regression. As already mentioned in previous pages, in vivo evidence of atherosclerosis regression in thoracic aorta by statin use has been first reported ten years ago (Corti et al., 2001) using MRI. More recently using dedicated carotid MRI protocol (Underhill et al., 2009) it has been demonstrated that intraplaque haemorrhage and statin therapy were key determinants of opposite changes in plaque burden: being intraplaque haemorrhage associated with accelerated plaque growth, whereas statin therapy was associated with plaque stabilization by slowing or halting lesion progression. According to these authors the phase of 16% to 49% of plaque induced vessel stenosis is probably a critical stage of the plaque natural history, whereas plaque regression has been associated with statin use.

In the following pages we describe the process of atherosclerosis regression as it has been documented in a group of selected statin treated subjects in a primary prevention setting during the last ten years in our echo-lab. To be included in this retrospective analysis the subjects should have had at least two B-mode ultrasound plaque imaging examinations of at least 2 years apart during an uninterrupted statin treatment. Twelve subjects have been found to match such criteria. These subjects have been treated with simvastatin or rosuvastatin at a dosage aimed obtaining a total cholesterol plasma level kept round 140 mg/dl. None of them have had any CV events during the study period. The most representative structural findings associated with plaques regression are presented in the following pages and proposed as reference structural changes to be routinely examined in patients for an office-based practice as an alternative to the more demanding and expensive MRI based analyses.

As largely reported in previous page, evidence exists on the possibility to identify subjects with preclinical atherosclerosis who can take advantage from its early detection by improving a safer life style and by statin use in particular. In fact, the possibility to monitor plaque dimension and structure changes along time with a completely noninvasive approach by using ultrasounds allows a safe and personalized treatment approach in the course of years, with an improved patient' and doctor' satisfaction. To recognize the great advancement in the field of primary prevention and of usefulness of early atherosclerotic disease detection by the way we are suggesting, a citation is worthy of David Blankenhorn's intuition and early demonstration of this possibility more than 30 years ago in California and summarized in the following lines from a paper (George Lyman Duff Memorial Lecture) co-authored with Howard Hodis (Blankenhorn DH & Hodis HN, 1994): "Coronary atherosclerosis is ubiquitous, but we know that some individuals develop more severe coronary atherosclerosis at an earlier age than others. A case finding and treatment strategy based on noninvasive imaging would benefit those with premature atherosclerosis who are not recognized with current risk factor screening until they develop symptoms. Screening for peripheral vessel changes indicative of high risk is possible and cost effective with procedures now available". The following cases we are going to describe closely match this position and add new evidence on the real possibility by the simple and totally noninvasive ultrasound exam to characterize carotid and femoral artery plaque structure and the profound changes induced by statin treatment (Fig 4 to 9).

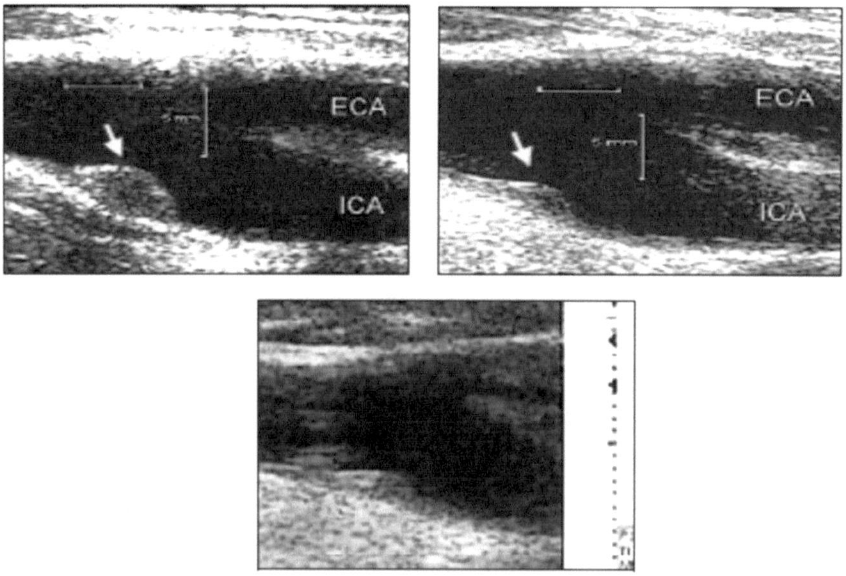

Fig. 4. *Upper left panel* - B-mode ultrasound of the right carotid artery bifurcation in a asymptomatic 50 y.o. man with hypercholesterolemia (280-300 mg/dl). A soft and lipid-rich atherosclerotic plaque (arrow) about 4 mm in thickness and 7 mm in length is present at the posterior wall of the carotid artery bifurcation associated with outward remodeling of the arterial wall. These charcteristics allow classification of the plaque as an advanced atherosclerotic plaque type IV lesion (see pag 12). *Upper right panel* - Imaging of the same artery after three years 20 mg simvastatin treatment and plasma total cholesterol level kept around 150 mg/dl. A marked reduction of plaque dimension is shown (arrow) associated with arterial wall reverse remodeling. *Lower panel:* imaging of the same artery (with same magnification) obtained three years after spontaneous statin treatment interruption. New plaque progression can be appreciated with an associated IMT increase. Legend: ECA = external carotid artery, ICA = internal carotid artery.

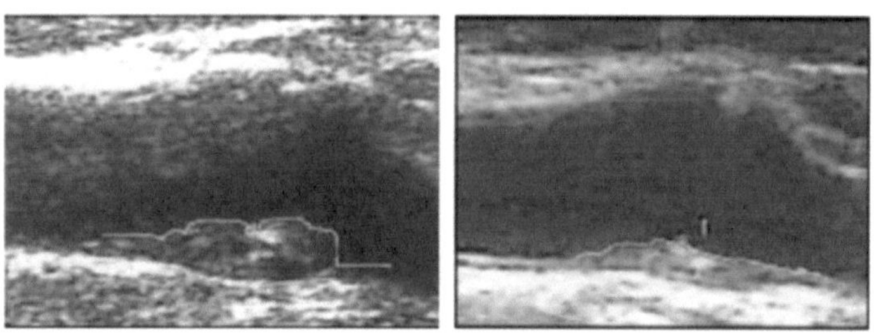

Fig. 5. B-Mode ultrasound (with plaque outlining) of the right carotid artery in a 66 y.o. man with hypercholesterolemia (250 mg/dl) followed-up for 4 years during statin therapy (rosuvastatin 10 mg/day). *Left panel*: Lipid rich plaque with a small (white) calcium deposit. *Right panel*: Same imaging 4 years later demonstrating plaque volume reduction with almost complete regression of the echolucent lipid-rich areas, leaving intact the small nucleus of calcium deposit within the plaque. Almost complete reverse remodelling of the posterior vessel wall also occurred.

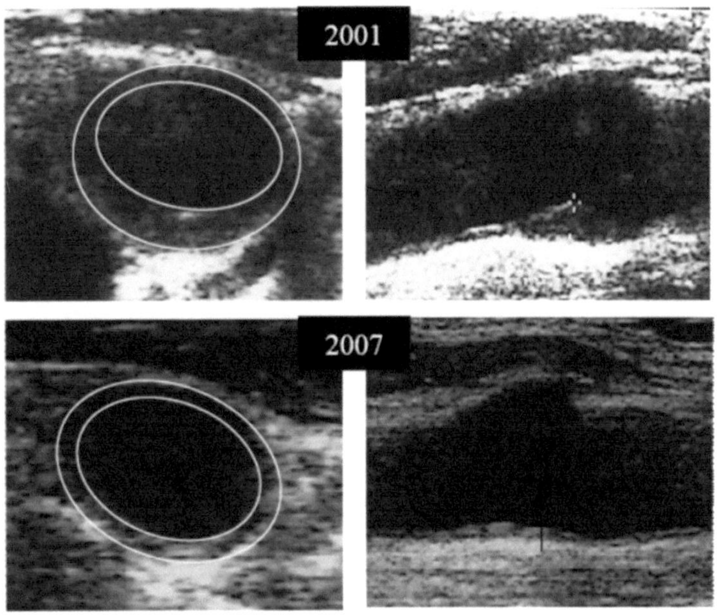

Fig. 6. B-Mode ultrasonography imaging in a short axis (left side) and long axis view (right side) of the right carotid artery in asymptomatic man with hypercholesterolemia (240 mg/dl) followed-up for 6 years during statin therapy.

Upper line: At first examination (age 59 years) a small echolucent plaque was present in the far field of common carotid artery, better appreciated in its extension in the high lightened short axis view. *Bottom line*: Same imaging showing a complete plaque regression after five years of Simvastatin (20 mg/day) treatment. No further examinations were performed during this period. Arterial reverse remodelling, better appreciated in the short axis view, also occurred in association with plaque regression. Cholesterol plasma levels have been kept around 140 mg/dl during the whole treatment period.

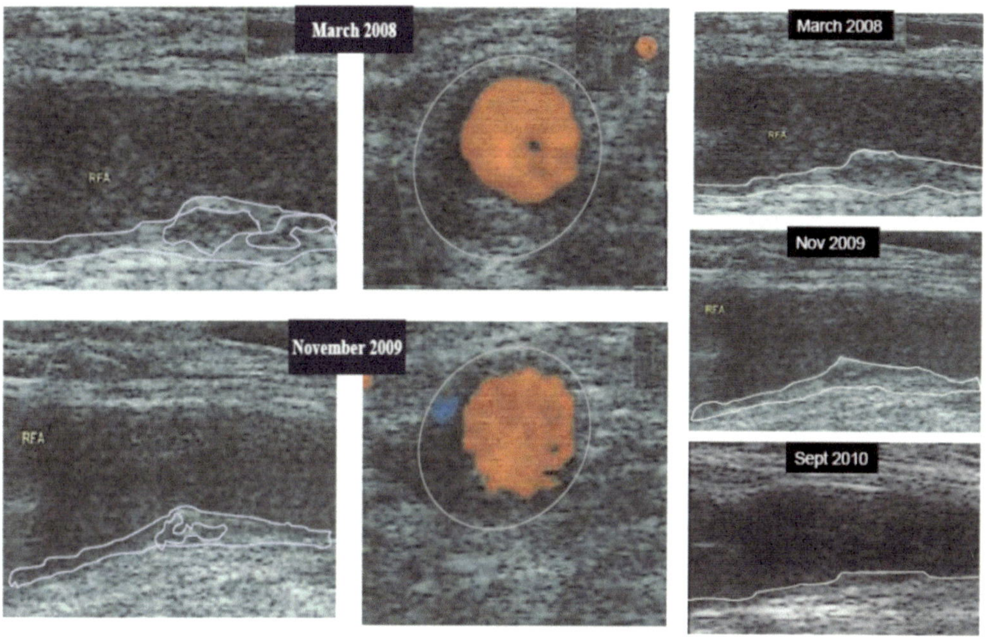

Fig. 7. *Left panel*: B-Mode ultrasonography imaging in a long- and short-axis view (with colour Doppler flow imaging) of femoral arteries in a 69 y.o. healthy man during a 20 months treatment period with rosuvastatin 20 mg/day and cholesterol plasma level kept around 140 mg/dl. Plaque volume reduction and inverse arterial remodelling haves occurred by statin treatment. Far field endothelial surface, total plaque area, and echo-lucent area within the plaques have been manually outlined for better understanding of the plaque structural changes. Plaque volume reduction and arterial reverse remodelling are better appreciated in the short axis view. *Right panel*: Further plaque reduction in the long axis view occurred after additional 10 months of statin treatment.

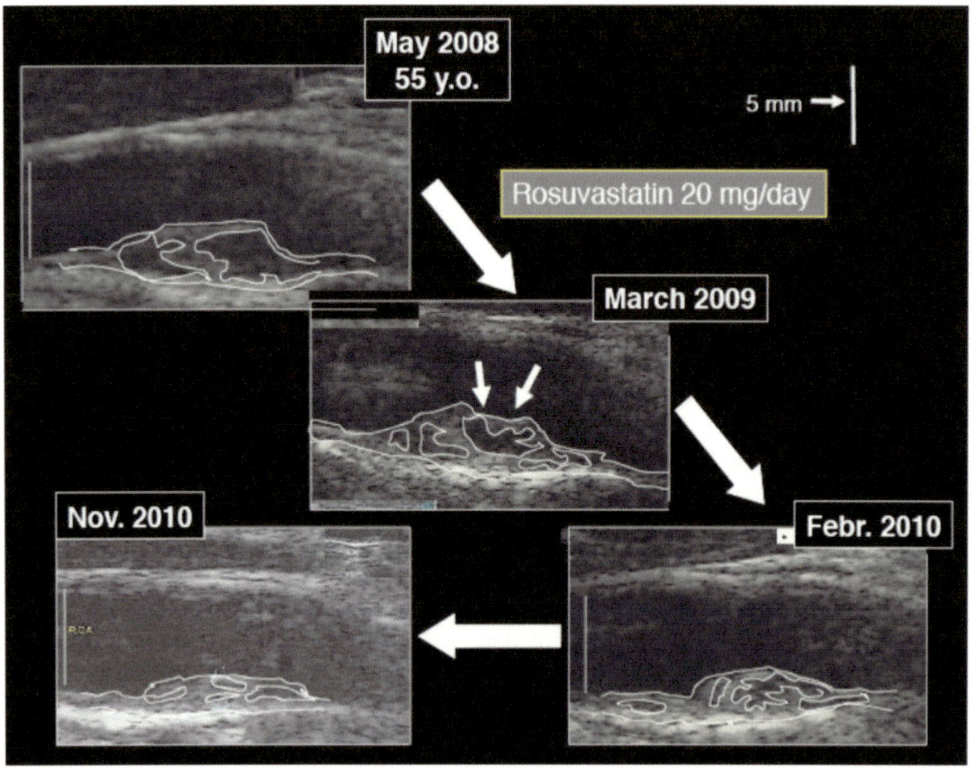

Fig. 8. Left carotid plaque monitoring during a 2.5 years follow-up period in a 55 y.o. subject during statin treatment (rosuvastatin 20 mg/day) with a reduction of cholesterol level from 200 mg/dl to around 140 mg/dl. with HDL Cholesterol increase from 50 to 75 mg/dl. The plaque border and the echolucent areas within the plaque have been outlined for a better understanding of the structural findings associated with plaque regression. At first imaging (May 2008) the plaque exhibits the characteristics of a rupture-prone (vulnerable/instable) plaque represented by the triad of a very thin fibrous cap combined with large echolucent (lipid/necrotic) core and positive (outward) arterial wall remodelling. An impressive volume reduction (~75%) occurred during the treatment period. In this case, the close temporal images' sequence allowed superior understanding of structural modifications associated with plaque regression and stabilization. According to these changes the following observations can be done: 1) The amount of baseline echolucent areas within the plaque predicts the regression potential by statin treatment, even to almost complete plaque regression when the echolucent area is predominant, 2) the reabsorbtion of these areas is progressive and is accompanied by plaque volume reduction and structural findings suggesting plaque stabilization (the arrows in the imaging of march 2009 indicate a partial plaque collapse due to early marked reduction of underlying echolucent area), 3) in association with plaque volume reduction a progressive reverse arterial wall remodelling also occurred, 4) the time interval needed for early regression appreciation appears to be 10 to 12 months. As occurred in this case, plaque regression appears to depend on "robust measures" such as marked reduction in plasma concentrations of LDL cholesterol and large increases in the reverse transport of lipids out of the plaque by an increased HDL-cholesterol.

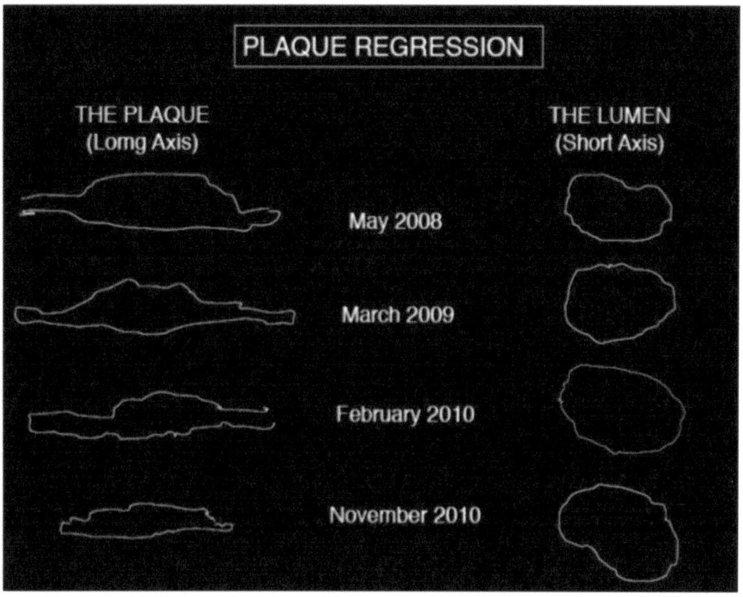

Fig. 9. Same case of the figure 8. Plaque and vessel luminal area (by manual outlining) in a long and a short axis view respectively, by B-mode ultrasound imaging of the carotid artery obtained during the study period. This analysis adds further information on the characteristics of the process of plaque reduction, vessel inverse remodelling and reduced vulnerability in this patient.

6. Conclusions

After arteriographic studies on atherosclerosis regression by lipid lowering drugs pioneered by Blankenorn in late seventhies, conclusive demonstration of the plaque lipid depletion hypothesis in human beings during lipid lowering therapy has been possible only in recent years using ultrasound and MRI. During the last few years the sonographic characteristics of carotid plaques have been thoroughly studied by sophisticated methods enabling semiquantitative analysis of their structure (Reiter et al., 2007). However, as in depth discussed in this chapter we think that the simple, non-invasive, relatively cheap and totally innocuous B-Mode ultrasound examination of carotid and/or femoral arteries represents the first choice and still largely unmet opportunity for atherosclerosis screening of asymptomatic subjects deemed at intermediate risk by traditional risk factors (fig 10).

As already discussed, due to the associated radiation risk, the use of CCS as a screening tool in primary prevention setting (usually requiring subsequent examinations) should be considered in specific circumstances only as alternative to arterial ultrasound scanning when this imaging modality is not available. Definite superiority of the B-mode ultrasound approach is greatly supported by the possibility to monitor the natural course of plaque structural changes and, of outmost importance, to assess the drugs' effect which we have observed to occur during statin use in a very short period of time, ten to twelve months apart.

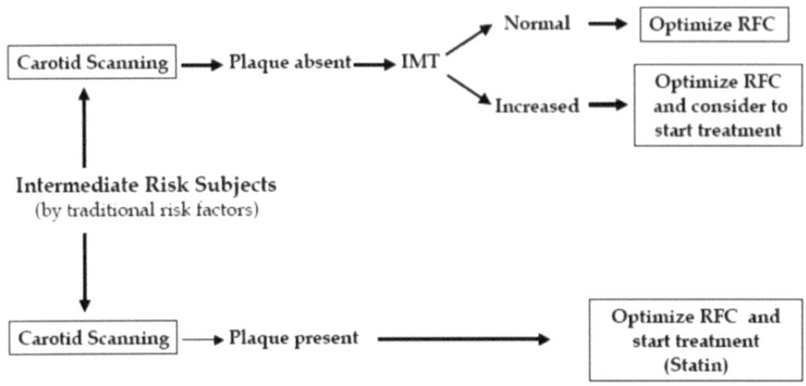

Fig. 10. Algorithm for cardiovascular risk assessment and as decision making approach using B-Mode ultrasound examination of carotid (and femoral) arteries for preclinical atherosclerosis screening in subjects deemed to be at intermediate risk by traditional risk factors. RFC = Risk factor control. (Modified by Gepner et al., 2007)

7. References

Aikawa, M., Rabkin, E.,& Okada, Y. (1998). Lipid lowering by diet reduces matrix metalloproteinase activity and increases collagen content of rabbit atheroma: a potential mechanism of lesion stabilization. *Circulation*. 97:2433–2444.

Allam, AH., Thompson, RC., Wann, LS., Miyamoto, MI., el-Halim, Nur., el-Din, A., el-Maksoud, GA., Al-Tohamy, Soliman M., Ibrahem, Badr. I., el-Rahman, Amer HA., Sutherland, ML., Sutherland, JD. ,& Thomas, GS. (2011). Atherosclerosis in Ancient Egyptian Mummies The Horus Study. *J Am Coll Cardiol Img*, 4, 315-27.

Amarenco, P. Lavalèe, PC., Labreuche, J., & Ducocq, G.(2010). Prevalence of Coronary Atherosclerosis in Patients With Cerebral Infarction. *Stroke* ,42: 22-291.

Aroon, D., Hingorani, Bruce. & Paty, M. (2009). Primary Prevention of Cardiovascular Disease: Time to Get More or Less Personal? *JAMA*, 302(19), 2144-2145.

Arsenault, BJ., Benoit, J., Arsenault, Philip Barter., DeMicco, David A., Weihang, Bao., Preston, Gregory M., LaRosa, John C., Grundy, Scott M., Deedwania, Prakash., Greten, Heiner., Wenger, Nanette K., Shepherd, James., Waters, David D., & Kastelein John J.P. (2011).TNT Study Investigators. Prediction of Cardiovascular Events in Statin-Treated Stable Coronary Patients by Lipid and Nonlipid Biomarkers. *J Am Coll Cardiol*, 57, 63-69.

Ayman, A., Hussein, AA., Uno, K., Wolski, K., Kapadia, S., Schoenhagen, P., Tuzcu, EM., Nissen, SE.,& Nicholls, SJ.(2011). Peripheral Arterial Disease and Progression of Coronary Atherosclerosis. *J Am Coll Cardiol* ,57,1220–5.

Bajaj, M.,& Ben-Yehuda, O. (2006). A big fat wedding: association of adiponectin with coronary vascular lesions. *J Am Coll Cardiol*, 48, 1163–5.

Barker, DJP. Fetal And Infant Origins Of Adult Disease. Published by the BMJ - London 1992.

Belcaro, G., Nicolaides, AN., Ramaswami, G., Cesarone, MR., De Sanctis, M., Incandela, L., Ferrari, P., Geroulakos, G., Barsotti, A., Griffin, M., Dhanjil, S., Sabetai, M., Bucci, M., & Martines, G. (2001). Carotid and femoral ultrasound morphology screening and cardiovascular events in low risk subjects: a 10-year follow-up study (the CAFES-CAVE study[1]). *Atherosclerosis*, 156, 379 -387.

Benn, M., Tybjærg-Hansen, A., Stender, F., Frikke-Schmidt, R.,& Nordestgaard, BG. (2011). Low-Density Lipoprotein Cholesterol and the Risk of Cancer: A Mendelian Randomization Study. *J Natl Cancer Inst*, 103(6), 508-519.

Berseghian,A. Gawande,D.& Bajaj,M. (2011). Adiponectin and Vulnerable Atherosclerotic Plaque. J *Am Coll Cardiol*, 57,761-70.

Blaha, M., Budoff, MJ.,& Shaw LJ. (2009). Absence of coronary artery calcification and all cause mortality, *J Am Coll Cardiol Img*, 2,692-700.

Blankenhorn, DH., Brooks, SH., Selzer, RH. &Barndt, JrR. (1978). The rate of atherosclerosis change during treatment of hyperlipoproteinemia. *Circulation*,57,355-361.

Blankenhorn, DH. (1978). Reversibility of latent atherosclerosis. Studies by Femoral Angiography in Humans. Mod Conc Cardiovasc Dis, 47, 79-84.

Blankenhorn, DH., & Hodis HN. (1994). George Lyman Duff Memorial Lecture. Arterial Imaging and Atherosclerosis Reversal. *Arterioscler Thromb.Vasc Biol*, 14, 177-192.

Brewer, Jr HB. (2011). The Evolving Role of HDL in the Treatment of High-Risk Patients with Cardiovascular Disease. The Journal of Clinical Endocrinology & Metabolism, March 9.

Brown, SM.& Goldstein JL.(1996). Heart Attacks: Gone with the Century?. *Science*,272:626.

Brown, BG., Zhao, XQ.,& Sacco, DE. (1993). Lipid lowering and plaque regression: new insights into prevention of plaque disruption and clinical events in coronary disease. *Circulation*. 87,1781–1791.

Brown, BG., Stukovsky, KH.,& Zhao, XQ. (2006). Simultaneous low density lipoprotein-C lowering and high-density lipoprotein-C elevation for optimum cardiovascular disease prevention with various drug classes, and their combinations: a meta-analysis of 23 randomized lipid trials. *Curr Opin Lipidol*. 17,631-6.

Brugts, J.,& Deckers, JW.(2010). Statin prescription in men and women at cardiovascular risk: to whom and when?. *Curr Opin Cardiol*, 25, 484-489.

Cheung, BMY. & Lam KSL.(2010). Is intensive LDL-cholesterol lowering baneficial and safe?. *The Lancet*, Vol 376, Issue 9753, 1622-1624.

Chhatriwalla, AF., Nicholls, SJ., Wang, TH., Wolski, K., Sipahi, I.,Crowe, T., Schoenhagen, P., Kapadia, S., Tuzcu, EM., & Nissen, SE. (2009). Low Levels of Low-Density Lipoprotein Cholesterol and Blood Pressure and Progression of Coronary Atherosclerosi. *J Am Coll Cardiol*, 53, 1110-5.

Cohen, JC., Boerwinkle, E., Mpsley, TH.,& Hobbs, HH.(2006). Sequence variations in PCSK9, Low LDL and Protection against Coronary Artery Disease. *N Engl J Med*, 354, 1264-72.

Collins R, Armitage J, Parish S, Sleigh P, Peto R; (2003). Heart Protection Stdy Collaborative Group. MRC/BHF Heart Protection Study of cholesterol-lowering with simvastatin in 5963 people with diabetes: a randomised placebo-controlled trial. *The Lancet*; 361:2005-16.

Helen M Colhoun, HM., Betteridge, JD., Durrington, PN., Hitman, GA., Neil, HAW., Livingstone, SJ., & Thomason, MJ., Mackness, MI., Charlton-Menys, V., Fuller, JH. (2004) The CARDS Study. *The Lancet*,346,685-696.

Corti, R., Fayad, ZA., Fuster, V., Worthley, SG., Helft, G., Chesebro, J., Mercuri, M.,& Badimon, JJ. (2001). Effects of Lipid-Lowering by Simvastatin on Human Atherosclerotic Lesions: A Longitudinal Study by High-Resolution, Noninvasive Magnetic Resonance Imaging. *Circulation* ,104, 249-252.

Corti, R., Fuster, V., Fayad, ZA., Worthley, SG., Helft, G.,Chaplin, WF., Mountwyler, J., Viles-Gonzales, JF., Chesebro, J., Mercuri, M.,& Badimon, JJ. (2005). Effects of Aggressive

Versus Conventional Lipid-Lowering Therapy by Simvastatin on Human Atherosclerotic Lesions. A Prospective, Randomized, Double-Blind Trial With High-Resolution Magnetic Resonance Imaging. *J Am Coll Cardiol,* 46,106–12.

Crisby, M., Nordin-Fredriksson, G., Shah, PK., Yano, J. Zhu, J.,& Nilsson J. (2001). Pravastatin Treatment Increases Collagen Content and Decreases Lipid Content, Inflammation, Metalloproteinases, and Cell Death in Human Carotid Plaques Implications for Plaque Stabilization. *Circulation,*103,926-933.

Cziraky, MJ., Watson, KE., & Talbert, RL. (2008). Targeting low HDL-cholesterol to decrease residual cardiovascular risk in the managed care setting. *J Manag Care Pharm,* 14(8 Suppl):23-28.

Cholesterol Treatment Trialist '(CTT) Collaboration'(2005). Efficacy and safety of more intensive lowering of LDL cholesterol: a meta-analysis of data from 170,000 participants in 26 randomized trials. *The Lancet,* 366,9493,1267-1278.

Davies, M.J.,(1998). Reactive Oxygen Species, Metalloproteinases, and Plaque Stability. *Circulation* 97: 2382-2383.

Davis, JR., Rudd, JH.,& Weissberg, PL. (2004). Molecular and Metabolic Imaging of Atherosclerosis. *J Nucl Med,* 45, 1898-1907.

De Vries, BMW., Hillebrands, J-H., Van Dam, GM., Tio, RA., De Jong, JS., Slart, RHJA.,& Zeebregts, CJ. (2011). Multispectral Near-Infrared Fluorescence Molecular Imaging of Matrix Metalloproteinases in a Human Carotid Plaque Using a Matrix-Degrading Metalloproteinase- Sensitive Activatable Fluorescent Probe. *J Am Coll Cardiol* ,57,10,1220–5.

Donnelly, P., Maurovich-Horvat, P., Vorpahl, M., Nakano, M., Kaple, RK., Warger, W., Tanaka, A., Tearney, G., Virmani, R.,& Hoffmann, U. (2010). Multimodality Imaging Atlas of Coronary Atherosclerosis. *J Am Coll Cardiol Img,* 3,8.

Donnelly, P., Maurovich-Horvat, P., Vorpahl, M., Nakano, M., Kaple, RK., Warger, W., Tanaka, A., Tearney, G., Virmani, R., & Hoffmann, U. (2010). Multimodality Imaging Atlas of Coronary Atherosclerosis. *J Am Coll Cardiol Img* ,3,8, 876-80.

Downs, JR., Clearfield, M., Tyroler, HA., Whitney, EJ., Kruyer, W., Langendorfer, A., Zagrebelsky, V., Weis, S., Shapiro, DR., Beere, PA., & Gotto, AM. (2001). Air Force/Texas Coronary Atherosclerosis Prevention Study (AFCAPS/TEXCAPS): additional perspectives on tolerability of long-term treatment with lovastatin. *Am J Cardiol,* 87(9),1074-9.

Eisenberg, MJ., Afilalo, J., Lawler, PR., Abrahamowicz, M., Richard, H.,& Pilote, L.(2011). Cancer risk related to low-dose ionizing radiation from cardiac imaging in patients after acute myocardial infarction. *CMAJ,* 183, 4.

Emerson, J. (2010). Safety of statin therapy: meta-analysis of data on cancer from 166,000 participants in 25 randomized trials. *European Heart Journa,l* Abstract Volume; Abstract 5035

Endres, M., Heuschmann, PU., Laufs, U., & Hakim, AM.(2011). Primary prevention of stroke: blood pressure, lipids and heart failure. *European Heart Journal,* 32,545-552.

Erbel, R., Möhlenkamp, S., Moebu,s S., Schmermund, A., Lehmann, N., Stang, A., Dragano, N., Grönemeyer, D., Seibel, R., Kälsch, H., Bröcker-Preuss, M., Mann, K., Siegrist, J., Jöckel, K-H., & Nixdorf, H. (2010). Recall Study Investigative Group. *J. Am. Coll. Cardiol,* 56, 1397-1406.

Erbel, R., Delaney, JA., Lehmann, N., McClelland, RL., Mohlenkamp, S., Kronmal, RA., Schmermund, A., Moebus, S., Dragano, N., Stang, A., Jockel, KH., & Budoff, MJ. (2008). On behalf of the Multi-Ethnic Study of Atherosclerosis and the Investigator Group of the Heinz Nixdorf Recall Study. Signs of subclinical coronary atherosclerosis in relation to risk factor distribution in the Multi-Ethnic Study of Atherosclerosis (MESA) and the Heinz Nixdorf Recall Study (HNR). *Eur Heart J*, 29,22,2782-2791.

Farmer, JA. & Liao J. (2011). Evolving Concept on the Role of High-Density Lipoprotein in Protection from Atherosclerosis. *Curr Atheroscler Rep*. Published on line:08 March 2011.

Farmer, J. & Liao, J. (2011). Evolving Concepts of the Role of High-Density Lipoprotein in Protection from Atherosclerosis. Current Atherosclerosis Reports, 3, 1-8.

Fowkes, FG., Murray, GD., Butcher, I. (2008). Ankle Brachial Index Collaboration; Ankle brachial index combined with Framingham Risk Score to predict cardiovascular events and mortality: A meta-analysis. JAMA;300:197-208.

Ford, ES., Ajani, UA., Croft, JB., & Critchly, JA.(2007). Explaining the Decrease in U.S. Deaths from Coronary Disease. *N Engl J Med* ,356, 2388-2398.

Freeman, LEB., Lauer, RM.,& Clark, WR. (2006). The Epidemiology of Childhood Cholesterol. Pediatric Prevention of Atherosclerotic Cardiovascular Disease. *Oxford University Press*,109-124.

Friedewald, VE., Giles, TD., Pool, JL., Yancy, CW., & Roberts WC. (2008). The Editor's Roundtable: Endotherlial Dysfunction in Cardiovascular Disease. *Am J Cardiol*, 102, 418-423

Genest, J., McPherson, R., & Frohlic, J., Anderson, T., Campbell, A. Carpentier, A., Couture, P., Dufour, R., Fodor, G., & Francis, GA. (2009). Canadian Lipid Guidelines. Canadian Journal of Cardiology retrieved from 2009 Canadian Cardiovascular Society/Canadian

guidelines for the diagnosis and treatment of dyslipidemia and prevention of cardiovascular disease in the adult – 2009 recommendations. *Can J Cardiol*, 25, 10,567-579.

Gepner, AD., Wyman, RA., Korkarz, C., Aesclimann, SE., & Stein, JH. (2007). An Abbreviated Carotid Intima-Media Thickness Scanning Protocol to Facilitate Clinica Screening for Subclinical Atherosclerosis. *J Am Soc Echocardiog*, 20, 1269-1275.

Gill, EA. (2010). Does Statin Therapy Affect the Progression of Atherosclerosis Measured by a Coronary Calcium Score?. *Curr Atheroscler Rep*. 2010,12,2,83-87.

Gisbertz, SS., Wouter, Derksen, WJM., De Kleijn, DPV.,Vink, A., Bots, ML., De Vries, MJP., Moll. FL.,& Pasterkamp G. (2011). The effect of alcohol on atherosclerotic plaque composition and cardiovascular events in patients with arterial occlusive disease. *Journal of Vascular Surgery*, 03,18.

Glagov, S., Weisenberg, E., Zarins, CK., Stankunavicius, R., & Kolettis, JI. (1987). Compensatory enlargement of human atherosclerotic coronary arteries. *N Engl J Med*, 316, 1371-1375.

Gordon, DJ.,& Rifkind, BM.(1989). High density lipoprotein- the clinical implications of recent studies. *N Engl J Med*,321,1311-6.

Gottlieb, I., Miller,J., Arbab-Zadeh, A., Dewey, M., Clouse, ME., Sara, L., Niinuma, H., Bush, D., Paul, N., Vavere, AL., Texter, J., Brinker, J., Lima, JAC.,& Rochitte, CE. (2010).The absence of coronary calcifications does not exclude obstructive coronary artery disease or the need for revascularisation in patients referred for conventional coronary angiography. *J Am Coll Cardiol* ,55,627–34.

Gorelick PB. Challenges of designing trials for the primary prevention of stroke. *Stroke* 2009;40(Suppl.3):S82-S84.

Greenberg, H. (2010). The global impact of the Framingham Heart Study. Editor's Introduction. *Prog Cardiovasc Dis*,53,10-14.

Greenland, P., & Gaziano, JM. (2003). Clinical practice. Selecting asymptomatic patients for coronary computed tomography or electrocardiographic exercise testing. *N Engl J Med*, 349,465-73.

Grundy, SM. (2004). Atherosclerosis Imaging and the Future of Lipid Management. *Circulation*, 110, 3509-3511.

Grundy, SM., Cleeman, JI., Merz, CNB., Brewer, B., Luther, T., Clark, B., Donald B. Hunninghake, DB., Pasternak, RC., Smith, SC., & Neil, J. (2004). Stone, for the Coordinating Committee of the National Cholesterol Education Program Endorsed by the National Heart, Lung, and Blood Institute, American College of Cardiology Foundation, and American Heart Association Implications of Recent Clinical Trials for the National Cholesterol Education Program Adult Treatment Panel III Guidelines. *Circulation*, 110, 227-239.

Hansson, GK. (2005). Inflammation, atherosclerosis, and coronary artery disease. *N Engl J Med*, 352, 1685-95.

Heart Protection Study Collaborative Group. C-reactive protein concentration and the vascular benefits of statin therapy: an analysis of 20 536 patients in the Heart Protection Study. (2002). *The Lancet*, 360,7-22.

Heinecke, J. (2011). HDL and Cardiovascular-Disease Risk. Time for a New Approach?. *N Engl J Med* , 364, 170-1.

Hermann, TS., Li, W.,& Dominguez, H., (2006).Quinapril treatment increases insulin-stimulated endothelial function and adiponectin gene expression in patients with type 2 diabetes. *J Clin Endocrinol Metab*,91,1001-8.

Hong, MK., Park, DW., Lee, CW., Lee, SW., Kim, YH., Kang, JK., Kim, JJ., Park, SW.,& Park, SJ. (2009). Effects of statin treatments on coronary plaques assessed by volumetric virtual hystology intravascular ultrasound analysis. *J Am Coll Cardiol Cardiovasc Interv*, 2(7),679-88.

Hurst, RT., Robert, F., Burke, RE., Wissner, E., Roberts, A., Kendall, CB., Lester, SJ., Somers, V., Goldman, ME., Wu, Q. & Khandheria, B. (2010). Incidence of Subclinical Atherosclerosis as a Marker of Cardiovascular Risk in Retired Professional Football Players *Am J Cardiol*, 105, 1107–1111.

Intensive lowering of LDL cholesterol with 80 mg versus 20 mg simvastatin daily in 12,064 survivors of myocardial infarction: a double-blind randomised trial Study of the Effectiveness of Additional Reductions in Cholesterol and Homocysteine (SEARCH) Collaborative Group. *The Lancet*, (2010), 376, 1658–69.

Jafri, H., Alsheikh-Ali, AA., & Karas,RH. (2010). Meta-analysis: Statin Therapy Does Not Alter the Association Between Low Levels of High-Density Lipoprotein Cholesterol and Increased Cardiovascular Risk. *Ann Intern Med*, 153,800-808.

Joy, T., & Hegel, RA.(2008). Is raising HDL a futile strategy for atherosclerosis-protection?. *Nat Rev Drug Discov*, 7,143-55.

Kathiresan, S., Martin Larson, MG., Keyes, MJ., J. Keyes, Michelle., Joseph, F., Polak, JF., Wolf, PA., D'Agostino, RB., Jaffer, FA., Clouse, EM., Levy, D., Manning, WJ., & O'Donnell, CJ. (2007). Assessment by cardiovascular magnetic resonance, electron beam computed tomography, and carotid ultrasonography of the distribution of subclinical atherosclerosis across Framingham risk strata. *Am J Cardiol*, 99, 310–4.

Kera, AV., Cuchel, M., De la Llera-Moya, M., Rodrigues, A., Megan, F., Burke, BA., Jafri, K., French, BC., Phillips, JA., Megan, L., Mucksavage, Wilensky RL., Mohler, ER., Rothblat, GH.,& Rader, DJ.(2011). Cholesterol efflux capacity, high-density lipoprotein function, and atherosclerosis. *N Engl J Med*, 364, 127-35.

Kim, WY., Danias, PG., Stuber, M., Flam, SD., Plein, S., Nagel, E., Langerak, S., Weber, OM., Pedersen, EM., Matthias, S., Botnar, RM.,& Manning, WY.(2001). Coronary magnetic resonance angiography for the detection of coronary stenoses. *N Engl J Med*, 345, 1863-9.

Kim, LG., Scott, RAP., Ashton, HA., & Thompson, SG. (2007). For the Multicentre Aneurysm Screening Study Group. A sustained mortality benefit from screening for abdominal aortic aneurysm. *Ann Intern Med* , 146, 699 -706.

Kivimäki, M., Magnussen, CG., Juonala, M., Kähönen, M., Kettunen, J., Loo, BM., Lehtimäki, T., Viikari, J.,& Raitakari,OT. (2011). Conventional and Mendelian randomization analyses suggest no association between lipoprotein (a) and early atherosclerosis: the Young Finns Study. *Int J Epidemiology*, 40,2,470-478.

Knopp, RH., D'Emden, M., Smilde, JG., & Pocock, SJ., the ASPEN Study Group. (2006). Efficacy and safety of atorvastatin the prevention of cardiovascular end points in subjects with type 2 diabetes: the Atorvastatin Study for Prevention of Coronary Heart Disease Endpoints in Non-Insulin-Dependent Diabetes Mellitus (ASPEN). *Diabetes Care*, 29,1478-1485.

Kooi, ME., Cappendijk, VC., Cleutjens, KBJM., Kessels, AGH., Kitslaar, PJEHM., Borgers, M., Frederik, PM., Daemen, MJAP.,& Van Engelshoven, JMA.(2003). Accumulation of ultrasmall superparamagnetic particles of iron oxide in human atherosclerotic plaques can be detected by in vivo magnetic resonance imaging. *Circulation*,107,2453-2458.

Korcarz, CE., DeCara, JM., Hirsch, AT., Mohler, ER., Pogue, B., Postley, J., Tzou, WS., & Stein JH. (2008). Ultrasound Detection of Increased Carotid Intima-Media Thickness and Carotid Plaque in an Office Practice Setting: Does It Affect Physician Behavior or Patient Motivation? *J Am Soc Echocardiogr*, 21, 1156-1162.

Lamina, C., Meisinger, C., & Heid, IM. (2006). Association of ankle brachial index and plaques in the carotid and femoral arteries with cardiovascular events and total mortality in a population-based study with 13 years of follow-up. *Eur Heart J*, 27, 2580 -2585.

Lavoie, AJ., Bayturan, O., Uno, K., Hsu, A., Wolski, K., Schoenhagen, P., Kapadia, S., Tuzcu, EM., Nissen, SE., & Nicholls, SJ. (2010). Plaque Progression in Coronary Arteries With Minimal Luminal Obstruction in Intravascular Ultrasound Atherosclerosis Trials. *Am J Cardiol*, 105,1679 -1683.

Lester, SJ., Eleid, MF., Khandheria, BK., & Hurst, RT. (2009). Carotid Intima-Media Thickness and Coronary Artery Calcium Score as Indications of Sublinical Atherosclerosis. *Mayo Clin Proc*, 84, 3, 229-233.

Laurer, MS. (2007) Screening for coronary heart disease; Has the time for universal imaging arrived? *Cleveland Clinic J Med* 74(9):645-654.

Makris, GC.(2011). The Management of Asymptomatic Carotid Plaque Disease: Our Assumptions When We Are Less Radical. Angiology, published on line before print Febr. 8.

Mamm, CW., Nef, HM., Rolf, A.,& Molmann, H.(2011). Calcium and C-Reactive Protein. Hot enough to Predict the Future. *J Am Coll Cardiol* ,13,1465-7.

McGill, HC. & McMahan CA. (2006). Pathology of Atherosclerosis in Youth and Cardiovascolar Risk Factors. Pediatric Prevention of Atherosclerotic Cardiovascular Disease. *Oxford University Press* , 3-26.

Mendis, S. (2010). The contribution of the Framingham Heart Study to the prevention of cardiovascular disease: a global perspective. *Prog Cardiovasc Dis*, 53,10-14.

Miayazaki, A., Hideki Sakuma, S., Morikawa, W., Takiue, T., Miake, F., Terano, T., Sakai, M., Hakamata H., Sakamoto, Y-I., Naito, M., Ruan, Y., Takahashi, K., Ohta, T., & Horiuchi, S. (1995). Intravenous injection of rabbit Apolipoprotein A- 1 inhibits the progression of atherosclerosis in cholesterol- fed rabbits. *Arterioscler thromb vasc biol* ,15,1882-1888.

Möhlenkamp, S., Lehmann, SN., Moebus, S., Schmermund, A., Dragano, N., Stang, A., Siegrist, J., Mann, K., Jöckel, K-H., & Nixdorf H.(2011). Recall Study Investigators. Quantification of Coronary Atherosclerosis and Inflammation to Predict Coronary Events and All-Cause Mortality. *J. Am. Coll. Cardiol*, 57, 1455-1464.

Möhlenkamp, S., Lehmann, SN., Greenland, P., Moebus, S., Kaisch, H., Schmermund, A., Dragano, N., Stang, A., Siegrist, J., Mann, K., Jöckel, K-H., Erbel, & Nixdorf, H.(2011). Recall Study Investigators. Coronary calcium score improves cardiovascular risk prediction in persons without indication for statin therapy. *Atherosclerosis*, 215,229-236.

Moguillansky, D., Leng, X., Carson, A., Lavery, L., Schwartz, A., Chen, X., & Villanueva, FS. (2011). Quantification of plaque neovascularization using contrast ultrasound: a histologic validation. *Eur Heart J*, 32(5), 646-653.

Naghavi, M., Libby, P., & Falk, E. (2003). From vulnerable plaque to vulnerable patient: A call for new definitions and risk assessment strategies: Part I. *Circulation*, 108, 1664 -72.

Naghavi M, Falk E, Hecht HS, Jamieson MJ, Kaul S, Berman D, Fayad Z, Budoff MJ, Rmberger JJ, Naqvi TZ, Shaw LJ, Faergeman O, Cohn J, Bahr R, Koenig W, Demirovic J, Arking D, Herrera VLM, Badimon J, Goldstein JA, Rudy R, Airaksinen J, Schwartz RS, Riley WA, Mendes RA, Douglas P, Shah PK and for the SHAPE Task Force. (2006). From Vulnerable Plaque to Vulnerable Patient—Part III: Executive Summary of the Screening for Heart Attack Prevention and Education (SHAPE) Task Force Report. Am J Cardiol;98:2H-15H.

Nakamura, H., Arakawa, K., Itakura, H., Kitabatake, A., Goto, Y., Toyota, T., Nakaya, N., Nishimoto, S., Muranaka, M., Yamamoto, A., Mizuno, M., & Ohashi, Y. (2006). For the MEGA Study Group. Primary prevention of cardiovascular disease with pravastatin in Japan (MEGA Study): a prospective randomised controlled trial. *The Lancet*. 368,9542,1155-63.

Napoli, C., Lerman, LO., De Nigris, F., Gossi, M., Balestrieri, ML., & Lerman, A. (2006). Rethinking Primary Porevention of Atherosclerosis-Related Diseases. *Circulation*, 114, 2517-2527.

Napoli, C., Lerman, LO., De Nigris, F., Grossi, M., Balestrieri, ML., & Lerman, A. (2006). Rethinking Primary Prevention of Atherosclerosis-Related Diseases. *Circulation*, 114, 2517-2527.

Nissen, SE., Tuzcu, EM., Schoenhagen, P., Brown, PG., Ganz, P., Vogel, RA., Crowe, T., Howard, G., Cooper, CJ., Brodie, B., Grines, CL.,& DeMaria, AN. (2005). REVERSAL Investigators. Statin Therapy, LDL Cholesterol, C-Reactive Protein, and Coronary Artery Disease. *N Engl J Med*, 352, 29-38.

Nissen, SE., Nicholls, SJ., Sipahi, I., Libby, P., Raichlen, JS., Ballantyne, CM., Davignon, J., Erbel, R., Fruchart, JC., Tardif, J-C., Schoenhagen, P., Crowe, T., Cain, V., Wolski, K., Goormastic,. & Tuzcu, E. (2006). For the ASTEROID Investigators. Effect of Very High-Intensity Statin Therapy on Regression of Coronary Atherosclerosis: The ASTEROID Trial. *JAMA*,295, (13):1556-1565.

Ogasawara, D., Shite, J., Shinke, T., Watanabe, S., Otake, H., Tanino, Y., Sawada, T., Kawamori, H., Kato, H., Miyoshi, N.,& Hirata, K. (2009). Pioglitazone reduces the necrotic-core component in coronary plaque in association with enhanced plasma adiponectin in patients with type 2 diabetes mellitus. *Circ J* 73,343–51.

Oliver, MF., Heady, JA., Morrios, JN., & Cooper, J.(1978). A co-operative trial in the primary prevention of ishemic heart disease using clofibrate. Report from the Committee of Principal Investigators. *Br Heart J*, 40(10), 1069-1118.

Otake, H., Shite, J., & Shinke, T.(2008). Relation between plasma adiponectin, high-sensitivity C-reactive protein, and coronary plaque components in patients with acute coronary syndrome. *Am J Cardiol*, 101,1–7.

Peto, R., Emberson, J., Landray, M., Baigent, C., Collins, R., Clare, R., & Califf, R. (2008). Analyses of Cancer Data from Three Ezetimibe Trials. *N Engl J Med*, 359, 1357-66.

Pignoli, P. (1984). Ultrasound B-Mode imaging of arterial wall thickness measurement. In: Atherosclerosis Reviews. *Raven Press*,12,177-184.

Pineiro, R., Iglesias, MJ., & Gallego, R.(2005). Adiponectin is synthesized and secreted by human and murine cardiomyocytes. *FEBS Lett*, 579, 5163–9.

Pischon, T., Mohlig, M., Hoffmann, K., Spranger, J., Weikert, C., Willich, SN., Pfeiffer, AF., & Boeing, H.(2007). Comparison of relative and attributable risk of myocardial infarction and stroke according to C-reactive protein and low-density lipoprotein cholesterol levels. *Eur J Epidemiol*, 22, 429-438.

Plantinga, Y., Dogan, S., Grobbee, DE., & Bots, ML.(2009). Carotid intima-media thickness measurement in cardiovascular screening programmes. *Eur J Cardiovasc Prev Rehabil*, 16, 6, 639-44.

Poli, A., Pignoli, P., Mora, G., Tremoli, E., & Paoletti, R. Arterial wall visualization with bio-sound. In: Non Invasive Access to Cardiovascular Dynamics, pag 140-3 ed. Rusconi C, Orlando G. Proceedings of tje XIII Congress of the European Society for Non Invasive Cardiovascular Dynamics. (April 22-25, 1985 - Brescia, Italy).

Puska, P. (2010). From Framingham to North Karelia. From descriptive epidemiology to public health action. *Prog Cardiovasc Dis*, 53,15-20.

Raman, SB., Winner, MW., Tran, T., Velayutham, M., Simonetti, OP., Baker, PB., Olesik, J., McCarthy, B., Ferketich, AK., & Zweier, JL.(2008). In Vivo Atherosclerotic Plaque Characterization Using Magnetic Susceptibility Distinguishes Symptom-Producing Plaques. *J Am Coll Cardiol Img*, 1, 49–57.

Ridker, PM., Cushman, M., Stampfer, MJ., Tracy, RP., & Hennekens, CH.(1997). Inflammation, aspirin, and the risk of cardiovascular disease in apparently healthy men. *N Engl J Med*, 336, 973-9. [

Ridker, PM. (2007). C-Reactive Protein and the Prediction of Cardiovascular Events Among Those at Intermediate Risk. Moving an Inflammatory Hypothesis Toward Consensus. *J Am Coll Cardiol* ,49,2129–38.

Ridker, PM., Danielson, E., Fonseca, FAH., Genest, J., Gotto, Jr., Kastelein, JJP., Koenig, W., Libby, P., Lorenzatti, AJ., MacFadyen, Nordestgaard, BG., Shepherd, J., Willerson, JT.,

& Glynn, RJ. (2008). For the JUPITER Study Group. Rosuvastatin to Prevent Vascular Events in Men and Women with Elevated C-Reactive Protein. *N Engl J Med,* 359, 2195-207.

Riera-Guardia, N., & Rothenbacher, D.(2008). The effect of thiazolidinediones on adiponectin serum level: a meta-analysis. *Diabetes Obes Metab,* 10, 367–75.

Roberts, WC, (2002) Getting More People on Statin. *Am J Cardiol* 90:683-684.

Rose, G., Blackburn, H., Keys, A., Taylor, HL., Kannel, WB., Paul, O., Reid, DD., & Stamler, J. (1974). Colon cancer and blood cholesterol. *Lancet,*1(7850), 181-183.

Rozanski, A., Gransar, H., Shaw, LJ., Kim, J., Miranda-Peats, L., Wong, ND., Rana, JS., Orakzai, R., Hayes, SW., Friedman, JD., Thomson, LEJ., Polk, D., Min, J., Budoff, MJ., & Berman, DS. (2011). Impact of Coronary Artery Calcium Scanning on Coronary Risk Factors and Downstream Testing: The EISNER (Early Identification of Subclinical Atherosclerosis by Noninvasive Imaging Research) Prospective Randomized Trial *J. Am. Coll. Cardiol,* 57, 1622-1632.

Rusconi, C. (2008). Cardiovascular Risk Assessment and Primary Prevention in the Era of Plaque Imaging. *European Cardiology,* (Touch Briefings).12-16

Rusconi, C., Raddino, R., Trichaki, E., Grassi, V., & Dei Cas, L. Plaque regression and arterial reverse remodeling by statins. An ultrasound follow-up study of carotid (and femoral) arteries in primary prevention setting. Abstract book: STROKE 2011, 16th-18th February 2011 Florence, Italy

Sawada, T., Shite, J., Shinke, T. (2010). Low plasma adiponectin levels are associated with presence of thin-cap fibroatheroma in men with stable coronary artery disease. *Int J Cardiol,* 142,250 - 6.

Scandinavian Simvastatin Survival Study Group (4S). Randomized trial of cholesterol lowering in 4444 patients with coronary heart disease: the 4S. *Lancet,* 344, 1983-9.

Scott, M., Grundy, James I., Cleeman, C., Bairey, Merz., Noel, H., Brewer, Bryan Jr., Luther, T., Clark, Donald., Hunninghake B., Pasternak, Richard C., Sidney, C., Smith, Jr.,& Stone, Neil J.(2004). Coordinating Committee of the National Cholesterol Education Program. Implications of recent clinical trials for the National Cholesterol Education Program Adult Treatment Panel III Guidelines.*J Am Coll Cardiol,* 44, 720-732.SEARCH Study. Am Heart J 2007;154:815-23.

Sever, P., Dahlöf, B., Poulter, N., Wedel H., Beevers, G., Caulfield, M., Collins, R., Sverre E Kjeldsen, S., Kristinsson, A., McInnes, G., Jesper Mehlsen, J., Nieminen, M., O'Brien, E., & Östergren, J. (2003). Prevention of coronary and stroke events with atorvastatin in hypertensive patients who have average or lower-than-average cholesterol concentrations, in the Anglo-Scandinavian Cardiac Outcomes Trial—Lipid Lowering Arm (ASCOT-LLA): a multicenter randomized controlled trial. *The Lancet,* 361, 9364, 1149 - 1158.

Sewar, A., Shaw, LJ., Blankstein, R., Hoffman, U., Cury, RC., Abbara, S., Brady, TJ., Budoff, MJ., Blumenthal, RS.,& Nasir, K. (2009). Diagnostic and prognostic value of absence of coronary calcification. *J Am Coll Cardiol Img,* 2,675-88.

Shepherd, J., Cobbe, SM., Ford, I., Isles, CG., Lorimer, AR., MacFarlane, PW., McKillop, JH., & Packard, CJ. (1995) Prevention of coronary heart disease with pravastatin in men with hypercholesterolemia. West of Scotland Coronary Prevention Study Group. *New Engl J Med,* 16,333(20),1301-7.

Shepherd, J., Blauw, GJ., Murphy, MB., Bollen, EL., Buckley, BM., Cobbe, SM., Ford, I.,

Gaw, A., Hyland, M., Jukema, W., Kamper, AM., Macfarlane, PW., Meinders, AE., Norrie, J., Packard, CJ., Perry, IJ., Stott, DJ., Sweeney, BJ., Twomey, C., & Westendorp, RGJ. (2002). Pravastatin in elderly individuals at risk of vascular disease (PROSPER): a randomised controlled trial. *Lancet,* 360, 1623–30.

Shuhei, N., Söderlund, S., Jauhiainen, M., & Taskinen, MR. (2010). Effect of HDL composition and particle size on the resistance of HDL to the oxidation. *Lipids Health Dis,*9,104-10.

Simon, A., Chironi, G., & Levenson, J. (2006). Performance of Subclinical Arterial Disease Detection as a Screening Test for Coronary Artery Disease. *Hypertension,* 48,392-396.

Smilde, TJ., van Wissen, S., Awollersheim, H., Trio, MD., Kastelein, JJP., & Stalenhoef, AFH. (2001). Effect of aggressive versus conventional lipid lowering on atherosclerosis progression in familial hypercholesterolemia (ASAP): a prospective, randomised, double-blind trial. *The Lancet,* 357, 577- 581.

Stamler, J., Daviglus,ML., Garside, DB., Greenland, P., Eberly, LE., Yang, L.,& Neaton, JD.(2006). Low-Risk Cardiovascular Status: Impact on Cardiovascular Mortality and Longevity. Pediatric Prevention of Atherosclerotic Cardiovascular Disease. *Oxford University Press,* 49-60.

Stary, HC., Chandler, AB., Glagov, S., Guyton, JR., Insull, W., Rosenfeld, ME., Schaffer, SA., Schwartz, CJ., Wagner, WD., & Wisseler, RW.(1994). A Definition of Initial, Fatty Streak, and Intermediate Lesions of Atherosclerosis. A Report From the Committee on Vascular Lesions of the Council on Atherosclerosis, *American Heart Association,* 89,2462-2478

Stein, JH., Korcarz, CE., Hurst, RT., Lonn, E., Kendall, CB., Mohler, ER., Najj, S., Rembold, CM., & Post, W. (2008). American Society of Echocardiography Carotid Intima-Media Thickness Task Force. Use of carotid ultrasound to identify subclinical vascular disease and evaluate cardiovascular disease risk: A consensus statement from the American Society of Echocardiography Carotid Intima-Media Thickness Task Force. Endorsed by the Society for Vascular Medicine. *J Am Soc Echocardiogr,*21,93-111.

Tabas, I., Williams, KJ.,& Boren, J. (2007). Subendothelial Lipoprotein Retention as the Initiating Process in Atherosclerosis. Update and Therapeutic Implications. *Circulation,* 116,1832-44.

Sosnowski, C., Janeczko-Sosnowska, E., Pasierski, T., Szulczyk, A., Dabrowski, R., Woźniak, J., Sumiński, A., & Ruzyłło, W. (2007). Femoral rather than carotid artery ultrasound imaging predicts extent and severity of coronary artery disease. *Kardiol Pol,* 65, 7, 760-6.

Temelkova-Kurktschiev, T. & Hanefeld M.(2004). The lipid triad in type 2 diabetes - prevalence and relevance of hypertriglyceridemia/low high density lipoprotein syndrome in type 2 diabetes. *Exp Clin Endocrinol Diabetes,* 112(2),75-9.

The SEARCH Collaborative Group. *SLCO1B* Variants and Statin-Induced Myopathy-A Genomewide Study.. *N Engl J Med,* 359,789-799.

Tomas, M., & Mann, J. (1998). Increased thrombotic vascular events after change of statin. *The Lancet,* 352, 1830-1831.

Tomiyama, H., & Yamashina, A. (2010). Non-Invasive Vascular Function Tests. Their Pathophysiological Background and Clinical Application. *Circ J;*74: 24-33.

Wissler, RW., & Vessellnovitch, D. (1977). Regression of atherosclerosis in experimental animals and men. *Mod Con. Cardiovasc Dis,* 46,27-32.

Underhill, HR., Yuan, C., Yamikh, VL., Chu, B., Oikawa, M., Polissar, NL., Schwarts, SM., Jarwick, GP., & Hatsukami, TS. (2009). Arterial Remodeling in subclinical carotid Artery Disease. *J Am Coll Cardiol img,* 2, 1381-1389.

Underhill HR, Yuan C. (2011). Carotid MRI: a tool for monitoring individual response to cardiovascular therapy? *Exp Rev Cardiovasc Ther,* 9, 63-80.

Valgimigli, M., Rodriguez-Granillo, GA., Garcia-Garcia, HM., Malagutti, P., Regar, E., de Jaegere, P., de Feyter, P., & Serruys, PW. (2006). Distance from opstium as an indipendent determinant of coronary plaque composition in vivo: an intrvascular ultrasound study based radiofrequency data analysis in humans. *Eur Heart,* 27(6), 655-63.

van Velzen, JE., Schuijf, JD., de Graaf, FR., Boersma, E., Pundziute, G., Spanó, F., Boogers, MJ., Schalij, MJ., Kroft, LJ., de Roos, AJ., Jukema, W., van der Wall, EE., & Bax, JJ. (2011). Diagnostic performance of non-invasive multidetector computed tomography coronary angiography to detect coronary artery disease using different endpoints: detection of significant stenosis vs. detection of atherosclerosis. *Eur Heart J,* 32, 637-645.

Virmani, R., Frank, D., Kolodgie, FD., Allen, P., Burke. Farb, A., Schwartz, SM., Strong, JP., Malcom, GT., McMahan, CA., Tracy, RE., Newman, WP., Herderick, EE., & Cornhill, JF. For the Pathobiological Determinants of Atherosclerosis in Youth Research Group. (1999). Prevalence and Extent of Atherosclerosis in Adolescent and Young Adults. Implications for Prevention From the Pathobiological Determinants of Atherosclerosis in Youth Study. *JAMA,*:281:727-73.

Virmani, R., Frank, D., Kolodgie, FD, Allen, P., Burke, Farb, A., & Stephen, M. (2000). Lessons From Sudden Coronary Death. A Comprehensive Morphological Classification Scheme for Atherosclerotic Lesions. *Arterioscler Thromb Vasc Biol;*20,1262-1275.

Virmani, R., Kolodgie, FD, & Burke, AP. (2005). Atherosclerotic plaque progression and vulnerability to rupture: angiogenesis as a source of intraplaque hemorrhage. *Arterioscler Thromb Vasc Biol,*;25:2054- 61.

Waters, DD., Guyton, JR., Herrington, DM., McGowan, MP., Wenger, NK., & Shear, C.(2004) For the TNT Steering Committee Members and Investigators. Treating to New Targets (TNT) Study: Does Lowering Low-Density Lipoprotein Cholesterol Levels Below Currently Recommended Guidelines Yield Incremental Clinical Benefit?. *Am J Cardiol,* 93,154–158.

Westover, MB., Bianchi, MT., Echman, MH., & Greenberg, SM. (2011). Statin Use Following Intracerebral Hemorrage: A Decision Analysis. *Arch Neurol,* 0: 20103491-2.

Wurtz, P., Soininen, P., Kangas, AJ., Makinen, VP., Groop, PH., Savolainen, MJ., Viikari, JS., Kahonen, M., Lehtimaki, T., Raitakari, OT., & Ala-Korpela, M. (2011). Characterization of systemic metabolic phenotypes associated with subclinical atherosclerosis. *Mol Biosyst,* 7(2),385-93.

Yerramasu, A., & Venuraju, S. Lahiri. (2011). Evolving role of cardiac CT in the diagnosis of coronary artery disease *Postgrad Med J,* 87, 180-188.

Yuan, C. (2008). Carotid Atherosclerosis and Magnetic Resonance Imaging. *J Am Coll Cardiol Img,* 1,58-60.

Yusuf, S., Hawken, S., & Ounpuu, S. (2004). INTERHEART Study Investigators: Effect of potentially modifiable risk factor associated with myocardial infarction in 52 countries (The INTERHART study): case-control study. *Lancet,* 364, 937-95.

7

Ultrasonic Imaging in Liver Disease: From Bench to Bedside

Celia Resende, Andréia Lessa and Regina C. S. Goldenberg
Universidade Federal do Rio de Janeiro
Brazil

1. Introduction

Hepatology is an excellent example of how results deriving from basic science influence our everyday clinical practice. This involves diagnostic procedures as well as therapeutic developments. The role of diagnostic imaging in the assessment of liver disease continues to gain in importance. Imaging of the liver has progressed rapidly during the past decade with continued advancement of current ultrasound, computed tomography, and magnetic resonance imaging. Refinement enabling better anatomic characterization of disease and significant strength from the addition of new techniques and high resolution images were seen. Improvements in ultrasound (US) scanners over the past few decades have been remarkable: advances such as color Doppler and harmonic imaging have increased image quality and accuracy. Ultrasound is usually the first imaging modality in the evaluation of liver disease because it is easy to perform, widely available, relatively inexpensive and is cost effective. US can detect morphological changes in the liver and characterize focal lesions (cystic or solid) with high accuracy. Color Doppler sonography is a well established method for assessment of the hepatic vasculature, offering hemodynamic and anatomical information.

2. Hepatic ultrasound in rodents

An important challenge in pre-clinical *in vivo* studies is to follow up the evolution of the disease induced in animal models without sacrifice them. In this context, noninvasive methods available for the diagnosis and prognosis of liver diseases bring a significant contribution for the progress of this field of study. Prior animal research may support the step forward to human clinical trials.

Rodents represent an important animal group used in experimental model of liver diseases. Steatosis, cirrhosis and some hepatic focal lesions can be induced in mice and rats by administration of toxins, among which carbon tetrachloride (CCL4), ally alcohol, retrorsine and 2-acetylaminofluorene (2-AAF), by surgical insult such as bile duct ligation or hepatic resection, and virus infection. The induced hepatopathies may present change in liver size, shape, position, or opacity and these parameters can be evaluated by ultrasound imaging.

US imaging is an ideal complementary diagnostic tool to evaluate the liver. Hepatic ultrasound can noninvasively examine the internal architecture of the liver parenchyma, biliary system, portal and hepatic vascular supply. Also, ultrasonography allows assessment of changes in liver echogenicity, which correlates with disease (Lessa et al., 2010); identifies focal verses diffuse disease processes (Lima et al., 2008); detects vascular and biliary abnormalities (Partington & Biller, 1995). Additionally, besides being a noninvasive method, US is innocuous, reliable, rapid, reproducible and inexpensive, with high accuracy in evaluating liver disease.

2.1 Scanning techniques for hepatic ultrasound in rodents

Tranquilization is always required. In our experience, animals are successfully anesthetized using Ketamine (0.5mL/kg) and Xilazin (1mL/kg) intraperitoneally or by inhalation of Isoflurane, USP. If possible, the rodent should be fasting for 12 hours. This preparation may prevent vomiting and aspiration during anesthesia and helps reducing the sonographic barriers of excessive gas in the stomach and intestine.

The ventral abdomen must be shaved or have the hair removed with a commercially available hair remover creme to reduce imaging artifacts in the ultrasonographic examination. A sound-conducting gel is applied and the US examination can be performed in rats using a multifrequencial linear transducer (7.5 to 12MHz) attached to a conventional ultrasound machine or can be performed in mice and in rats using mechanical sector high resolution transducers (30 MHz and 40 MHz) in a dedicated ultrasound equipment for small animals (Vevo 770 - Visualsonics - Canada).

The animals are positioned in dorsal recumbence on a rectangular table for liver, hepatic artery and portal vein scanning. The liver is assessed by placing the transducer just distal to the last right costal cartilages and angling its beam cranially, obtaining multiple transversal and longitudinal scans (Fig. 1A-D). The hepatic artery and portal vein are scanned in the longitudinal views.

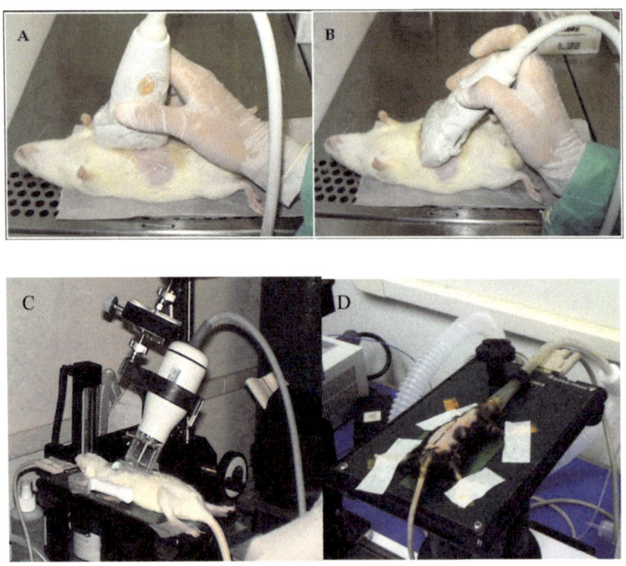

Fig. 1. Liver scanning: [1.A] Longitudinal scans are made by angling the transducer beam from right to left; [1.B] Transversal scans are made by angling the transducer beam from cranial to caudal; [1.C] High resolution mechanical sector transducer; [1.D] Dedicated ultrasound table with inhalatory anesthesia system.

2.2 The normal hepatic ultrasound

In order to standardize normal US parameters, our research group has examined 276 healthy Wistar rats. Such as described in small animals, the liver is bounded cranially by the concave highly echogenic curvilinear structure of the diaphragm-lung interface. It is bordered caudally by the fluid and gas reverberations in the fundus and body of the stomach to the left, and the pylorus and right kidney to the right. The anatomy divides the rat liver in four lobes: the right lateral lobe, middle, left lateral and caudate lobes, which in turn have independent portal and arterial vascularization and a separate biliar drainage. The right lateral lobe is subdivided into two segments, anterior and posterior, the last one adjacent to the right kidney and placed behind the inferior vena cava. The left lateral lobe is located on the left, in front of the stomach. In the midline, the caudate lobe is located dorsally and the median lobe lies ventrally.

The liver has homogeneous parenchyma with medium level echogenicity and straight hepatic surface as normal characteristics (Fig. 2A) (Dias et al., 2008; Lessa et al., 2010; Manheimer et al., 2009). In the 276 rats we examined, the transverse diameter of the liver measures from 3.5 to 3.8 cm and the portal vein caliber between 1.5 mm and 1.6 mm. The hepatic parenchyma is less echogenic than the right renal cortex in the great majority of rodents. Similar echogenicity in both organ parenchymas is observed in less than 5% of them (Lessa et al., 2008). The ultrasonographer should attempt to obtain images of the liver adjacent to the right kidney (longitudinal scan) (Fig. 2B). These images have to be made with proper control settings to prevent an incorrect diagnosis of diffuse hepatic disease. The hepatic parenchyma contains variably sized circular and tubular anechoic structures that represent the hepatic and portal veins (Partington & Biller, 1995).

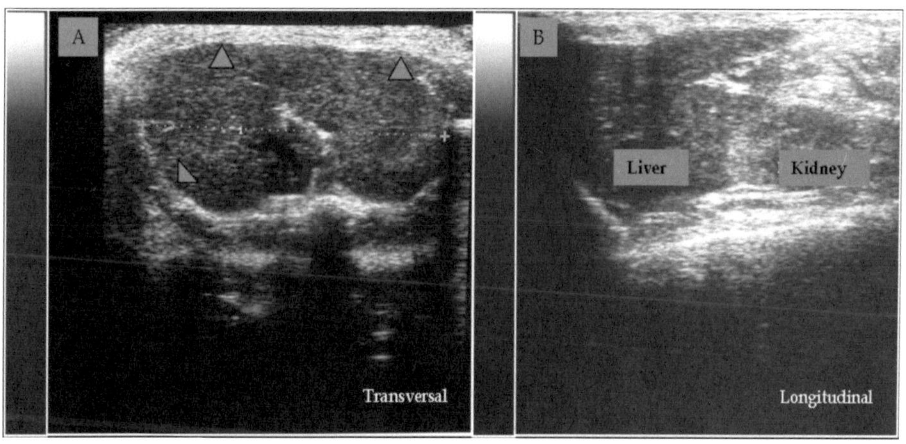

Fig. 2. Liver sonograms of a healthy rat: [2.A] Transversal sonogram shows homogeneous liver parenchyma, with medium level echogenicity and a regular hepatic surface (arrowheads); [2.B] Longitudinal sonogram presents right renal cortex more echogenic than liver parenchyma.

The caudal vena cava and the portal vein are parallel and run longitudinally. The portal vein caliber is measured in the mid-point of the main portal vein (Fig. 3A). Intrahepatic bile ducts are not identified routinely with ultrasound. Rats do not have gallbladder but mice do have it. The spleen has a homogeneous parenchyma (Fig.3B).

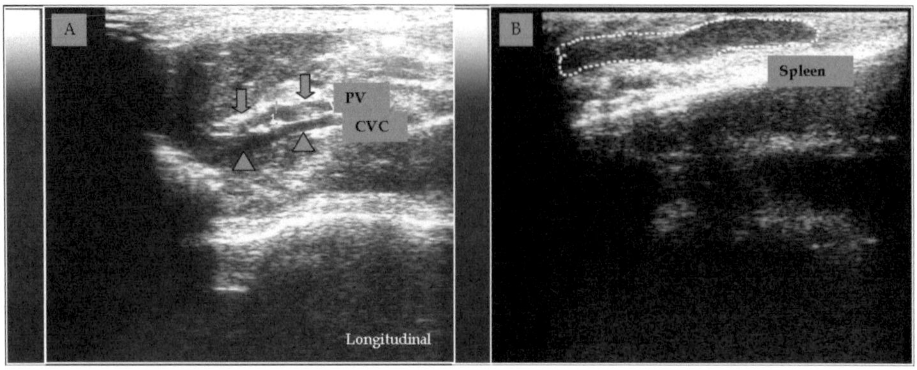

Fig. 3. [3.A] Longitudinal sonogram: portal vein (PV) (arrows) and the caudal vena cava (CVC) (arrowheads) in a healthy rat; [3B] Spleen sonogram: measurement of its area.

In high resolution ultrasound equipment specially designed to evaluate small animals the liver parenchyma and the relationship between liver/kidney echogenicity in rodents can be accurately examined. The portal vein caliber of the mice measures around 1.0 mm and the hepatic artery around 0.2 mm. This equipment allows to use the Doppler method to evaluate vascular resistance. The hepatic artery has a normal low resistance flow with the resistive index (RI) measuring around 0.50 (Fig. 4A-C). Resistive index (RI) is calculated using the peak systolic velocity (S) and end diastolic velocity (D) measurements as follows:

$$RI=\frac{S-D}{S}$$

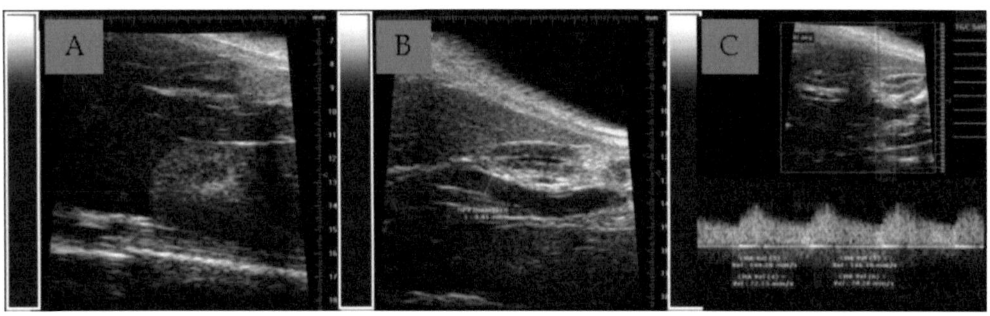

Fig. 4. [4.A] Longitudinal scan: normal liver parenchyma less echogenic than the renal cortex. [4B] Longitudinal scan: normal portal vein (PV) - caliber: 0.85 mm. [4C] Doppler spectrum: normal low resistance flow of the hepatic artery with high diastolic flow.

2.3 Difuse hepatic disease

Difuse hepatic disease may cause a change in the echogenicity of hepatic parenchyma (Dias et al., 2008; Lessa et al., 2010). Increased echogenicity is identified as hepatic echogenicity equal or greater than the renal cortex and similar to the spleen (Lessa et al., 2010; Lima et al., 2008; Partington & Biller, 1995). Diseases that may cause an increase in hepatic echogenicity include cirrhosis, hepatic steatosis, steroid hepatopathy, lymphosarcoma, and long-term cholangiohepatitis (Partington & Biller, 1995).

In 2005, Lee et al. demonstrated that B-mode mean grey level has a close correlation with fatty change and it is useful for the diagnosis of liver fibrosis (Lee et al., 2005). In 2008, it was described that US revealed steatosis based on liver echogenicity relative to the kidney and could detect focal lesions up to 0.5 mm in a rat model of NASH (non-alcoholic steatohepatitis) with cirrhosis (Lima et al., 2008).

In 2010, our group determined the reliability of US findings in the assessment of fatty liver disease and cirrhosis in rats in comparison to histological results by following up a rat model of hepatic disease induced by dual exposure to CCl_4 and ethanol (Lessa et al., 2010). In brief, ultrasound analysis was performed after 4, 8 and 15 weeks of liver injury induction, following the scanning techniques for hepatic ultrasound in rodents described above. Ultrasonographic findings were analyzed based on our previous observations and on criteria for US diagnosis in humans according to the following classification:

A. Liver echogenicity (Fig. 5) - four patterns: (0) homogeneous liver parenchyma with medium level echogenicity and a regular hepatic surface; (1) diffusely increased parenchymal echogenicity, reduced visualization of the diaphragm and small peripheral vessels with no change on liver surface; (2) discrete coarse and heterogeneous parenchymal echogenicity, dotted or slightly irregular liver surface; (3) extensive coarse and heterogeneous parenchymal echogenicity, irregular or nodular hepatic surface with underlying regenerative nodules;

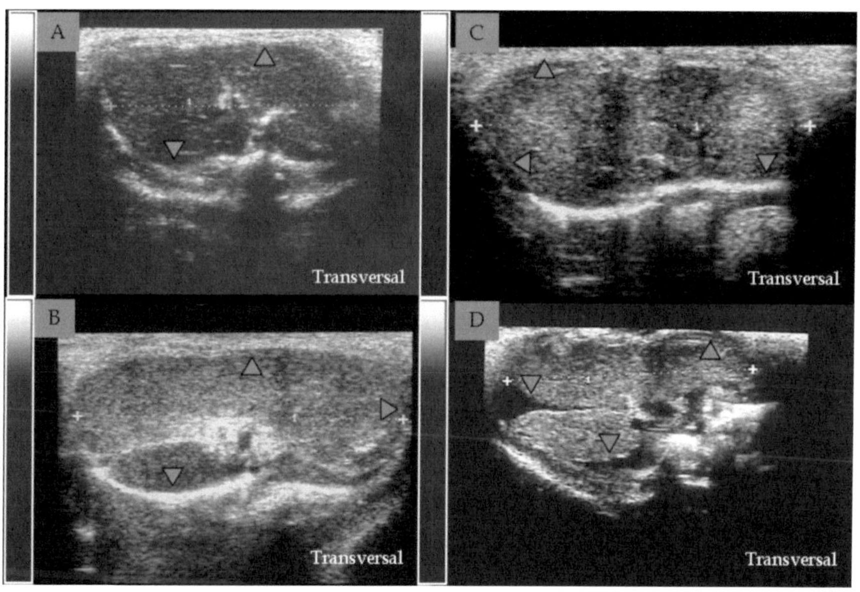

Fig. 5. Liver echogenicity patterns:
[5A] Pattern 0
[5B] Pattern 1
[5C] Pattern 2
[5D] Pattern 3

B. Inversion of the echographic relationship between the liver and the renal cortex (Fig. 6). This finding was considered to be positive if the echogenicity of the liver parenchyma was greater or equal to the right renal cortex, instead of lesser than it;

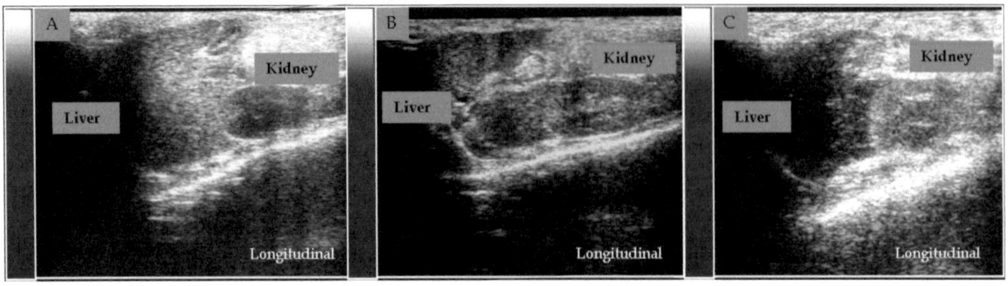

Fig. 6. Relationship between liver and right kidney echogenicities: Longitudinal scan [6A] Liver is less echogenic than right renal cortex; [6B] Hepatic echogenicity is equal to the right renal cortex in a cirrhotic liver; [6C] Hepatic parenchyma is more echogenic than right renal cortex in a steatotic liver.

C. Increased portal vein caliber (PVC). PVC was considered to be abnormal if equal or greater than 2.1 mm;
D. Presence of ascites;
E. Spleen area;
F. Doppler waveforms of the hepatic artery shows an increase in the resistive index due to the difficult inflow related to the presence of diffuse liver disease.

The liver parenchymal echogenicity changes correlates to the time of injury induction. The first pattern of liver echogenicity (pattern 0) is identified in normal rats. The pattern 1 correlates to fatty liver without/with minimal fibrosis. The pattern 2 corresponds to steatosis associated to different degrees of fibrosis and pattern 3 correlates to cirrhosis.

Cirrhosis may present nodules from macronodular regeneration (Lessa et al., 2010; Partington & Biller, 1995). As these nodules are most commonly isoechoic, their identification by ultrasound is difficult (Biller et al., 1992).

The hepatic echogenicity increases due to the presence of fatty infiltration and/or fibrosis, changing the relation between liver and right renal cortex (Biller et al., 1992). In our experience, this inversion had high sensitivity (90%), specificity (100%), positive and negative predictive values (100% and 76.9% respectively), and accuracy (92.5 %) for the detection of hepatic steatosis (Lessa et al., 2010), which is compatible with the findings described in the literature (Biller et al., 1992; Palmentiere et al., 2006).

Rats with mild hepatic steatosis can appear to be normal in US examination (Lessa et al., 2010). The US has been reported to have sensitivity of 90-91% for the detection of moderate to marked steatosis, but its sensitivity decreases to 30–64% when fatty liver is mild (Biller et al., 1992; Palmentiere et al., 2006). In addition, it is important to exclude kidney diseases when using this approach (Biller et al., 1992).

The evaluation of portal hypertension is important to access the severity of the disease. One of its most important signs is the widening of the portal vein (Fig.7). The PVC presented statistically significant differences ($p<0.001$) between cirrhotic and non-cirrhotic rats. The increase in its caliber, which was greater or equal to 2.1mm, can be considered a relevant ultrasound parameter, with sensitivity of 100% and specificity of 90.5 % (Lessa et al., 2010). Additionally, a 50% increase in PVC after cirrhosis induction can be another good parameter for advanced hepatic fibrotic change (Mannheimer et al., 2009).

Among the imaging diagnostic methods, the ultrasound is considered ideal for the study of ascites, which can be observed even when mild. Considering diffuse hepatic disease, the presence of ascites invariably corresponds to cirrhosis (Fig. 8)

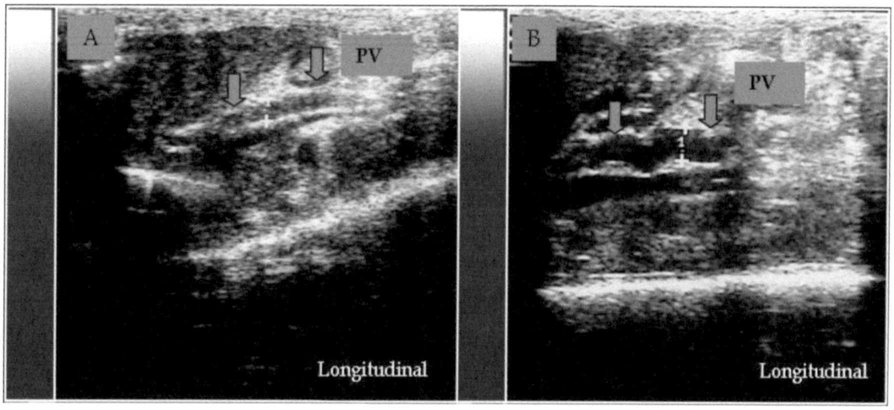

Fig. 7. Portal vein caliber (PVC): Longitudinal scans - [7A] Straight and thin portal vein (caliber=1.4 mm) in a healthy rat (arrows); [7B] Tortuous and dilated portal vein (caliber=2.2 mm) in a cirrhotic rat (arrows).

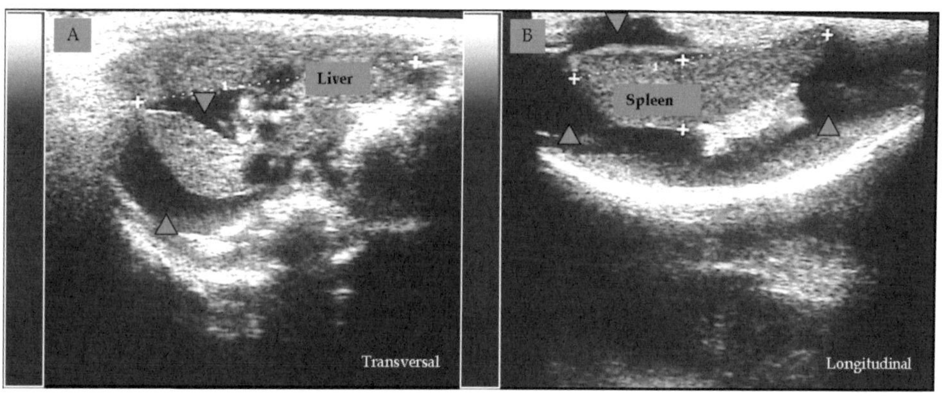

Fig. 8. [8A] Transversal liver sonogram shows a small cirrhotic liver with marked ascites; [8B] Longitudinal sonogram presents a great amount of ascites surrounding the spleen.

2.4 Focal liver lesions

Focal hepatic lesions are more easily detected by ultrasound when these lesions have a different echogenicity than the surrounding normal liver. Focal hepatic diseases include cysts, hematomas, abscess, granulomas, regenerative nodules, primary and metastatic neoplasms (Partington & Biller, 1995). US usually detects and characterize these lesions.

Regenerative hepatic nodules are benign reorganized masses of hepatic tissue that contain lipid, blood-filled sinusoids, lymphocytes and areas of atrophied or necrotic hepatocytes. These nodules are most commonly isoechoic and can be multiple and variably sized (Fig. 9).

Primary hepatic neoplasia may appear as solitary or multiple focal lesions that can be hypo, iso or hyperechoic in relation to normal liver. Also it can appear as a very large, moderately circumscribed or infiltrating mass. The US appearance of liver neoplasia is not specific for the histopathological cell type (Partington & Biller, 1995).

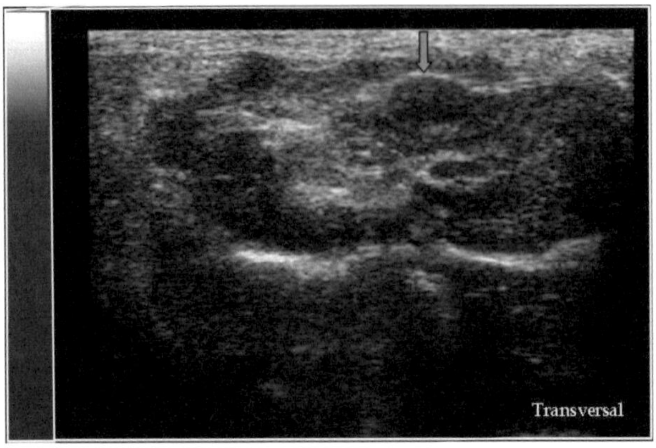

Fig. 9. Transversal sonogram shows a cirrhotic liver with an isoechoic regenerative nodule (arrow).

3. Human liver ultrasound imaging

The liver is the largest abdominal organ weighting 1.5 kg and lying in the right side of the upper abdomen under the right hemidiaphragm and extending across the midline to the left hypochondrium. The parenchymal echoes are a mid-grey and consist of a uniform, sponge-like pattern interrupted by the vessels. In transverse sections the wedge shape of the liver is seen, tapering to the left (Fig.10A). The caudate lobe is seen as an extension of the right lobe in transverse sections and as an almond-shaped structure posterior to the left lobe in longitudinal views (Fig.10B). In the longitudinal sections the liver has a triangular shape, the right lobe larger than the left (Fig. 10C).

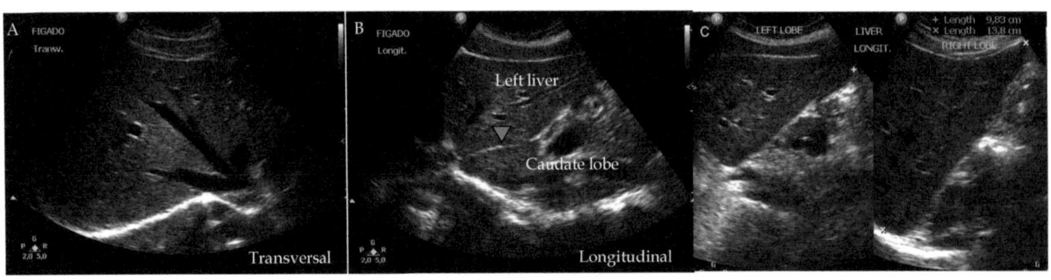

Fig. 10. [A] Transversal section of normal liver with the hepatic veins draining into the inferior vena cava. [B] Longitudinal scan of the left and caudate lobe being separated by the fissure of the ligamentum venosum (arrowhead); [C] Longitudinal scan of the liver: normal left lobe and right lobe.

3.1 Technique

The liver is best imaged with the patient supine or in a right anterior oblique position. Intercostal imaging is always required, in which case the transducer is placed parallel to the adjacent ribs to avoid acoustic shadowing. Multiplanar imaging of the liver is obtained. Sagittal, transverse, coronal and subcostal oblique views are required. A 5-2 MHz curved array transducer with appropriate gain and depth settings permits adequate visualization of the entire liver. A wide field of view in the near field is essential for good liver imaging. The liver should be imaged in real-time in the sagittal and transverse or oblique planes. The left lobe is usually best imaged with the patient supine and the transducer placed in an anterior subxiphoid position. Real-time imaging during suspended deep inspiration allows the most superior aspects of the left lobe to be visualized. The right lobe usually requires an intercostal or subcostal oblique approach with the patient supine and in the left-side-down decubitus position. Certain regions are more difficult to image such as the high dome and the lateral aspect of the right lobe of the liver, usually best imaged from subcostal oblique and intercostal planes in suspended inspiration. The patient should be fasting for at least 6 hours prior to the exam to limit bowel gas and so that the gallbladder is not contracted.

3.2 Focal liver lesions

Liver masses are increasingly being identified due to the widespread use of imaging modalities. The majority of these lesions are detected incidentally in asymptomatic patients. Characterization of a liver mass on sonography is based on the appearance of the mass on gray scale imaging as well as on vascular information that may be obtained on Doppler examination.

3.2.1 Hepatic cysts

Simple cysts are usually described as congenital lesions, but are probably better considered developmental, since their frequency increases with age. Simple hepatic cysts are usually solitary, have a thin epithelial lining, and contain watery fluid. Their size varies from less than 1 cm to more than 20 cm in diameter. Simple cysts are found 4 times more frequently in females than males. Symptoms are rare, but may occur from mass effect, rupture, hemorrhage or infection. The classic sonographic findings are well known: a well defined, anechoic lesion with a well-demarcated, thin wall and good distal sonic enhancement (Fig. 11A). Thin septations are frequent, and should not suggest a different diagnosis. Occasionally there may occur cyst hemorrhage or infection when it will contain internal echoes and septations, a thickened wall and may appear solid (Fig. 11B). If thick septae or nodules are seen, differential diagnosis of biliary cystadenomas and cystic metastases must be considered. Acquired cysts are usually secondary to trauma, inflammation or parasitic infection and are indistinguishable from primary cysts. Cyst ablation with alcohol or surgical excision can be performed if indicated.

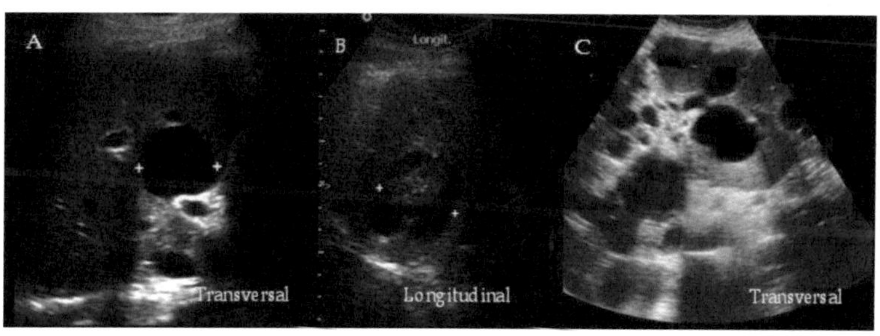

Fig. 11. [A] Hepatic cyst: a well defined, anechoic lesion with a thin wall and good distal enhancement; [B] Hemorrhagic cyst - a well defined cystic lesion with internal amorphous echoes and septation; [C] Polycystic liver disease: multiple anechoic cysts of varying sizes, thin walls and posterior distal enhancement. Note that some cysts contain internal echoes with fluid/fluid level due to internal hemorrhage.

Polycystic renal disease is a relatively common congenital condition and has an autosomal dominant mode of inheritance. Liver cysts are associated with this condition in approximately 57% to 74% (Levine et al., 1985). The most common presentation is hepatomegaly. The ultrasound appearance of multiple cysts of varying sizes, thin walls and posterior acoustic accentuation is characteristic (Fig. 11C). Hemorrhage or infection in the cysts may produce internal echoes. Acoustic accentuation beyond each cyst may produce the impression of an abnormal liver parenchymal texture. There may be cysts in other organs like pancreas, spleen, ovaries and lungs. Usually they do not require any treatment and complications are rare including hemorrhage, rupture or infection.

3.2.2 Biliary hamartomas (von Meyenburg Complexes)

Bile duct hamartomas are small focal developmental lesions composed of groups of dilated intrahepatic bile ducts with a collagenous stroma. They are benign liver malformations that are detected incidentally in 0.6 to 5.6% of reported autopsy series (Redston & Wanless, 1996). Commonly they are documented on sonograms as bright echogenic foci with distal ringdown or comet tail artifacts, diffusely distributed until the periphery of the liver (Fig. 12A-B) that could be related to the presence of tiny cysts beyond the resolution of the ultrasound equipment or to the cholesterol crystals within the dilated tubules. They may also appear as well-defined small hypoechoic solid nodules (Fig. 12C-D).

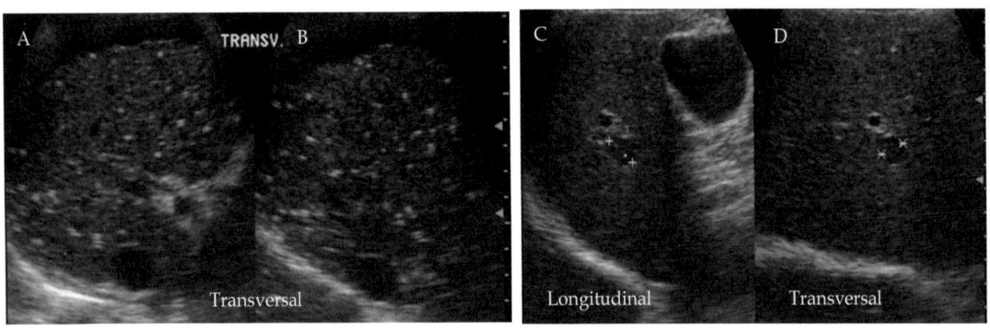

Fig. 12. Biliary hamartomas: [A-B] multiple bright echogenic foci some of them with distal ringdown or comet tail artifacts, diffusely distributed until the periphery of the liver; [C-D] Small hypoechoic nodule that on MRI was confirmed to be von Meyenburg complex.

3.2.3 Hydatid disease

The liver is the most frequently involved organ in hydatid disease but other sites may be involved, such as the lungs, the bones, the brain and the peritoneal cavity. In the liver the right lobe is more frequently involved where they form slow-growing cysts. Lewall & McCorkell (1985) proposed four groups of sonographic features of hepatic hydatid disease: solitary cysts containing sand; cysts with detached endocyst secondary to rupture; cysts with daughter cysts; and densely calcified masses. The distinction between simple and hydatid cysts may be one of the following features: wall calcification, debris consisting of sand and the two layers of the wall resulted from detachment and collapse of the inner germinal layer from the exocyst. The development of daughter cysts produces a characteristic appearance.

3.2.4 Hepatic abscess

Liver abscesses are frequently related to direct extension from the biliary tract infection in patients with suppurative cholangitis and cholecystitis or to complications of an intra-abdominal infection with direct portal venous system spread to the liver, such as diverticulitis or appendicitis. They may also be present in the liver as a result of blunt or penetrating trauma or through the hepatic artery in patients with osteomyelitis and subacute bacterial endocarditis. No cause can be found in approximately 50% of the cases of hepatic abscesses (Wilson & Withers, 2005).

Sonographically, pyogenic liver abscess has a variable appearance. Typically, pyogenic abscesses are poorly defined, irregularly marginated, and primarily hypoechoic. Irregular areas of increased echogenicity are frequent (Fig.13A-B). Bright punctate echoes often represent gas within the abscess. On occasion, a diffusely hyperechoic appearance may be noted, related to large amounts of gas from gas-forming organisms (Fig. 13C-D). Fluid-fluid interfaces, internal septations and debris can be observed. The abscess wall can vary from well-defined to irregular and thick. Diffuse microabscesses may occasionally cause a confusing sonographic pattern of increased irregular hepatic echogenicity. The differential diagnosis of pyogenic liver abscess includes complicated hepatic cysts with hemorrhage, hematoma, amebic infection and necrotic neoplasm.

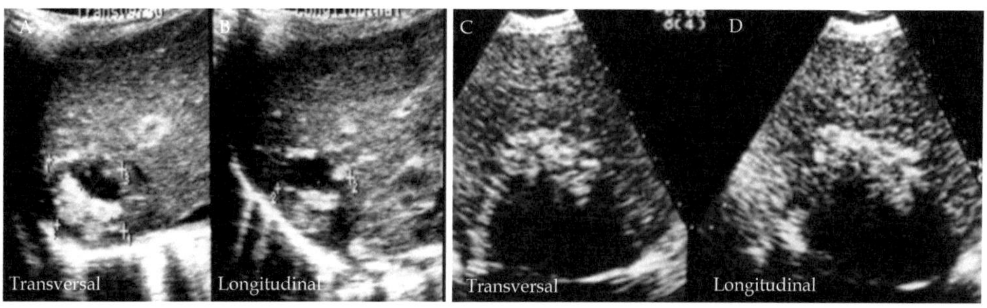

Fig. 13. [A-B] Hepatic abscess - Thick wall fluid collection with hyperechoic heterogeneous internal echoes; [C-D] Gas forming abscess - diffusely irregular hyperechoic lesion with posterior accoustic attenuation.

Entamoeba histolytica primarily infects the colon. Transmission is by the fecal-oral route. Amebic liver abscess is the most common non-enteric complication of amebiasis. The most common presenting symptom is pain. An amebic abscess may be indistinguishable from a pyogenic abscess. Sonographic features include lack of a significant wall echo, symmetric oval or round configuration, hypoechogenicity compared to normal liver with a homogeneous pattern of internal echoes, increased sound transmission and subcapsular location (Fig. 14). Ralls et al. (1987a) in a review of 112 amebic lesions described two sonographic patterns that were more prevalent in amebic abscesses: round or oval shapes in 82% versus 60% of pyogenic abscess and hypoechoic appearance with fine internal echoes at high gain in 58% versus 36% of pyogenic abscesses. The majority of hepatic amebic abscesses disappear with amebicidal drugs (Ralls et al., 1987b).

3.2.5 Cavernous hemangioma

Cavernous hemangiomas are the most frequently encountered benign tumor of the liver and are seen in 1 to 4% of the population as an incidental finding. These lesions are most

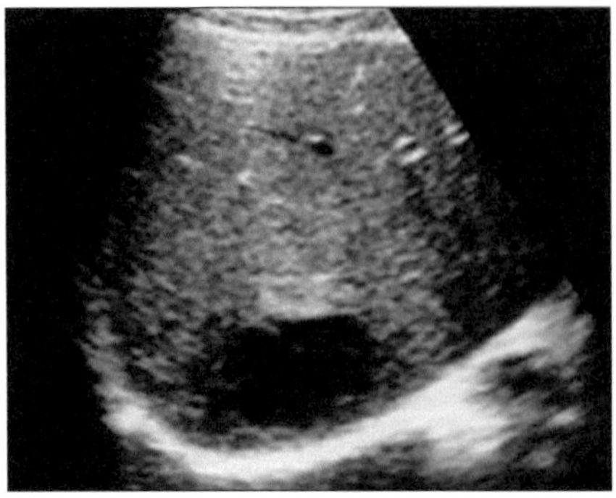

Fig. 14. Amebic abscess: lack of significant wall echo, round hypoechoic liver lesion with increased sound transmission and subcapsular location.

commonly seen in women with a female/male ratio of 5:1 (Snover, 2009). Hemangiomas are composed of dilated endothelial-lined vascular channels, infiltrated by varying degrees of fibrous stroma.

The typical hemangioma is a uniformly well circumscribed hyperechoic mass less than 3 cm in diameter. These lesions are often small and can be multiple (Fig. 15A-B). The increased echogenicity has been related to the numerous interfaces between the walls of the cavernous sinuses and the blood within them. In the setting of hepatic steatosis or cirrhosis, however, they may appear hypoechoic. Although this lesion is hyperechoic, in many cases hemangiomas will exhibit posterior acoustic enhancement because the dilated, fluid-filled sacs of blood do not attenuate sound. An atypical but not uncommon sonographic appearance of the hemangioma is a lesion with an echogenic rim and an internal hypoechoic pattern (Wilson & Withers, 2005) (Fig.15C-D). Larger lesions tend to be heterogeneous with central hypoechoic foci corresponding to fibrous collagen scars, large vascular spaces, or both. Calcification is rare. Hemangiomas only rarely demonstrate internal flow on Doppler studies, due to the multidirectionality and slow velocity of flow. There are potentially significant lesions that may mimic the morphology of a hemangioma on ultrasound and produce a single mass or multiple masses of uniform increased echogenicity such as metastases from a colon primary tumor; small hepatocellular carcinomas (HCC) may show this morphology. Caturelli et al. (2001) in a prospective evaluation of 1982 patients with newly diagnosed cirrhosis found that 50% of echogenic liver lesions suggestive of

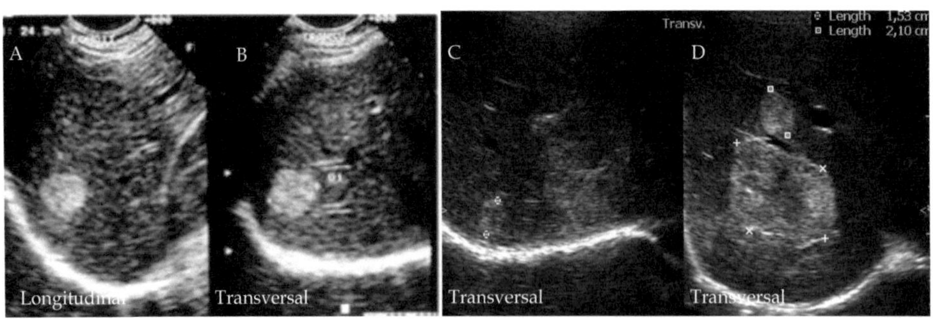

Fig. 15. Hemangioma: [A-B] Typical hemangioma: hyperechoic round lesion at the posterior segment of the right lobe of the liver with posterior acoustic enhancement; [C-D] Multiple hemangiomas: Multiple echogenic lesions with central hypoechoic areas.

hemangiomas had the diagnosis of HCC. These results emphasize the importance to prove the diagnosis of all masses with this morphology in high-risk patients.

3.2.6 Focal nodular hyperplasia

Focal nodular hyperplasia (FNH) is the second most commonly encountered benign liver lesion and is seen most often as an incidental observation in a young adult female. FNH is not an actual neoplastic tumor but represents instead a hyperplastic response to an underlying vascular malformation in the liver. Histologically, it is made up of normal liver components, including hepatocytes and Kupffer cells. FNH is a hypervascular lesion, often showing a central stellate vascularity and a large and tortuous feeding artery. On sonography, FNH is often a subtle liver mass that is difficult to differentiate in echogenicity from the adjacent liver parenchyma (Fig.16A-B). The lesions may be slightly hypoechoic, isoechoic, or slightly hyperechoic than the surrounding liver. Use of color and power Doppler US may add information concerning the vascularity of the suspected FNH. In addition, use of US contrast media to characterize FNH has been reported. These lesions usually produce a contour abnormality to the surface of the liver or may displace the normal blood vessels within the parenchyma. The central scar may be seen on gray-scale sonograms as a hypoechoic linear or stellate areas within the central portion of the mass. Well-developed peripheral and central blood vessels are seen to course within the central scar with either a linear or stellate configuration (Fig.16C-D). Spectral interrogation usually shows predominantly arterial signals centrally.

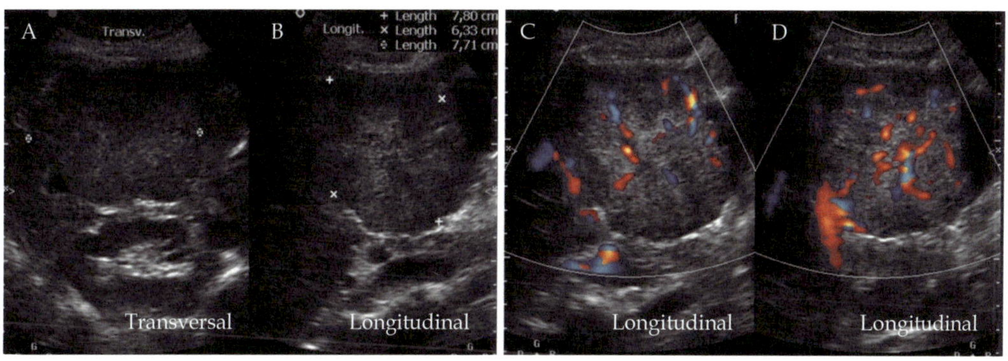

Fig. 16. Focal Nodular Hyperplasia. [A-B] Isoechoic large lesion in the right lobe deforming the contour of the liver with a subtle hypoechoic central area; [C-D] Color Doppler showing stellate pattern blood vessels within the central scar.

3.2.7 Hepatic adenoma

Hepatic adenomas (HA) are less common than FNH, benign neoplasms, usually solitary and well encapsulated, ranging in size from 8 to 15 cm, which have a small risk for malignant transformation into hepatocellular carcinoma, as well as a propensity for hemorrhage and rupture. The majority of these lesions occur in young women taking oral contraceptives. The risk of developing HAs is related to both the duration of use and dose of hormones. These lesions regress when oral contraceptives are discontinued (Fig.17A-F). Other populations noted to have an increased incidence of HAs include individuals with type I glycogen storage disease. In these patients, hepatic adenomas tend to be multiple. The sonographic appearance is nonspecific. Although in 70% to 80% of cases, HAs present as a solitary and large hyperechoic lesion with central anechoic areas, corresponding to zones of internal hemorrhage, they can be isoechoic or complex masses. It is difficult to distinguish hepatic adenoma from FNH. Color Doppler evaluation can be helpful, demonstrating peripheral and intratumoral vessels showing increased venous structures within the center of the mass and a paucity of arterial vessels (Fig.17G-H). These lesions are substantially less vascular than most FNH (Wilson & Withers, 2005).

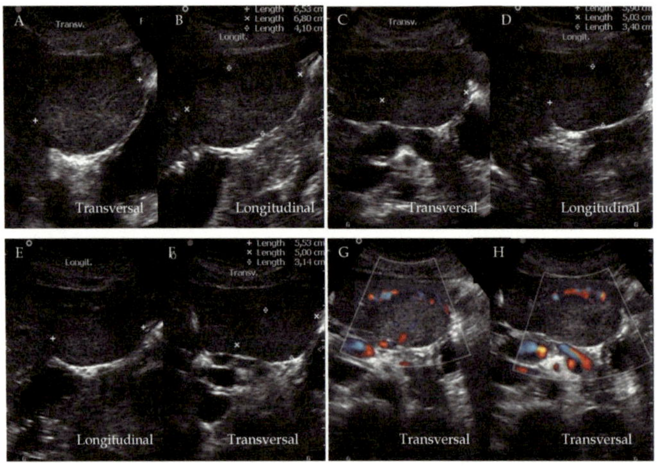

Fig. 17. Hepatic Adenoma: [A-F] Isoechoic lesion in the left lobe of the liver that diminished in size as oral contraceptives were discontinued (A-B: 1st exam, C-D: 2nd exam, E-F: 3rd exam-every two months); [G-H] Color Doppler showing predominantly peripheral vessels.

3.2.8 Hepatocellular carcinoma

Hepatocellular carcinoma (HCC) is the commonest primary liver cancer, comprising 80% of primary liver malignancies in the United States. The majority of HCC patients (95% in the western, 60% in Asian countries) will develop the disease on the ground of preexisting liver cirrhosis. Alcoholic cirrhosis-related HCC has a lower frequency (10% of autopsied patients) than HBV or HCV (Parkin et al., 2005). Although α-fetoprotein (AFP) is a known and specific tumor maker for HCC, it is not suitable for the screening and surveillance of HCC because of its poor predictive value and low sensitivity. The use of imaging modalities is essential for the screening, diagnosis and treatment of HCC. US plays a major role among them, because it provides real-time and noninvasive observation by a simple and easy technique. The development of digital technology has led to the detection of blood flow by color Doppler US, and the sensitivity for detecting tumor vascularity has shown remarkable improvement with the introduction of microbubble contrast agents. Screening generally consists of serologic testing for alpha-fetoprotein and/or hepatitis B and C, often coupled with sonography of the liver. Some studies showed that surveillance based on US and AFP every 6-12 months improved the survival of patients (Bolondi et al., 2001; Sangiovanni et al., 2004). Pathologically HCC occurs in three forms: 1. Solitary tumor; 2. Multiples nodules; 3. Diffuse infiltration. Sonographic findings in HCC are variable, and may cause difficulty in distinguishing advanced HCC from metastatic disease. This is less of a problem in screening programs, where HCCs less than 5 cm are often detected. In these small lesions, sonographic findings are not as diverse. About 75% of small HCCs (<5 cm) are hypoechoic (Fig.18A-B). As HCCs enlarge, they tend to develop hypoechoic peripheral rims. With further progression, lesions become more numerous and heterogeneous. Some hepatocellular carcinomas, even small lesions, undergo fatty metamorphosis, causing increased echogenicity and potential confusion with hemangioma. Hepatocellular carcinomas arising in normal livers are uncommon. Fibrolamellar HCC, which accounts for 2% of hepatocellular carcinoma, but 25% to 50% of HCC in young adults, often arises as a single well-circumscribed lesion with lobulated margins in an otherwise normal liver. Other features may include a "central scar" and a high prevalence of calcification. Vascular invasion is common and should suggest the diagnosis of HCC. HCC invades portal veins more frequently than hepatic veins. Intravascular tumor is usually reflective and expands the vessel, but positive differentiation from blood thrombus depends on detecting arterial Doppler signals from within the thrombus (Fig. 18C-F); only venous signals are found in blood thrombus as it is recanalized. HCC has a characteristic hypervascular appearance with centripetal blood flow, and a basket pattern is one of the typical findings of HCC by color Doppler imaging (Tanaka et al., 1990). Using microbubble contrast agents HCC shows as a highly vascular lesion in the overwhelming majority of patients studied.

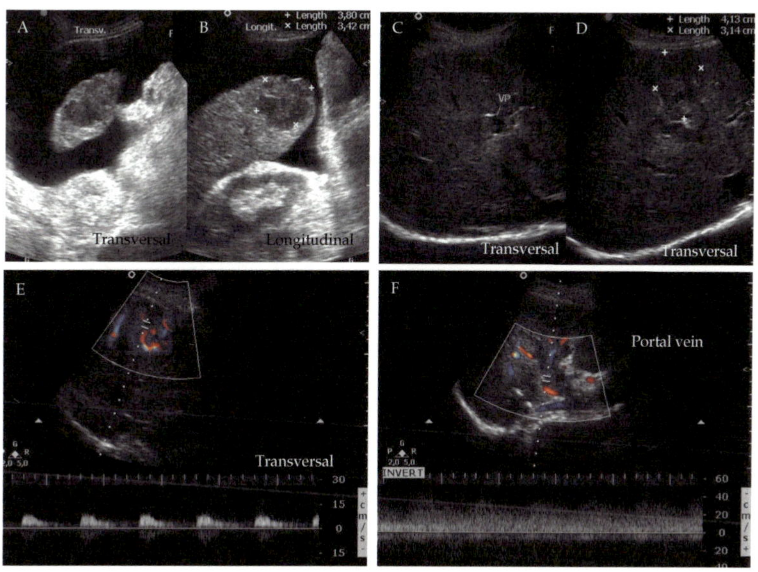

Fig. 18. Hepatocellular Carcinoma: [A-B] Lobulated hypoechoic lesion in the periphery of the right lobe; [C-F] Hipoechoic lesion in segment IV with portal tumoral thrombus. Note on color Doppler that the lesion has intra and peripheral vascularity (E) and that there is arterial flow inside the portal vein (F).

3.2.9 Cholangiocarcinoma

Cholangiocarcinoma arises from the bile ducts, and account for about 10% of all primary liver cancers. Cholangiocarcinoma is associated with hemochromatosis, ulcerative colitis, Caroli disease and choledochal cyst. Cholangiocarcinoma has two forms, peripheral cholangiocarcinoma (PCC) and hilar cholangiocarcinoma, also known as Klatskin tumor, when it involves the confluence of the left and right hepatic ducts at the porta hepatis. In the

United States, PCC is 3 times more common than hilar cholangiocarcinoma. The prevalence is equal in Japan. PCC is usually a large tumor, while hilar cholangiocarcinoma presents earlier with ductal obstruction and jaundice, and is usually not associated with a large mass. Hemochromatosis is associated with both PCC (9% of patients) and HCC (18% of patients). The sonographic findings in PCC are variable. In general, cholangiocarcinomas are hard to visualize with all modalities. Some investigators report predominance of hypoechoic lesions, and others predominantly hyperechoic lesions. Our experience suggests that slightly hypoechoic lesions are more frequent. Portal venous invasion is frequent. Sonography is generally superior to multiphase helical CT in demonstrating masses associated with hilar cholangiocarcinomas. Dilatation of the biliary tree can be followed down to the point of obstruction, where it may be possible to detect a solid, poorly reflective mass which, if large enough, can be seen to have a heterogeneous internal echo pattern and ill-defined margins (Fig.19).

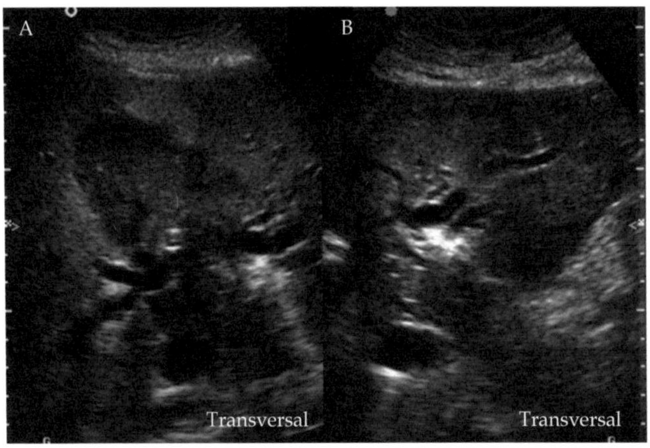

Fig. 19. Cholangiocarcinoma: large hilar hypoechoic mass with right and left intrahepatic bile ducts dilatation.

3.2.10 Metastatic disease

In the United States, metastatic disease is by far the most common significant focal liver lesion. Metastases are 18 to 20 times more common than hepatocellular carcinoma (HCC) and produce symptoms 10 times more frequently. In one large autopsy series (Edmonson, 1987), 38% of all patients with carcinoma had hepatic metastases. The most common carcinomas metastasizing to the liver include, in order of decreasing frequency: gallbladder, colon, stomach, pancreas, breast and lung. Metastatic disease is multifocal in approximately 90% of patients. Most metastases to the liver are blood-borne via the hepatic artery or portal vein. The portal vein provides direct access to the liver for tumor cells originating from the gastrointestinal tract and probably accounts for the high frequency of liver metastases from organs that drain into the portal circulation. Virtually any sonographic appearance may occur in liver metastasis. The following sonographic appearances of metastatic liver disease have been described: echogenic, hypoechoic, target, calcified, cystic and diffuse. Hypoechoic halos are common. The presence of a hypoechoic halo surrounding a liver mass has been regarded as an ominous sign with a high association with malignancy, particularly metastatic disease. Wernecke et al. (1992) described the importance of the hypoechoic halo in the differentiation of malignant from benign focal hepatic lesions. Its identification has a positive and negative predictive value of 86% and 88%, respectively. Echogenic metastases tend to arise from a gastrointestinal origin or from HCC (Fig.20A). While it must be emphasized that sonographic appearance is a poor predictor of the primary tumor, certain patterns may be suggestive. For example, large to moderate-sized hyperechoic metastases, especially those with microcalcifications, should suggest the possibility of a colonic primary. A target or bull's eye appearance with varying rings of hypo- and hyperechogenicity are common (Fig. 20B). Ill-defined infiltrative disease with focal nodularity is another fairly frequent pattern. Metastasis and HCC may be impossible to distinguish sonographically, although the presence of underlying liver disease favors HCC. Invasion of the portal or hepatic veins suggests hepatocellular carcinoma, rather than metastasis. Most liver metastases that are hypoechoic are hypovascular. Colon, lung, breast, and gastric cancers are the most common causes of hypovascular liver metastases (Fig.20C). The most common causes of hypervascular hepatic metastases include neuroendocrine tumors (eg, carcinoid, pheochromocytoma, and islet cell tumors), renal cell carcinoma, melanoma, choriocarcinoma, and thyroid carcinoma. Breast carcinoma and, rarely, pancreatic adenocarcinoma can also cause hypervascular metastases.

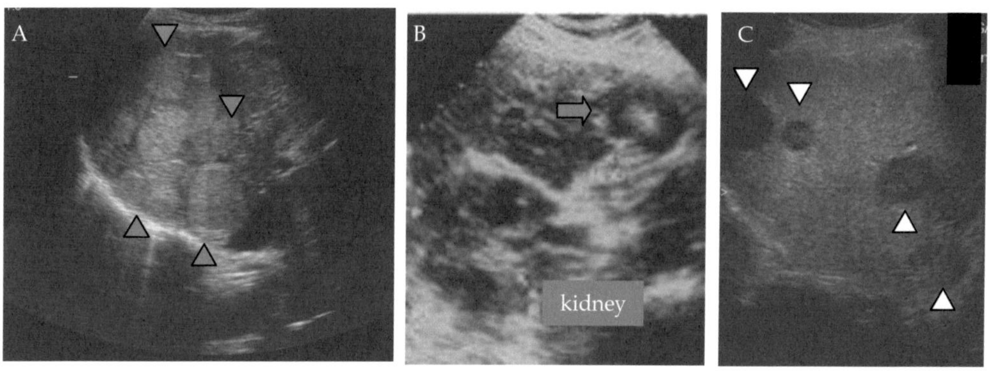

Fig. 20. Metastases: [A] Multiple echogenic nodular lesions due to HCC metastases (gray arrowheads); [B] Bull's eye appearance and another echogenic lesion secondary to colon carcinoma (arrow); [C] Multiple hypoechoic nodular lesions; metastases from cholangiocarcinoma (white arrowheads).

3.3 Diffuse liver disease

Recent innovations in imaging technology and contrast media development have augmented the role of radiology in the detection, characterization, and follow up of diffuse liver diseases. Although biopsy still remains the gold standard for establishing the diagnosis of diffuse liver disease, imaging is used to narrow the differential diagnosis, to follow up patients in which the diagnosis has been made, to detect complications, and to monitor response to therapy.

3.3.1 Fatty liver

Hepatic steatosis or fatty changes is an acquired, reversible disorder of metabolism and can result from a variety of pathologic processes including increased production or mobilization of fatty acids (e.g., hyperalimentation, starvation, obesity, steroid use, diabetes mellitus, and gastrointestinal bypass surgery) or decreased hepatic clearance of fatty acids from hepatocellular injury (e.g., alcoholic liver disease, hepatitis, drug-induced liver disease, and liver transplantation). The distribution of steatosis can be quite variable, ranging from focal to regional to diffuse. Histopathologically, the hallmark of all forms of fatty liver is the accumulation of fat globules within the hepatocytes. If accompanied by inflammation but not associated with alcohol abuse, the condition is called nonalcoholic steatohepatitis. Probably the most common cause of a fatty liver is obesity. Correction of the primary abnormality will usually reverse the process, although it is now recognized that fatty infiltration of the liver is the precursor for significant chronic disease in a percentage of patients.

Diffuse steatosis is common. It has been detected in up to 7% of abdominal CT examinations, and a relatively recent autopsy series found significant steatotic changes in 7% of nonobese patients and 29% of obese patients (El-Hassan et al., 1992; Wanless & Lentz, 1990). Generally, patients with steatosis are asymptomatic, although some individuals may present with abnormal liver function tests or right upper quadrant pain, the latter probably due to distention of Glisson's liver capsule from hepatomegaly. In patients with pure hepatic steatosis without coexistent hepatocytic injury, weight reduction or stopping the underlying etiologic factor usually reduces the amount of fatty change.

Sonography of fatty infiltration may be varied. Mild steatosis is detected when there is minimal diffuse increase in hepatic echogenicity with normal visualization of diaphragm and intrahepatic vessels (Fig.21A). Moderate steatosis is seen as moderate increase in hepatic echogenicity with slightly impaired visualization of intrahepatic vessels and diaphragm (Fig.21B). Severe steatosis is diagnosed when there is marked increase in echogenicity with poor penetration of the posterior segment of the right lobe of the liver and poor or nonvisualization of hepatic vessels and diaphragm (Fig.21C-D), the so-called bright liver on ultrasound (Taylor et al., 1986). Significant findings include hepatomegaly, decreased sonographic visualization of portal and hepatic veins and an unusual "fine" liver texture (Zwibel, 1995;).

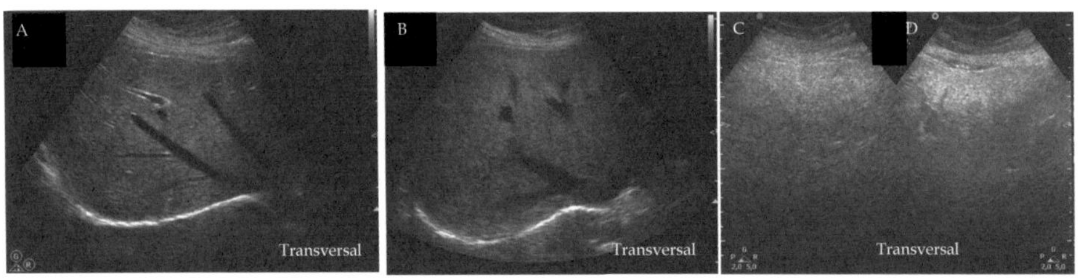

Fig. 21. Diffuse steatosis: [A] Mild steatosis: minimal diffuse increase in hepatic echogenicity with normal visualization of diaphragm and intrahepatic vessels; [B]Moderate steatosis: moderate increase in hepatic echogenicity with slightly impaired visualization of intrahepatic vessels and diaphragm; [C-D] Severe steatosis: marked increase in hepatic echogenicity with nonvisualization of hepatic vessels and diaphragm.

3.3.2 Focal steatosis and focal sparing

Hepatic fatty change is not always uniform but can present as a focal or regional area of steatosis in an otherwise normal liver (focal steatosis) or as subtotal fatty change with sparing of certain areas (focal sparing) (Baker et al., 1985). Both processes are common and may cause considerable diagnostic confusion, especially in the workout of primary or metastatic malignant liver disease (Baker et al., 1985). Aberrant blood supply to those areas has been demonstrated to be the underlying etiology for nonuniform change (Arai et al., 1988). In individuals with focal fatty sparing, it is assumed that the spared regions do not have a normal portal blood supply and therefore do not receive lipid-rich blood from the gut. Because of their underlying vascular aberrance, most of these spared areas have a characteristic location. For example, focal fatty sparing of the medial segment of the left liver lobe results from blood supply through the gastric veins, whereas aberrant blood supply from the internal thoracic artery has been established in some lesions around the falciform ligament (Matsui et al., 1995). Other characteristic locations include areas adjacent to the gallbladder fossa, the subcapsular region, and the porta hepatis. Islands of normal liver parenchyma may appear as hypoechoic masses within a dense, fatty infiltrated liver (Fig.22).

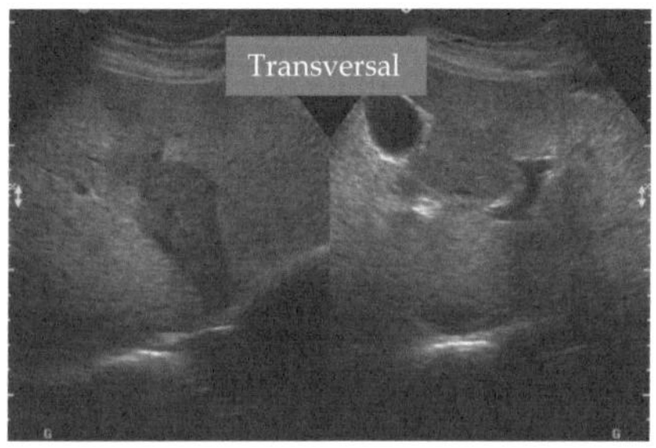

Fig. 22. Multifocal steatosis: multifocal increase in echogenicity of the liver parenchyma, sparing the segment IV that appears hypoechoic.

Less clear is why the same areas that can present as focal fatty sparing also have focal fatty infiltration. It is hypothesized that decreased delivery of unknown substances from the portal vein and relative ischemia from the paucity of portal blood supply are the main causative factors. In focal fatty infiltration, regions of increased echogenicity are present within a background of normal liver parenchyma and may present as a pseudonodular lesion (Fig.23). On imaging, several observational clues assist with correct identification of focal fatty change or focal spared areas:

1) typical periligamentous and periportal location,
2) lack of mass effect,
3) sharply angulated boundaries,
4) nonspherical shape,
5) absence of vascular displacement or distortion, and
6) lobar or segmental distribution.

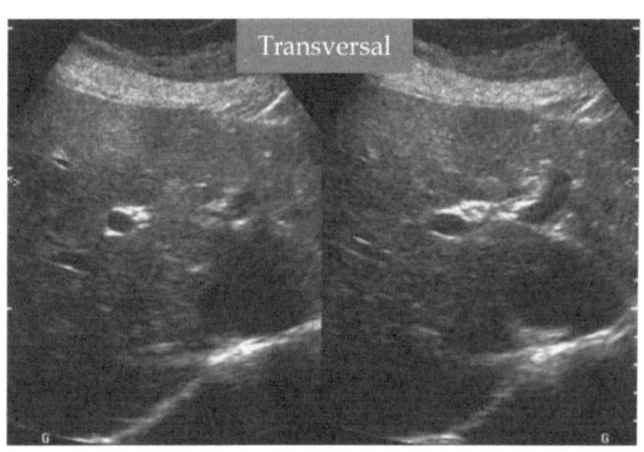

Fig. 23. Pseudonodular steatosis: Echogenic nodule (white arrow) in segment IVB anterior to the bifurcation of the portal vein that was confirmed to be a focal nodular steatosis in the MRI exam.

3.3.3 Cirrhosis

Cirrhosis is defined by the World Health Organization (WHO) as a diffuse process characterized by fibrosis and the conversion of normal liver architecture into structurally abnormal nodules. Liver cirrhosis is caused by diffuse fibrosis and regenerating nodules that result from liver cell necrosis and degeneration. It is characterized by architectural distortion and the development of a spectrum of nodules, ranging from benign regenerating nodules to HCC (Brown et al., 1997). In cirrhosis, in its early stages, the liver may appear normal. With progression of the disease, nodularity of the liver surface and generalized heterogeneity of the hepatic parenchyma can be seen. The porta hepatis and interlobar fissure frequently appear widened due to shrinkage of the right lobe and the medial segment of the left lobe, with concomitant enlargement of the caudate lobe and the lateral segment of the left lobe. The gross morphologic appearance of the cirrhotic liver is categorized by the size of the parenchymal nodules: micronodular, macronodular, or mixed. Micronodular cirrhosis is characterized by regenerative nodules of relatively uniform small size, ranging from 0.1 to 1.0 cm in diameter. This pattern is most commonly seen in chronic alcoholic cirrhosis. In macronodular cirrhosis, the parenchymal nodules are larger, coarser, and more variable in size, up to 5.0 cm in diameter. The most common cause of macronodular cirrhosis is chronic viral hepatitis.

The sonographic patterns associated with cirrhosis are:

1. Volume redistribution - In the early stages of cirrhosis, the liver may be enlarged, whereas in the advanced stages, the liver is often small, with relative enlargement of the caudate and the left lobe, and reduction of the size of the right lobe (Fig.24A). A ratio of caudate lobe to right lobe can be derived from a transverse scan of the liver immediately below the portal vein bifurcation: this is less than 0.6 in normal subject and greater than 0.65 in cirrhosis, with 100% specificity but sensitivities of 84% and 43% in two different series (Giorgio et al., 1986; Harbin et al., 1980);
2. Coarse echotexture - Increased echogenicity and coarse echotexture are frequent observations in diffuse liver disease (Fig.24B);
3. Nodular surface - Irregularity of the liver surface (Fig.24C);
4. Regenerative and dysplastic nodules - Regenerative nodules tend to be isoechoic or hypoechoic with a thin echogenic border. They may give a generalized granularity to the liver echotexture in forms of micronodular cirrhosis (Fig.24D). The larger nodules of macronodular disease may give an ultrasonically recognizable surface nodularity. Dysplastic nodules are considered premalignant.

Other ultrasound findings in cirrhosis are related to the complications associated with hepatocellular failure and portal hypertension: these include ascites, splenomegaly, the development of collateral venous channels and other abnormalities of the portal venous system.

3.4 Portal hypertension

Portal hypertension develops when increased resistance to portal flow and/or increased portal blood flow occur. Normal portal vein pressure is 5 to 10 mm Hg (14cm H2O). Portal hypertension is defined by a wedged hepatic vein pressure or direct portal vein pressure of more than 5 mm Hg greater than inferior vena cava pressure, splenic vein pressure of greater than 15 mm Hg, or portal vein pressure of greater than 30 cm H2O. They result in enlargement of the extrahepatic portal vessels, the development of spontaneous portosystemic collaterals and slow portal vein flow. Portal hypertension can be classified in

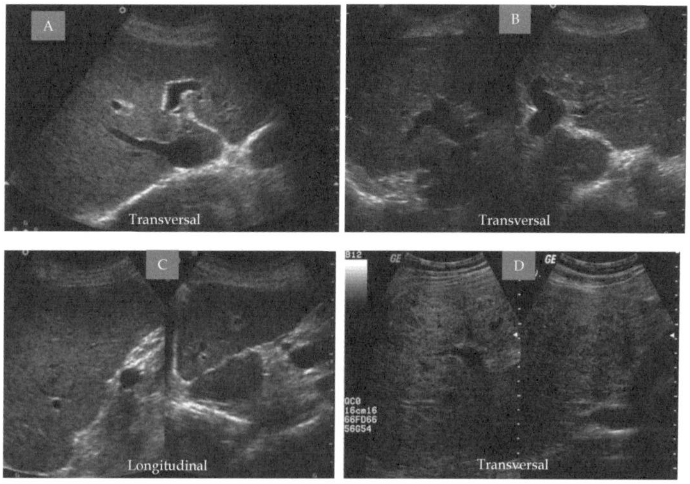

Fig. 24. Cirrhosis: [A] Volume redistribution with enlargement of the left and caudate lobes; [B] Volume redistribution with coarse echotexture; [C] Longitudinal scans showing lobulated contour; [D] Multiple small hypoechoic nodules along the entire liver parenchyma (regenerative).

several ways. We find that the easiest method is to divide it into intrahepatic, extrahepatic, and hyperdynamic. Extrahepatic portal hypertension can be subdivided into prehepatic (portal vein thrombosis, compression, and stenosis) and posthepatic (hepatic vein or inferior vena cava [IVC] thrombosis, compression, or stenosis). The extrahepatic presinusoidal portal hypertension should be suspected in any patient who presents with clinical signs of portal hypertension - ascites, splenomegaly and varices - and a normal liver biopsy. Thrombosis of the portal venous system occurs in children secondary to umbilical vein catheterization, omphalitis and neonatal sepsis. In adults, the causes of portal vein thrombosis include trauma, sepsis, HCC, pancreatic carcinoma, pancreatitis, portacaval shunts, splenomegaly and hypercoagulable states. Hyperdynamic refers to conditions that cause arterial portal fistulas or arteriovenous malformations. Extrahepatic portal hypertension and hyperdynamic portal hypertension are much less common than the intrahepatic category. Intrahepatic portal hypertension is subdivided into presinusoidal and postsinusoidal. The intrahepatic presinusoidal causes of portal hypertension include hepatic fibrosis, sarcoidosis, schistosomiasis, and lymphoma. Postsinusoidal includes cirrhosis and venoocclusive disease (Ralls, 1990).

Cirrhosis is the most common cause of intrahepatic portal hypertension. It causes hepatocellular death and parenchymal degeneration and regeneration. This results in bridging fibrosis that affects the central venules that drain the sinusoids, as well as the sinusoids themselves. The fibrosis causes increased resistance to blood flow. Initially, portal vein flow volume is maintained, but at a higher portal pressure. As the process progresses, the resistance to inflow in the liver equalizes with resistance to flow in portosystemic collaterals. At this point, portal flow starts to be diverted into the collaterals. As portal inflow to the liver decreases, hepatic arterial flow increases, and the arteries become larger and more tortuous. Eventually, resistance to arterial inflow reaches a point where arterial flow starts to shunt into the portal vein system. This initially produces portal vein flow reversal in isolated peripheral portal vein branches. But as more and more peripheral

branches reverse, flow in the major branches and eventually the main portal vein reverses (Ralls, 1990).
There are several sonographic findings of portal hypertension. Dilatations of the portal, mesenteric and splenic veins are all potential indicators of elevated pressures. Weinreb (1982) found 13 mm as the cutoff for upper limit of normal portal vein diameter. In general, an unusually large portal vein is a good sign of portal hypertension, but a normal size portal vein certainly does not exclude the diagnosis. Lack of caliber variation of the splenic and mesenteric vein during respiration is another parameter that has been investigated. This approach had a sensitivity of 80% and specificity of 100% in diagnosing portal hypertension (Bolondi et al., 1982).
A variety of Doppler techniques have been used to evaluate patients with suspected portal hypertension. Simple measurements of portal vein velocity are one such approach. Zirone et al. (1992) found a sensitivity of 88% and a specificity of 96% using a mean portal vein velocity cutoff of 15 cm/sec. Although there is general agreement that portal vein velocities usually decrease with portal hypertension, the expected values in control subjects and cirrhotic patients vary considerably. Mean portal venous flow velocity is approximately 15 to 18 cm/sec. Sources of variability include interobserver variability, intermachine variability, presence of variable collateral pathways (especially recanalized umbilical veins), and variations caused by differences in patient positioning, different phases of respiration, states of fasting, exercise status and cardiac output. These variations probably also account for the fact that portal velocities tend to decrease as portal pressures increase, but the correlation is not statistically significant (Choi et al., 2003; Haag et al., 1999). As portal hypertension develops, the flow in the portal vein loses its ondulatory pattern and becomes monophasic (Fig.25A-B). As the severity of portal hypertension increases, flow becomes biphasic and finally hepatofugal (Fig.25C). The ratio of portal vein cross-sectional area and portal velocity has been called the congestion index and has also been used to diagnose portal hypertension. Moriyasu et al. (1986) described this index based on the assumption that portal vein cross-sectional area will increase and the portal velocity will decrease in the setting of portal hypertension, resulting in a quotient that increases dramatically. In this study, it was shown that the congestion index was 2.5 times higher in patients with cirrhosis and portal hypertension than in control subjects. Normal values were described to be up to 0.099 cm x sec. The sensitivity of congestion index measurements ranges from 67% to 95% (Haag et al., 1999; Moriyasu et al., 1986).

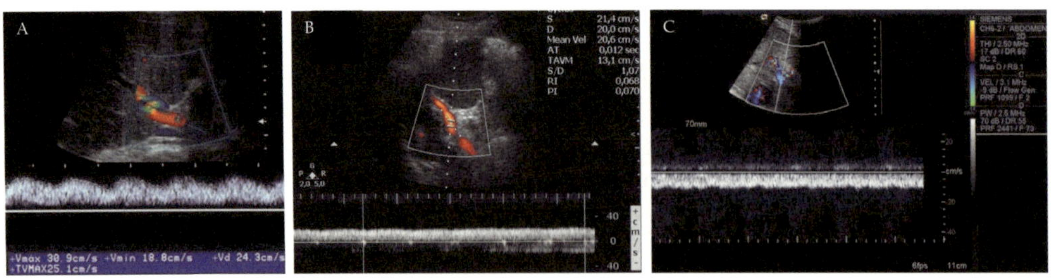

Fig. 25. Portal vein flow: [A] Ondulatory normal pattern; [B] Loss of ondulatory flow, mantaining the normal hepatopetal flow; [C]Hepatofugal portal vein flow as seen with the blue color inside the vein and the graphs below the baseline.

Alterations in the hepatic venous waveform can also occur with cirrhosis and portal hypertension. In general, the normal pulsatility of hepatic veins is either blunted or completely eliminated in patients with cirrhosis (Fig.26A-C). In fact, complete loss of any pulsatility has been shown to correlate with a higher Child-Pugh score and decreased survival rate (Ohta et al., 1995). The mechanism for this loss of hepatic vein pulsatility is unclear, but is likely related to hepatic vein loss of compliance due to hepatic fibrosis or stenosis, which can be caused by impression on the hepatic veins by regenerating nodules (Lorenz & Winsberg, 1996).

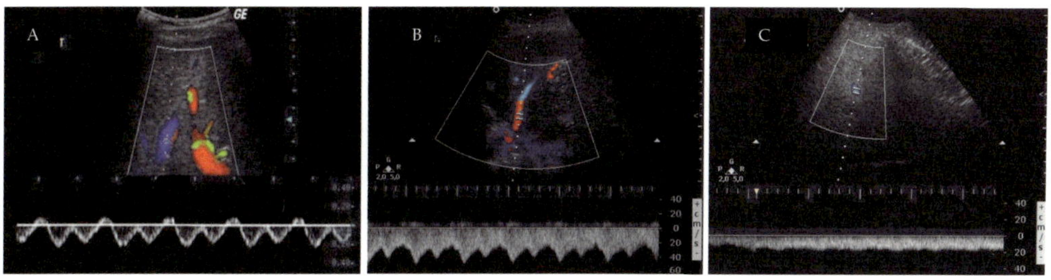

Fig. 26. Hepatic vein flow: [A] Normal triphasic flow; [B] Biphasic flow; [C] Monophasic (portalized) flow.

Although measurement of vessel diameters and velocities and calculation of various indices have shown promise in certain studies, the most reliable and widely used approach for the diagnosis of portal hypertension is the detection of portal systemic collaterals. The left gastric vein is the most prevalent portal systemic collateral present in 80% to 90% of patients with portal hypertension (Burcharth, 1979; Nunez et al., 1978) and its presence implies an increased risk for variceal hemorrhage. Sonographically, the left gastric vein is identified as a vessel communicating with the superior aspect of the portal or splenic vein in the region of the confluence (Fig. 27). The left lobe of the liver serves as an acoustic window, and when the left lobe is small, it may be difficult to visualize this vein. It extends superiorly and to the left and typically travels immediately anterior to the bifurcation of the celiac axis. The upper limit of normal for the vein diameter is 5 to 6 mm (Lafortune et al., 1984; Wachsberg & Simmons, 1994). Unfortunately, dilatation of the left gastric vein above a diameter of 6 mm occurs in only 25% of patients with portal hypertension, and it is not necessarily present for variceal hemorrhage to occur (Wachsberg & Simmons, 1994). On the other hand, the left gastric collateral was the only portal systemic collateral visualized in approximately 75% of patients. Other tributaries of the portal system can function as portal systemic collaterals and include short gastric veins and branches of the superior and inferior mesenteric veins. Identification of hepatofugal flow in any of these vessels is adequate to establish the diagnosis of portal hypertension.

Normally, the umbilical vein is an obliterated fibrous remnant that runs in the ligamentum teres. It can be identified in some patients as a hypoechoic band running within the fat of the ligamentum teres. It extends from the umbilicus to the most anterior aspect of the umbilical segment of the left portal vein. In individuals with no portal hypertension, no flow is present in the obliterated umbilical vein, and the fibrous remnant measures less than 3 mm (Gibson et al., 1989). In the setting of portal hypertension, the umbilical vein recanalizes and develops hepatofugal flow. The recanalized umbilical vein is best seen by scanning the left lobe of the liver and identifying the umbilical segment of the left portal vein. The umbilical vein itself travels inferiorly from the umbilical segment of the left portal vein and exits the liver where it extends inferiorly along the abdominal wall to the umbilical area (Fig.28A-B). From there, it extends further inferiorly to communicate with the inferior epigastric veins. Ultimately, it communicates with the iliofemoral system and in this way diverts blood back to the systemic circulation. Although these 2 collaterals are the easiest and most productive to analyze, there are other collaterals that can be detected sonographically, albeit with more difficulty in some cases. These include short gastric, splenorenal, splenoretroperitoneal, superior mesenteric, and inferior mesenteric collaterals.

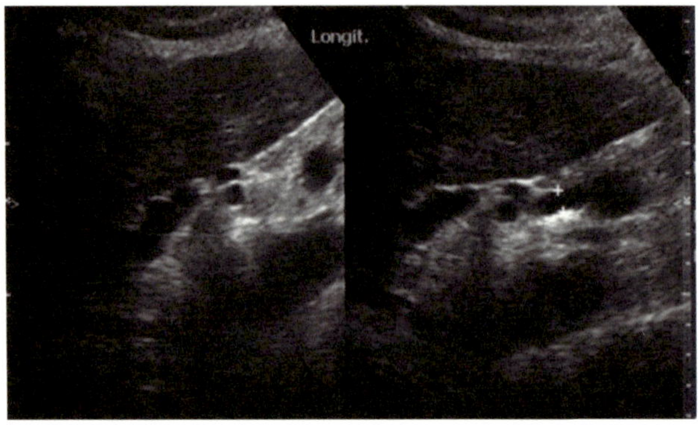

Fig. 27. Left gastric vein: Dilated left gastric vein in a longitudinal scan below the left lobe of the liver.

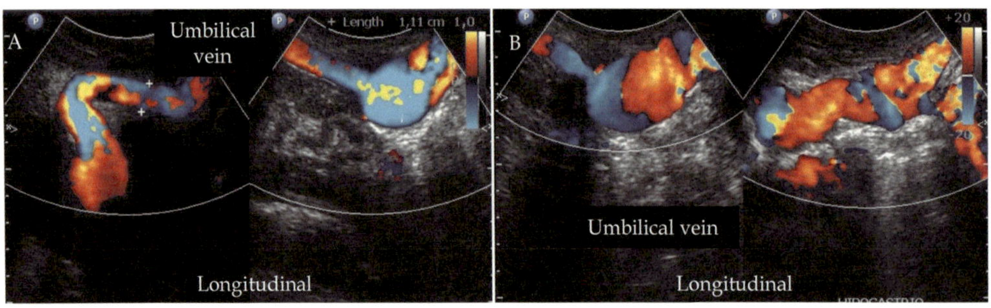

Fig. 28. Umbilical vein: [A-B] Recanalized umbilical vein from the falciform ligament to the anterior abdominal wall in the umbilical area going down to the hypogastrium.

Splenorenal collaterals are large spontaneous porto-systemic shunts from the splenic hilum or capsule to the left renal vein. It is often difficult to trace these collaterals from the splenic vein to the renal vein in continuity. Many times, the detection of multiple collaterals around the splenic hilum and an enlarged left renal vein is enough to make the presumptive diagnosis of a splenorenal collateral (Fig.29A-B). Splenoretroperitoneal collaterals may communicate with perivertebral vessels or gonadal vessels. Superior mesenteric collaterals communicate with pancreaticoduodenal veins and retroperitoneal/perivertebral veins. Inferior mesenteric collaterals communicate with retroperitoneal veins and hemorrhoidal veins. As mentioned earlier, as portal hypertension progresses, flow reversal occurs in isolated peripheral portal vein branches (Ralls, 1990; Wachsberg et al., 2002). It is very important to realize that most patients with portal hypertension maintain antegrade flow in the main portal vein. In addition to reversed flow, slow flow that alternates between antegrade and retrograde is another sign of portal hypertension.

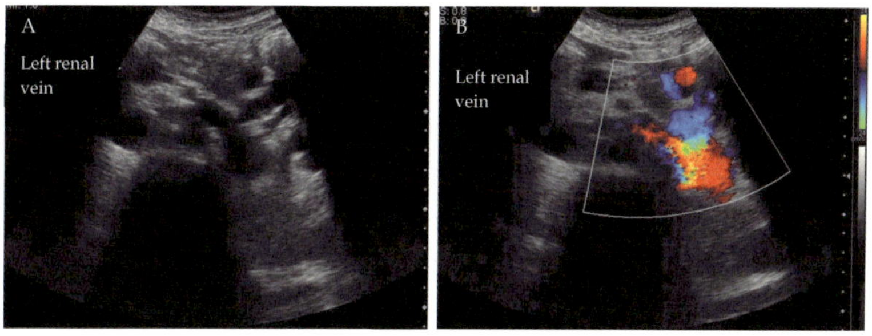

Fig. 29. Splenorenal shunt: [A] Dilated left renal vein; [B] Splenorenal shunt: splenic flow in blue going to the renal vein in red.

Portal vein thrombosis has been associated with chronic hepatitis, hepatocellular carcinoma, metastatic liver disease, carcinoma of the pancreas, chronic pancreatitis, septicemia, trauma, splenectomy, portocaval shunts and hypercoagulable states. Sonographic findings of portal vein thrombosis is best visualized in B-mode image and confirmed with color Doppler and include echogenic thrombus within the lumen of the vein, portal vein collaterals, expansion of the caliber of the vein and cavernous transformations. Cavernous transformation of the portal vein refers to numerous wormlike vessels at the porta hepatis, which represent periportal collateral circulation. Acute thrombus may appear relatively anechoic and may be overlooked unless Doppler interrogation is performed. Malignant thrombosis of the portal vein has a high association with HCC and is often expansive. Doppler sonography is useful in distinguishing between benign and malignant portal vein thrombi in patients with cirrhosis. Both benign and malignant thrombi may demonstrate continuous blood flow. Pulsatile arterial flow has been found to be 95% specific for the diagnosis of malignant portal vein thrombosis (Fig.18F). The sensitivity was only 62% because many malignant thrombi can be hypovascular (Dodd et al., 1995).

The normal hepatic artery in a fasting patient has a low resistance Doppler flow profile with an expected RI ranging from 0.55 to 0.7 (Fig.30A). During systole, the velocity is approximately 30-60 cm/sec; while during diastole, it normally slows to approximately 10-20 cm/sec, which is normally less than the velocity of the portal vein flow. The systolic acceleration time is typically less than 0.07 s. Liver disease may manifest in the hepatic artery as abnormally elevated (RI >0.7) or decreased (RI <0.55) resistance. High resistance is a nonspecific finding that may be seen in the postprandial state, patients of advanced age, and diffuse peripheral microvascular compression or disease, as seen in chronic hepatocellular disease including cirrhosis, hepatic venous congestion, cold ischemia (posttransplantation) and any stage of transplant rejection (Martínez-Noguera et al., 2002). The effect of cirrhosis on hepatic arterial microcirculation is complex and variable. Arterial resistance has been shown to be decreased, normal, or increased in cirrhotic patients (Vassiliades et al., 1993). Some aspects of the disease process, such as inflammatory edema, arterial compression by regenerative nodules and arterial compression by stiff noncompliant (fibrotic) parenchyma, have been thought to increase resistance (Fig.30B) (Alpern et al., 1987; Sacerdoti et al., 1995). Other aspects, such as the "hepatic arterial buffer response" (compensatory small artery proliferation and increased numbers of arteriolar beds) and arteriovenous shunting, are thought to decrease resistance (Lautt & Greenway, 1987). The overall balance of these factors presumably dictates the observed resistance, and it has been shown that hepatic arterial RI is not useful for diagnosing cirrhosis or predicting its severity (Lim et al., 2005; Vassiliades et al., 1993). It is important to compare the resistive indexes to those from prior examinations of the same patient.

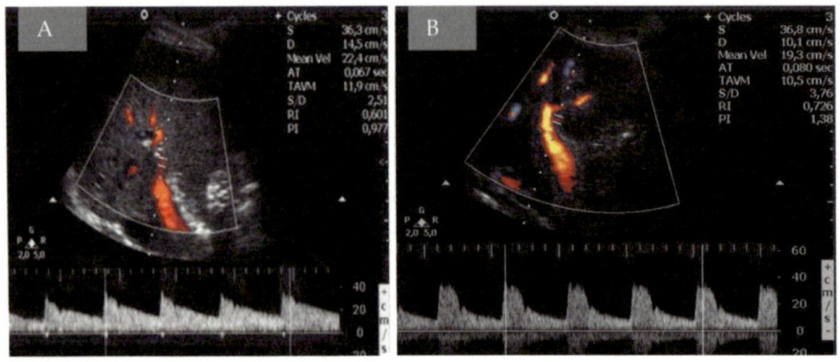

Fig. 30. HEPATIC ARTERY: [A] Normal low resistance flow in hepatic artery; [B] High resistance flow seen in the hepatic artery of the cirrhotic patient.

3.5 Liver transplantation

Liver transplantation has rapidly advanced from an experimental therapy to a mainstream treatment option for a wide range of acute and chronic liver diseases. Indications for liver transplant have evolved to include previously contraindicated conditions such as hepatocellular carcinoma and alcohol-related liver disease. Cirrhosis from chronic hepatitis C infection remains the most common indication today. The progressive improvement in survival from liver transplantation over the past few years has been due to a combination of factors, including better patient selection, improved organ preservation, developments in surgical technique, modern immunosuppressive agents and improved postoperative management. Overall posttransplant outcomes have steadily improved, with unadjusted 5-year patient survival rates of 77% among patients transplanted with MELD (Model for End-Stage Liver Disease) score between 15 and 20, and 72% for those with MELD scores between 21 and 30 (Merion, 2010). Ultrasound plays an important role in patient selection and management, being used in the pre-operative, operative and postoperative periods.

4. Conclusion

In conclusion, US imaging is an ideal complementary diagnostic tool to evaluate the liver from bench to bedside. Hepatic US can examine the internal architecture of the liver parenchyma, biliary system, portal and hepatic vascular supply. US can be regarded as a noninvasive method valid for follow-up studies of experimental hepatic diseases in rodents for pre-clinical drug or cell based therapy. Also, is the test of choice for assessment and follow-up of patients with suspected diffuse or focal hepatic disease, portal hypertension and screening for vascular and biliary complications following liver transplantation.

5. References

Alpern, M.B.; Rubin, J.M.; Williams, D.M. & Capek, P. (1987). Porta hepatis: duplex Doppler US with angiographic correlation. *Radiology,* Vol. 162, (January 1987), pp. 53–56.

Arai, K.; Matsui, O.; Takashima, T.; Ida, M. & Nishida, Y. (1988). Focal spared areas in fatty liver caused by regional decreased portal flow. *AJR American Journal of Roentgenology*, Vol. 151, No. 2, (August 1988), pp. 300–302.

Baker, M.K.; Wenker, J.C.; Cockerill, E.M. & Ellis, J.H. (1985). Focal fatty infiltration of the liver: diagnostic imaging. *Radiographics*, Vol. 5, No. 6, (November 1985); pp. 923–929.

Biller, D.S.; Kantrowitz, B. & Miyabayashi, T. (1992). Ultrasonography of diffuse liver disease. A review. *Journal of Veterinary Internal Medicine*, Vol. 6, No. 2, (March-April 1992), pp. 71-76.

Bolondi, L.; Gandolfi, L.; Arienti, V.; Caletti, G.C.; Corcioni, E.; Gasbarrini, G. & Labò, G. (1982). Ultrasonography in the diagnosis of portal hypertension: diminished response of portal vessels to respiration. *Radiology*, Vol. 142, No. 1, (January 1982), pp. 167-172.

Bolondi, L.; Sofia, S.; Siringo, S.; Gaiani, S.; Casali, A.; Zironi, G.; Piscaglia, F.; Gramantieri, L.; Zanetti, M. & Sherman, M. (2001). Surveillance programme of cirrhotic patients for early diagnosis and treatment of hepatocellular carcinoma: a cost effectiveness analysis. *Gut*, Vol. 48, No. 2, (February 2001), pp. 251-259.

Brown, J.J.; Naylor, M.J. & Yagan, N. (1997). Imaging of hepatic cirrhosis. *Radiology*, Vol. 202, No. 1, (January 1997), pp. 1–16.

Burcharth, F. (1979). Percutaneous transhepatic portography. Technique and application. *AJR American Journal of Roentgenology*, Vol. 132, No. 2, (February 1979), pp. 177-182.

Caturelli, E.; Pompili, M.; Bartolucci, F.; Siena, D.A.; Sperandeo, M.; Andriulli, A.; Bisceglia, M. (2001). Hemangioma-like lesions in chronic liver disease: Diagnostic evaluation in patients. *Radiology*, Vol. 220, No. 2, (August 2001), pp. 337-342.

Choi, Y.J.; Baik, S.K.; Park, D.H.; Kim, M.Y.; Kim, H.S.; Lee, D.K.; Kwon, S.O.; Kim, Y.J. & Park, J.W. (2003). Comparison of Doppler ultrasonography and the hepatic venous pressure gradient in assessing portal hypertension in liver cirrhosis. *Journal of Gastroenterology and Hepatolology*, Vol. 18, No. 4, (April 2003), pp. 424-429.

Dias, J.V.; Paredes, B.D.; Mesquita, L.F.Q.; Carvalho, A.B.; Koslowski, E.O.; Lessa, A.S.; Takiya, C.M.; Resende, C.M.C.; Coelho, H.S.M.; Campos-de-Carvalho, A.C.; Rezende, G.F.M. & Goldenberg, R.C.S. (2008). An ultrasound and histomorphological analysis of experimental liver cirrhosis in rats. *Brazilian Journal of Medical and Biological Research*, Vol. 41, No. 11, (November 2008), pp. 992-999, ISSN 0100-879X.

Dodd, G.D.; Memel, O.S.; Baron, R.L.; Eichner, L. & Santiguida, L.A. (1995). Portal vein thrombosis in patients with cirrhosis. Does sonographic detection of intrathrombus flow allow differentiation of benign and malignant thrombus? *AJR American Journal of Roentgenology*, Vol. 165, No. 3, (September 1995), pp. 573-577.

Edmonson, H.A. & Craig, J.R. (1987). Neoplasms of the liver, In: *Diseases of the Liver*, L. Shiff & E.R. Shiff, (Eds.), 1147-1150, Lippincott, Philadelphia, USA.

El-Hassan, A.Y.; Ibrahim, E.M.; Al-Mulhim, F.A.; Nabhan, A.A. & Chammas, M.Y. (1992). Fatty infiltration of the liver: analysis of prevalence, radiological and clinical features and influence on patient management. *British Journal of Radiology*, Vol. 65, No.777 , (September 1992), pp.774-778.

Gibson, R.N.; Gibson, P.R.; Donlan, J.D. & Clunie, D.A. (1989). Identification of a patent paraumbilical vein by using Doppler sonography: importance in diagnosis of portal hypertension. *AJR American Journal of Roentgenology*, Vol. 153, No. 3, (September 1989), pp. 513-516.

Giorgio, A.; Amoroso, P.; Lettieri, G.; Fico, P.; De Stefano, G.; Finelli, L.; Scala, V.; Tarantino, L.; Pierri, P. & Pesce, G. (1986). Cirrhosis: value of caudate to right lobe ratio in diagnosis with US. *Radiology*, Vol. 161, No. 2, (November 1986), pp. 443-445.

Haag, K.; Rossle, M.; Ochs, A.; Huber, M.; Siegerstetter, V.; Olschewski, M.; Berger, E.; Lu, S. & Blum, H.E. (1999). Correlation of duplex sonography findings and portal pressure in 375 patients with portal hypertension. *AJR American Journal of Roentgenology*, Vol. 172, No. 3, March 1999), pp. 631-635.

Harbin, W.P.; Robert, N.J. & Ferrucci, J.T. (1980). Diagnosis of cirrhosis based on regional changes in hepatic morphology: a radiological and pathological analysis. *Radiology*, Vol. 135, No. 2, (May 1980), pp. 273-83.

Lafortune, M.; Marleau, D.; Breton, G.; Viallet, A.; Lavoie, P. & Huet, P.M. (1984). The portal venous system measurements in portal hypertension. *Radiology*, Vol. 151, No. 1, (April 1984), pp. 27-30.

Lautt, W.W. & Greenway, C.V. (1987). Conceptual review of the hepatic vascular bed. *Hepatology*, Vol. 7, No. 5, (September-October 1987), pp. 952–963.

Lee, G.P.; Jeong, W.I.; Jeong, D.H.; Do, S.H.; Kim, T.H. & Jeong, K.S. (2005). Diagnostic evaluation of carbon tetrachloride-induced rat hepatic cirrhosis model. *Anticancer Research*, Vol. 25, No. 2A, (March/April 2005), pp.1029-38.

Lessa, A.S.; Rezende, G.F.M. & Resende, C.M. (2008). Ultra-sonografia na avaliação de um modelo experimental de esteatose e cirrose em ratos Wistar. *Radiologia Brasileira*, Vol. 41, No. 2, (March/April 2008), pp. 98.

Lessa, A.S.; Paredes, B.D.; Dias, J.V.; Carvalho, A.B.; Quintanilha, L.F.; Takiya, C.M.; Tura, B.R.; Rezende, G.F.M.; Campos de Carvalho, A.C.; Resende, C.M. & Goldenberg, R.C. (2010). Ultrasound imaging in an experimental model of fatty liver disease and cirrhosis in rats. *BMC Veterinary Research*, Vol. 6, (January 2010), pp. 1-10. Available from: http://www.biomedcentral.com/1746-6148/6/6

Levine, E.; Cook, L.T. & Granthem, J.J. (1985). Liver cysts in autosomal-dominant polycystic kidney disease. Clinical and computed tomographic study. *AJR American Journal of Roentgenology*, Vol. 145, No. 2, (August 1985), pp. 229-233.

Lewall, D.B. & McCorkell, S.J. (1985). Hepatic echinococcal cysts: Sonographic appearance and classification. *Radiology*, Vol. 155, No. 3, (June 1985), pp. 773-775.

Lima, V.M.; Oliveira, C.P.; Alves, V.A.; Chammas, M.C.; Oliveira, E.P.; Stefano, J.T. Mello, E.S.; Cerri, G.G.; Carrilho, F.J. & Caldwell, S.H.J. (2008). A rodent model of NASH with cirrhosis, oval cell proliferation and hepatocellular carcinoma. *Hepatology*, Vol. 49, No. 6, (December 2008), pp. 1055-1061.

Lim, A.K.; Patel, N.; Eckersley, R.J.; Kuo, Y.T.; Goldin, R.D.; Thomas, H.C.; Cosgrove, D.O.; Taylor-Robinson, S.D. & Blomley, M.J. (2005). Can Doppler sonography grade the severity of hepatitis C-related liver disease? *AJR American Journal of Roentgenology*, Vol. 186, No. 6, (June 2005), pp. 1848–1853.

Lorenz, J. & Winsberg, F. (1996). Focal hepatic vein stenoses in diffuse liver disease. *Journal of Ultrasound in Medicine*, Vol. 15, No. 4, (April 1996), pp. 313-316.

Mannheimer, E.G.; Quintanilha, L.F.; Carvalho, A.B.; Paredes, B.D.; Carvalho, F.G.; Takyia, C.M.; Resende, C.M.; Rezende, G.F.M.; Campos-de-Carvalho, A.C., Schanaider, A. & Goldenberg, R.C.S. (2011). Bone marrow cells obtained from cirrhotic rats do not improve function or reduce fibrosis in a chronic liver disease model. *Clinical Transplantation*, Vol. 25, No. 1, (January 2011), pp. 54-60.

Martínez-Noguera, A.; Montserrat, E.; Torrubia, S. & Villalba, J. (2002). Doppler in hepatic cirrhosis and chronic hepatitis. *Seminars in Ultrasound, CT, and MR*, Vol. 23, No. 1, (February 2002), pp. 19–36.

Matsui, O.; Kadoya, M.; Takahashi, S.; Yoshikawa ,J.; Gabata, T.; Takashima, T. & Kitagawa, K. (1995). Focal sparing of segment IV in fatty livers shown by sonography and CT: correlation with aberrant gastric venous drainage. *AJR American Journal of Roentgenology*, Vol. 164, No. 5, (May 1995), pp. 1137–1140.

Merion, R.M. (2010). Current Status and Future of Liver Transplantation. *Seminars in Liver Disease*, Vol. 30, No. 4, (November 2010), pp. 411-421.

Moriyasu, F.; Nishida, O.; Ban, N.; Nakamura, T.; Sakai, M.; Miyake, T. & Uchino, H. (1986). Congestion index of the portal vein. *AJR American Journal of Roentgenology*, Vol. 146, No. 4, (April 1986), pp. 735-739.

Nunez, D. Jr; Russell, E.; Yrizarry, J.; Pereiras, R. & Viamonte, M. Jr. (1978). Portosystemic communications studied by transhepatic portography. *Radiology*, Vol. 127, No. 1, (April 1978), pp. 75-79.

Ohta, M.; Hashizume, M.; Kawanaka, H.; Akazawa, K.; Tomikawa, M.; Higashi, H.; Kishihara, F.; Tanoue, K. & Sugimachi, K. (1995). Prognostic significance of hepatic vein waveform by Doppler ultrasonography in cirrhotic patients with portal hypertension. *American Journal of Gastroenterology*, Vol. 90, No. 10, (October 1995), pp. 1853-1857.

Palmentieri, B.; De Sio, I.; La Mura, V.; Masarone, M.; Vecchione, R.; Bruno, S.; Torella, R. & Persico, M. (2006). The role of bright liver echo pattern on ultrasound B-mode examination in the diagnosis of liver steatosis. *Digestive and Liver Disease*, Vol. 38, No. 7, (July 2006), pp. 485-489.

Parkin, D.M.; Bray, F.; Ferlay, J. & Pisani, P. (2005). Global cancer statistics, 2002. *CA: A Cancer Journal for Clinicians*, Vol. 55, No. 2, (March-April 2005), pp. 74–108.

Partington, B.P. & Biller, D.S. (1995). Hepatic Imaging with radiology and ultrasound. *Veterinary Clinics of North America: Small Animal Practice*, Vol. 25, No. 2, (March 1995), pp. 305-335.

Ralls, P.W.; Barnes, P.F.; Radin, D.R.; Colletti, P. & Halls, J. (1987). Sonographic features of amebic and pyogenic liver abscesses: A blinded comparison. *AJR American Journal of Roentgenology*, Vol. 149, No. 3, (September 1987), pp. 499-501.

Ralls, P.W.; Barnes, P.F.; Johnson, M.B., De Cock, K.M.; Radin, D.R. & Halls, J. (1987). Medical treatment of hepatic amebic abscess: Rare need for percutaneous drainage. *Radiology*, Vol. 165, No. 3, (December 1987), p. 805-807.

Ralls, P.W. (1990). Color Doppler sonography of the hepatic artery and portal venous system. *AJR American Journal of Roentgenology*, Vol. 155, No. 3, (September 1990), pp. 517-525.

Redston, M.S. & Wanless, I.R. (1996). The hepatic von Meyenburg complex: Prevalence and association with hepatic and renal cysts among 2843 autopsies. *Modern Pathology*, Vol. 9, No. 3, (March 1996), p. 233-237.

Sacerdoti, D.; Merkel, C.; Bolognesi, M.; Amodio, P.; Angeli, P. & Gatta, A. (1995). Hepatic arterial resistance in cirrhosis with and without portal vein thrombosis: relationships with portal hemodynamics. *Gastroenterology*, Vol. 108, No. 4, (April 1995), pp. 1152–1158.

Sangiovanni, A.; Del Ninno, E.; Fasani, P.; De Fazio, C.; Ronchi, G.; Romeo, R.; Morabito, A.; De Franchis, R.; Colombo, M. (2004). Increased survival of cirrhotic patients with a hepatocellular carcinoma detected during surveillance. *Gastroenterology*, Vol. 126, No. 4, (April 2004), pp. 1005-1014.

Snover, D.C. (2009). Non-neoplastic liver disease, In: *Sternberg's diagnostic surgical pathology*, E.C. Mills, D. Carter, J.K. Greeson, (Eds.), 1167-1191, Lippincott Williams & Wilkins, Philadelphia, USA.

Tanaka, S.; Kitamura, T.; Fujita, M.; Nakanishi, K. & Okuda, S. (1990). Color Doppler flow imaging of liver tumors. *AJR American Journal of Roentgenology*, Vol. 154, No. 3, (March 1990), pp. 509-514.

Taylor, K.J.W.; Riely, C.A.; Hammers, L.; Flax, S.; Weltin, G.; Garcia-Tsao, G.; Conn, H.O.; Kuc, R. & Barwick, K.W. (1986). Quantitative US attenuation in normal liver and in patients with diffuse liver disease: importance of fat. *Radiology*, Vol. 160, No. 1, (July 1986), pp. 65–71.

Vassiliades, V.G.; Ostrow, T.D.; Chezmar, J.L.; Hertzler, G.L. & Nelson RC. (1993). Hepatic arterial resistive indices: correlation with the severity of cirrhosis. *Abdominal Imaging*, Vol. 18, No. 1, (1993), pp. 61–65.

Wachsberg, R.H. & Simmons, M.Z. (1994). Coronary vein diameter and flow direction in patients with portal hypertension: evaluation with duplex sonography and correlation with variceal bleeding. *American Journal of Gastroenterology*, Vol. 162, No. 3, (March 1994), pp. 637-641.

Wachsberg, R.H.; Bahramipour, P.; Sofocleous, C.T. & Barone, A. (2002). Hepatofugal flow in the portal venous system: pathophysiology, imaging findings, and diagnostic pitfalls. *Radiographics*, Vol. 22, No. 1, (January-February 2002), pp. 123-140.

Wanless, I.R. & Lentz, J.S. (1990). Fatty liver hepatitis (steatohepatitis) and obesity: an autopsy study with analysis of risk factors. *Hepatology*, Vol. 12, No. 5, (November 1990), pp. 1106–1110.

Weinreb, J.; Kumari, S.; Phillips, G. & Pochaczevsky R. (1982). Portal vein measurements by real time sonography. *AJR American Journal of Roentgenology*, Vol. 139, No. 3, (September 1982), pp. 497-499.

Wernecke, K.; Vassallo, P.; Bick, U.; Diederich, S. & Peters, P.E. (1992). The distinction between benign and malignant liver tumors on sonography: Value of a hypoechoic halo. *AJR American Journal of Roentgenology*, Vol. 159, No. 5, (November 1992), pp. 1005-1009.

WHO: The World Health Report 2004 - changing history - deaths by cause, sex and mortality stratum in WHO regions, estimates for 2002, Published 2004, Accessed December 15 2010, Available from: http://www.who.int/whr/2004/annex/topic/en/annex_2_en.pdf.

Wilson, S.R. & Withers, C.E. (2005). The liver. In: *Diagnostic ultrasound*, C.R. Rumack, J.A. Wilson, J.W. Charboneau, (Eds.), 77-145, Elsevier Mosby, St Louis, USA.

Zironi, G.; Gaiani, S.; Fenyves, D.; Rigamonti, A.; Bolondi, L. & Barbara, L. (1992). Value of measurement of mean portal flow velocity by Doppler flowmetry in the diagnosis of portal hypertension. Journal of Hepatology, Vol. 16, No. 3, (November 1992), pp. 298-303.

Zwiebel, W.J. (1995). Sonographic diagnosis of diffuse liver disease. Seminars in Ultrasound, CT and MRI, Vol. 16, No. 1, (February 1995), pp. 8–15.

8

Techniques of Linear Endobronchial Ultrasound

Malay Sharma, Vishal Arya and CS RameshBabu
Jaswant Rai Speciality Hospital
Meerut, U.P.
India

1. Introduction

Endobronchial ultrasound (EBUS) visualizes structures within and adjacent to the airway (1). Most operators do not follow any standard positions of imaging during EBUS and use the computed tomography scan as a roadmap for imaging of the lymph nodes. A small window angle (50 to 75 degrees) in linear EBUS as compared with linear endoscopic US (130 to 180 degrees) makes visualization of the anatomic ultrasound landmarks difficult with EBUS. For better orientation, it is useful to recognize key anatomic landmarks and their relationship to the airways, apart from observing the position of the probe while performing EBUS. In this section we describe the mediastinal and parabronchial anatomy of different parts of the respiratory tract which is practically important during EBUS.

2. The ten commandments of imaging

2.1 Instrument and comparison of available scopes

Two types of scopes are available. Broadly the major difference is in the diameter and field of view. The diameter of pentax scope is larger than Olympus scope (7.4 mm vs 6.9 mm.) The field of vision and depth in imaging of the pentax scope is larger (field of vision 75° vs 50°, depth 5 cm vs approximately 2 cm)

2.2 Indication of EBUS

The main indications are evaluation of benign and malignant mediastinal lymphadenopathy. The role of linear EBUS for T staging of lung cancer is not yet defined. Limited assessment of M staging and loco regional spread of lung cancer is possible.

2.3 Alternative modalities of imaging and tissue sampling

Majority of lymph nodes can be seen by EBUS and EUS both while doing endoscopic imaging. The choice to do FNA by EBUS or EUS rest on the experience of the endosonographer. Some endosonographer are more experienced in EBUS while others are more experienced in EUS. However for persons who are experienced in both it may be difficult to choose between the two for FNAC if both are approachable.

2.4 Optimization of the imaging

a. The ultrasound waves are high frequency sound waves.

b. Ultrasound beam loses strength of the beam over time or distance travelled and the echoes that return from deeper structures are weak compared to those returning from the close structures. This phenomenon is called attenuation.
c. Attenuated waves need to be amplified before analysis. The echoes that come from deep within the body are more attenuated and need more amplification to make a smooth image. This is done by Time-Gain Compensation (TGC). The images thus amplified contain echoes of approximately equal strength from all the depths of tissue.
d. The waves make image. Images have resolution. The ability of the beam to differentiate two objects is called spatial resolution. Higher spatial resolution shows two points as separate while low spatial resolution shows them as a single blurred point.
e. Resolution has two main dimensions. Analysis along the length is called axial resolution, analysis along the breadth is called lateral resolution.
f. Axial resolution is determined by the frequency. Axial resolution is most important in determination of quality. High frequency shortens the pulse length and gives a better axial resolution. The frequency is inversely proportional to the penetration depth. At 5 M Hz ultrasound penetrates approximately 6 cm while at 10 M Hz the penetration field of ultrasound is about 3 cm.
g. Lateral resolution is determined by focal length. Lateral resolution differentiates between two points lying horizontal to the ultrasound beam. It is determined by the width of the Ultrasound beam. Changing focus of the beam to the level of investigation gives optimum lateral resolution at the point of focus.
h. Image depends on resolution. Changing frequency improves axial resolution while changing the focus improves lateral resolution.

So optimization of image is done by following techniques.

1. Choose the correct frequency 2. Focus the area

2.5 Orientation of imaging

The cranial caudal convention for longitudinal abdominal imaging and linear EBUS varies throughout the world. Endosonographers and radiologists all over the world do not yet have a universal convention on the demonstration of images in linear EBUS so far as cranial and caudal is concerned. In UK, USA and France the patient's cranial (head) and caudal (feet) are to the right and left of the screen respectively. In Japan and Germany the direction is reversed. We will follow the cranial to right and caudal to left convention for our presentation.

2.6 Providing anaesthesia

Some professionals prefer local anaethesia for EBUS. Others prefer general anaethesia.

2.7 Position of patient. Supine, left lateral or sitting. To each his own

Most of the conventional bronchoscopist use two hands to maneoure the scope. The EBUS operator who hold the echoendoscope in both hands cannot get used to manipulating the knobs of the ultrasound screen. The left lateral position of EBUS allows the operator to intermittently remove the right hand for manipulation of the screen.

2.8 Artifacts in imaging

There are two main artifacts during imaging from tracheobronchial tree. The artifacts of cartilage gradually disappear as the scope is advanced more distally into the tracheabronchial tree. Mirror image artifact is created by vessels.

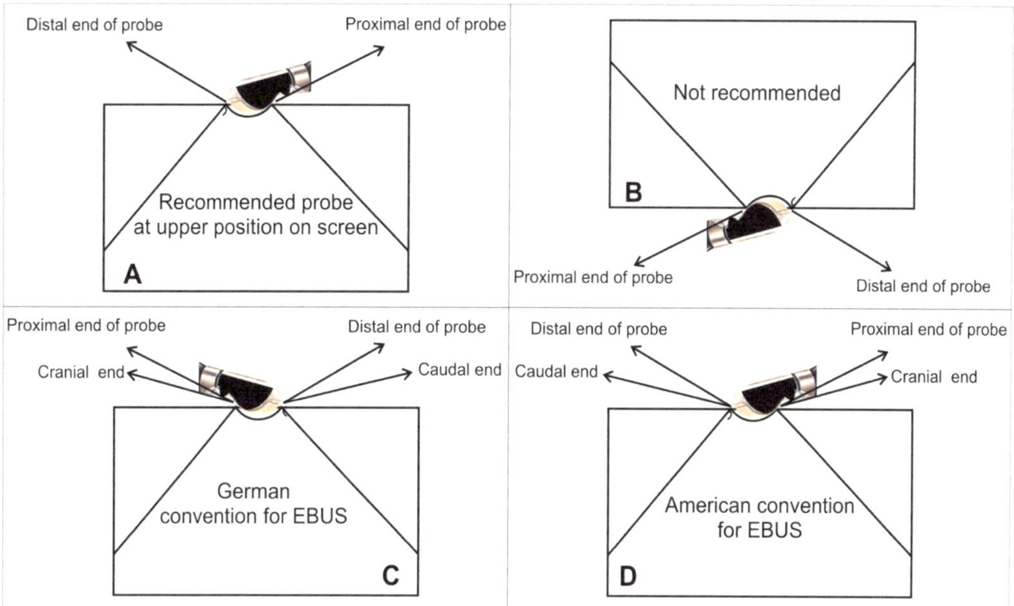

Fig. 1. Fig. A. The standard method of screening for EBUS requires positioning of the probe in the upper part of screen. Fig B. Keeping the probe in the lower part of the screen is generally not recomonded Fig. C & D. show the different convention of imaging followed by operators all over the world.

2.9 Air is the enemy water is the friend

There are two methods of establishing contact. Simple apposition of the probe against the wall may be enough to establish contact and use of balloon is not usually required with pentax scope. Generally the limited range of imaging 50° vs 75° requires contact with a balloon in Olympus EBUS scope.

2.10 There are three main movements of echoendoscope

2.10.1 In and out movement

In and out movements are done to position the scope at the desired cm landmark of imaging and is the key movement for changing the position.

2.10.2 Clockwise or anticlockwise rotation

In a linear EBUS scope where the imaging is in a longitudinal axis clockwise or anticlockwise rotation is the key movement for changing the view. Rotation changes the field totally in a linear scope only. Rotation alone brings no change in view in a radial EUS scope.

2.10.3 Angulations of scope, up or down

Angulations of scope, up or down is required for achieving close contact with the wall of trachea.

3. The CM landmarks in EBUS during imaging from mediastinum

While doing EBUS the operator generally enters the trachea approximately at 15 cm distance from the incisor. The trachea is about 10 cm long so the carina is generally reached when the scope lies at about 25 cm distance. The left bronchus is about 5 cm long and the lower end of left main stem bronchus is reached at an approximate distance of 30 cm. Similarly the 30 cm distance is the lower limit of reach in the right bronchus which includes 2.5 cm of right main stem bronchus and 2.5 cm of intermediate bronchus. The diameter of EBUS scope generally does not allow any further negotiation beyond the reach of intermediate bronchus on the right and left main stem bronchus on the left side. While doing imaging from the respiratory tract an additional cm landmark of importance is upper border of arch of aorta which lies at about 22cm distance. The lower border of arch of aorta lies at about 23 to 24 cm. The lower border of azygos vein and the upper border of left pulmonary artery lie approximately at 25 cm distance.

The trachea lies in front of esophagus which commences at the level of the cricoid cartilage at about 15 cm distance from incisor teeth. For the purpose of description, the esophagus can be divided into cervical (CE) from cricoid to 18 cm, upper thoracic [TE (U)] from 18-25 cm, till approximately the tracheal bifurcation), mid thoracic [TE (M)] from 25-32 cm, till approximately below the subcarinal area and lower thoracic [TE (L)] from 32-38 cm segments. While doing imaging from the trachea certain cm landmark of importance are upper border of arch of aorta (23cm), the lower end of trachea (25 cm), lower border of arch of aorta (25 cm), the lower border of azygos vein (25 cm), the upper border of left pulmonary artery (25 cm) and the upper border of left atrium (30 cm). While pushing the EBUS scope into esophagus the crux of diaphragm is seen at 40 cm.

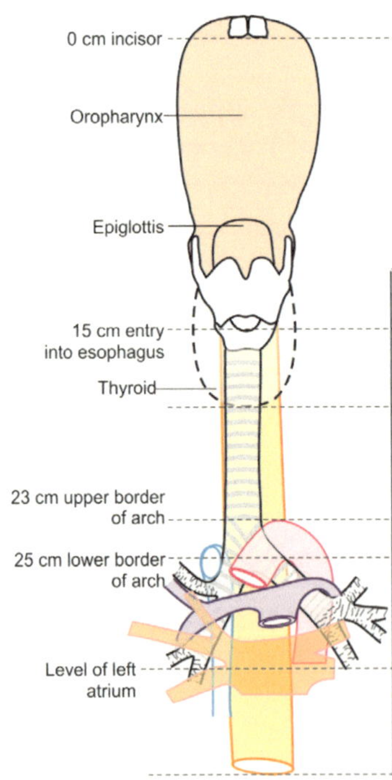

VS	DS	Cm from incisor	Part of eso-phagus
Thyroid	SP	15 to 18	CE
GV Neck	SP	18 to 23	TE(U)
AA	Arc. AV	23 to 25	
	DA, AV, TD	25 to 32	TE(M)
LA, RIPV	DA, AV, TD	32 to 38	TE(L)

Fig. 2. This figure shows the important CM landmarks while imaging with EBUS scope.

4. Applied anatomy of mediastinum

4.1 The compartments of mediastinum

It is important to have a brief idea of mediastinum before discussing the mediastinal structures. For descriptive purposes, the mediastinum is arbitrarily subdivided by a transverse plane that passes through the sternal angle and the lower border of the fourth thoracic vertebra. The superior mediastinum is above this plane and is limited superiorly by the superior thoracic aperture; the inferior mediastinum is below the plane, and the diaphragm limits it inferiorly. The inferior mediastinum is further compartmentalized based on its relation to the pericardial sac: the sac and its contents compose the middle mediastinum; between the sac and the sternum is the anterior mediastinum; between the vertebral bodies and the pericardial sac is the posterior mediastinum. The contents of the posterior mediastinum include the esophagus; the descending thoracic aorta and its branches; the veins of the azygos system and the thoracic duct.

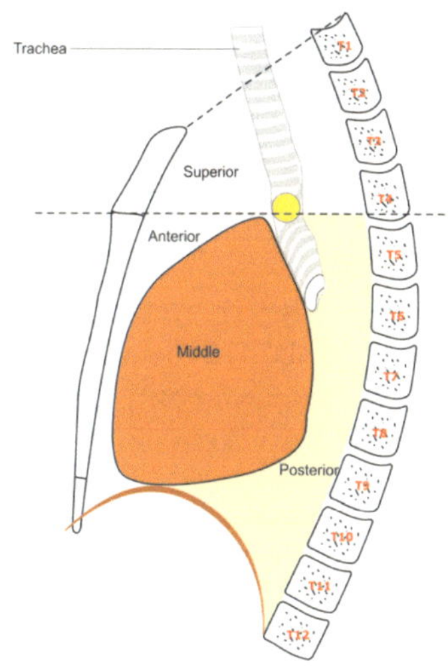

Fig. 3. The compartments of mediastinum are shown.

4.2 The trachea

The trachea is about 10 cm long and present from 15 to 25 cm distance from incisor. It is kept patent by a series of cartilages embedded transversely in its wall.The posterior wall of trachea is flat where the ends of cartilage bar are united by trachealis muscle and fibroelastic tissue. This surface is applied to esophagus. The cervical part of trachea is about 3-4 cm in length and is related to lobes of the thyroid gland before it enters superior mediastinum where it lies in midline. The division of the trachea into principal bronchi takes place behind the ascending aorta, to the right of, and below, the arch of the aorta, approximately at the level of sternal angle (level of fourth thoracic spine). The lower end of the trachea is displaced slightly to the right of the midline by the arch of the aorta, which occupies the angle between the trachea and the left bronchus.

On the right, the superior lobar bronchus branches off the principal bronchus before the later enters the hilum. The remaining main stem intermediate bronchus, gives off, more distally, the middle lobe bronchus, which runs forward and downward. The intermediate bronchus continues as inferior lobar bronchus.The left principal bronchus gives off the superior lobar bronchus as soon as it has entered the hilum, and the remaining main stem becomes the bronchus of the inferior lobe.

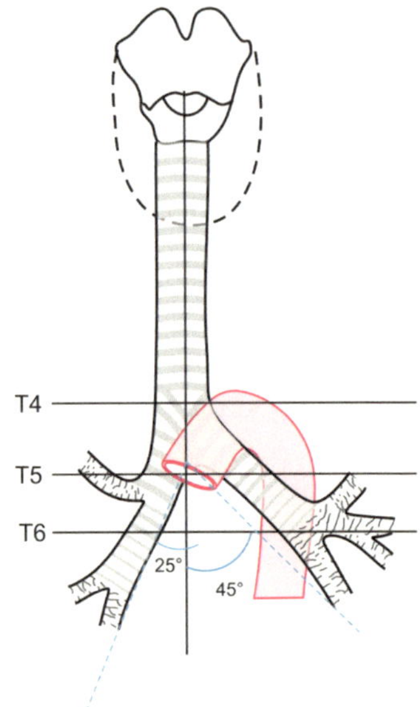

Fig. 4. The right principal bronchus is wider, shorter (about 2.5 cm) and more vertical than the left, leaves the trachea at an angle of about 25° and enters the right lung opposite the T5 vertebra. The left principal bronchus is narrower and more transverse than the right, leaves the trachea at an angle of about 45°, is nearly 5 cm long and enters the root of the left lung opposite the T6 vertebra.

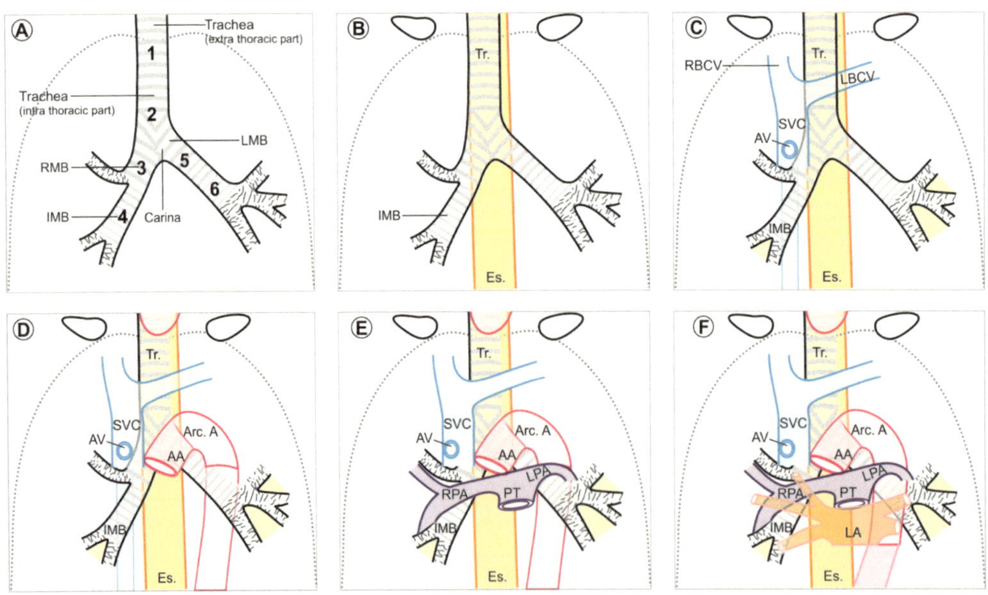

Fig. 5. The relationship of trachea to esophagus and paratracheal vascular structures

The figure 5 A shows six different positions (which will be discussed in later part of chapter) of imaging by Endobronchial ultrasound. 1 Imaging from the upper trachea, 2. Imaging from the lower trachea, 3. Imaging from the right main bronchus, 4. Imaging from Intermediate bronchus, 5. Imaging from upper part of left bronchus, 6. Imaging from the distal part of left bronchus. **Fig. B. to F** shows the relationship of parabonchial & vascular structures to trachea. **Fig. B** relationship of tracheobronchial tree to esophagus. **Fig. C.** relationship of tracheobronchial tree to azygos vein and superior vena cava. **Fig. D.** relationship of tracheobronchial tree to arch of aorta. **Fig. E.** relationship of tracheobronchial tree to pulmonary trunk and the two branches of pulmonary trunk. **Fig. F.** relationship of tracheobronchial tree to left atrium and the draining veins of the left atrium.

4.3 The right bronchus

The right bronchus passes behind the ascending aorta and the superior vena cava towards the root of lung. Two structures are related to anterior wall of right main bronchus, in the upper part the ascending aorta lies anteromedially and the superior vena cava is placed anterolaterally. The right pulmonary artery lies in close relationship with the intermediate bronchus. The right pulmonary artery initially lies first below and medial to intermediate bronchus, then in front of it and finally lies lateral and behind the intermediate bronchus. The azygos vein lies behind the right bronchus for some length and then arches over it to drain into superior vena cava.

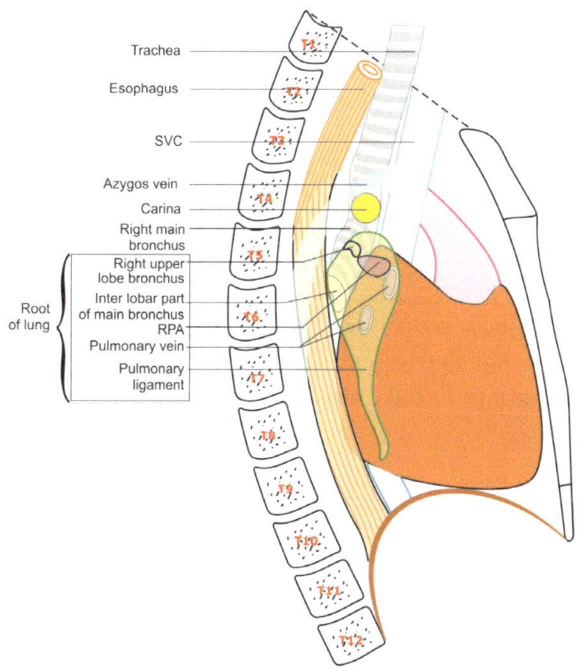

Fig. 6. The mediastinal surface of right lung is seen in this figure which shows relations of right bronchus. The right main bronchus is related anteriorly to superior vena cava and the azygos vein goes posterior to right main bronchus. It is important to note that azygous vein passes behind the root of lung and can be seen in posterior relation of right main bronchus as well as the intermediate bronchus.

4.4 The left bronchus

The left bronchus, in its course toward the hilus, passes through the loop formed by the arch of the aorta, emerging from behind the ascending aorta and passing downward and to the left in front of the descending aorta before it enters the lung. Two structures are placed in anterior wall of left bronchus. The arch of aorta lies close to upper part of left main bronchus and the left pulmonary artery ascends over its anterior surface just distal to the arch of the aorta.

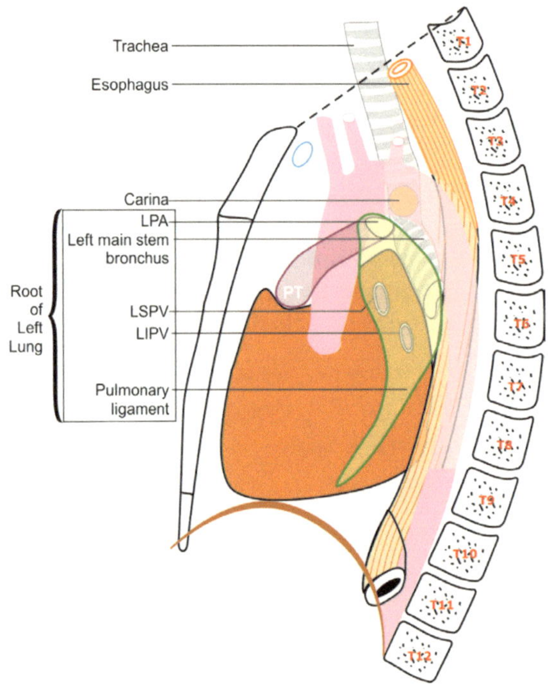

Fig. 7. The mediastinal surface of left lung is seen in this figure which shows relations of left bronchus. The left main bronchus is related anteriorly to ascending aorta in the upper part and the left pulmonary artery in the lower part. The descending aorta and esophagus lies behind the left bronchus.

4.5 The root of lung and pulmonary ligament

The roots of the lungs are posterior to the upper part of the pericardial sac. Most posterior in the upper part of each root is the bronchus, in front of it are the pulmonary artery and, in an even more anterior plane, the superior pulmonary vein. The arrangement of the pulmonary artery, pulmonary vein and bronchus in right and left lung root is slightly different. The left pulmonary artery is located above, rather than directly in front of, the left bronchus.

Usually, two bronchi the upper lobe bronchus and the bronchus intermedius are seen at the right hilum when the entire lung is removed. In the left hilum, only one bronchus is seen. The pulmonary ligament is the inferior redundant part of the pleura that surrounds the root of the lung and provides the dead space in which the root of the lung may move up and down during respiration.

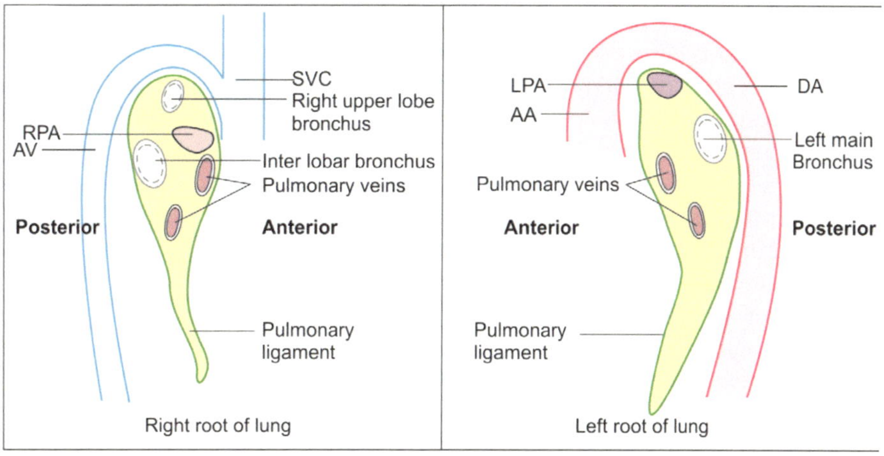

Fig. 8. It is important to know the relations at the root of the lung as the endosonographer is looking at structures from inside out. The relationship of the structures can be imagined after placing the scope inside the bronchus. Generally the veins lie most anteriorly. The artery lie behind the vein and the bronchus is the posterior most structure in the root of lung. The relations of structure at root of lung are different for right and left lung.

4.7 The aorta

As soon as the ascending aorta emerges from the pericardial sac, it begins to arch backward, and the segment that runs in a nearly sagittal plane in the superior mediastinum is known as the arch of the aorta. The arch of aorta begins behind manubrium sterni and runs first upwards backwards to the left and in front of trachea. It is then directed backwards on the left side of trachea and continues downwards on the left side of T4 vertebra and at the lower border of T-4 continues as descending aorta. The left common carotid the left subclavian and the brachiocephalic arteries arise from the convexity of arch. They are crossed anteriorly by the left brachiocephalic vein just above the convexity of arch of aorta.

The space below the concavity of arch of aorta is sometimes called as subaortic tunnel. The bifurcation of pulmonary trunk the right pulmonary artery and the left bronchus lies in this inferior concavity. The trachea and esophagus fit into the slight concavity that faces to the right.

4.8 The esophagus

For most of the length the esophagus lies in the posterior mediastinum, with the descending thoracic aorta posteriorly to its left. On its right side, it is covered by mediastinal pleura. The right pulmonary artery, the left principal bronchus, the transverse and oblique sinuses of the pericardium and the left atrium lie anterior to the esophagus.

4.9 The pulmonary trunk, the right pulmonary artery and left pulmonary artery

The pulmonary trunk (length approximately 5 cm) lies a little to the left of midline in the chest and divides into left and right branches. The left pulmonary artery immediately leaves the pericardial sac and just outside the pericardial sac is connected to the arch of the aorta by the ligamentum arteriosum. The upper border of the left pulmonary artery lies at a little higher level than the upper border of right pulmonary artery. The RPA runs horizontally behind the ascending aorta and superior vena cava before it leaves the pericardial sac in the concavity of the arch of the aorta. The right pulmonary artery emerges from the sac posterior to the superior vena cava and crosses the intermediate bronchus distal to the origin of the superior lobe bronchus. Soon after leaving the pericardial sac both right and left pulmonary arteries arch over the respective principal bronchi as they enter the hila of the lungs. The relationship of these pulmonary artery to the bronchus is more or less fixed and it gives a fair idea of the position to the endosonographer. The left pulmonary artery crosses the left principal bronchus and at the hilum, is superior to it, whereas the right pulmonary artery crosses the intermediate bronchus, having given off a major branch to the upper lobe before it enters the hilum. The ascending aorta, SVC and upper right pulmonary vein lie anterior to RPA. The esophagus and right bronchus lie posterior to RPA. The left bronchus and descending aorta lie posterior to LPA.

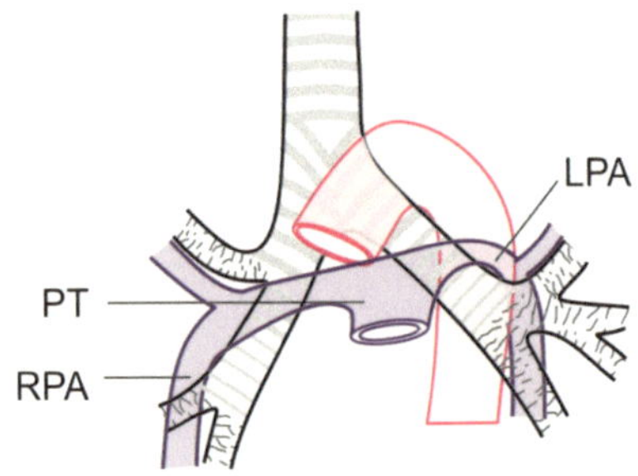

Fig. 9. The bifurcation of the pulmonary trunk takes place on the left of the ascending aorta in the concavity of the aortic arch. As a result the RPA (length approximately 2-3 cm) is longer than LPA and much of it is covered by serous pericardium.

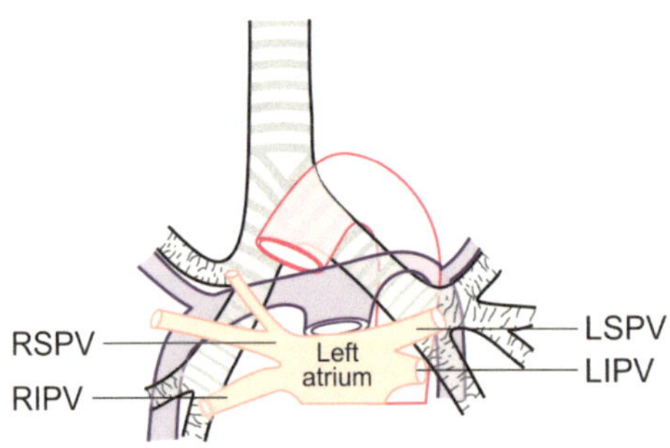

Fig. 10. The left atrium forms the lower boundary of subcarinal space. The veins coming to the left atrium have no intrapericardial course. The right superior pulmonary vein passes behind superior vena cava. Right inferior pulmonary vein crosses the esophagus.

4.10 The pulmonary veins and the left atrium

The left atrium has two portions. The posterior half of the chamber, into which the four pulmonary veins empty and the anterior half. There are four pulmonary veins, two each (superior and inferior), on the right and left sides. On the left side the superior and inferior veins drain the upper and lower lobes of the lung, respectively. The superior pulmonary vein is the most anterior structure, and the inferior pulmonary vein is the most inferior structure in the root of the lung. Thus on both sides, the principal order of the structures in an anteroposterior direction in root of lung is vein, artery, bronchus. The inferior pulmonary veins lie below the bronchus on both sides, and below them is the pulmonary ligament into which they can expand. The right inferior pulmonary vein crosses the esophagus and the right superior pulmonary vein crosses right pulmonary artery and right bronchus. On the right side the superior vein crosses behind the superior vena cava; and the inferior vein crosses behind the right atrium before they pierce the pericardial sac over the left atrium. The left inferior pulmonary vein cross the descending aorta.

Stations of EBUs Imaging

Structure	Station-1	Station-2	Station-3	Station-4	Station-5	Station-6
Respiratory Landmark	Upper Trachea	Lower Trachea	Right Main Stem Bronchus	Right Intermediate Bronchus	Left Upper Bronchus	Left Lower Bronchus
Main Arteries	BT, LCC, LSCA	Arch of Aorta SVC	RPA	RPA	LPA, DA	LPA
Main Veins	LBCV, RBCV	AV, SVC	SVC	RPV	–	LPV
Group of Lymph Node	2R, 2L, 3a, 3p	4R, 4L, 5 & 6	7, 10R	7, 8, 11R	7, 10L	7, 8, 11L
Vertebral Landmark	T-3	T-4	T-5 Upper Border	T-5	T-6	T-6
Other Structures	Thymus	Thymus	–	Chambers of Heart	–	Chambers of Heart

Table 1. The Imaging of the peribronchial structures can be done from six stations. Although there is no sharp boundary between the six stations, the structures mentioned at each station are generally seen in the positioned mentioned in the table.

5. Technique of imaging by EBUS scope

This evaluation can be done in patients referred for EBUS on an outpatient basis, under conscious sedation using midazolam and oral xylocaine spray. A linear EBUS scope (Pentax EB-1970UK) with 100° field of view, 45° forward oblique angle, a window angle of 75° and a distal end optic width of 7.4 mm was used for the purpose of description in this chapter. Imaging was done after endoscopic visualization from intrathoracic part of trachea and bronchus from six positions. Clockwise or anticlockwise rotation was done after apposition against the wall to change the axis of imaging. Cranial side left and caudal side right imaging convention was followed.

5.1 Imaging from upper trachea

Imaging is done 5 cm above carina where a clockwise and anticlockwise rotation from anterior wall of trachea to 90° on either side will show the right and left lateral tracheal walls and 180° rotation will show the esophagus behind the posterior wall of trachea (Fig 11 & 12). The presence of air in trachea and cartilage in the wall create prominent artifacts during imaging (Fig. 13 & 14).

On clockwise rotation, the brachiocephalic veins are seen joining near the right anterolateral wall of trachea to form the superior vena cava. The lower border of left brachiocephalic vein forms the upper boundary of station 2R and superior vena cava forms the posterior boundary of station 3a.

On anti clockwise rotation, the upper margin of the arch of aorta is seen from which the origin of left common carotid artery (left posterior boundary of station 3a), left subclavian artery and brachiocephalic trunk can be seen (Fig 11). Brachiocephalic trunk crosses to the right side of trachea, the left common carotid artery runs close to left wall of trachea and the left subclavian artery goes close to apex of lung where it creates mirror image artifact (Fig. 15 & 16). The transverse plane through the superior border of aortic arch makes lower border of the station 2L on the left and a transverse plane through the lower border of brachiocephalic vein forms lower border of 2R lymph nodes on the right side (Figures 17 & 18).

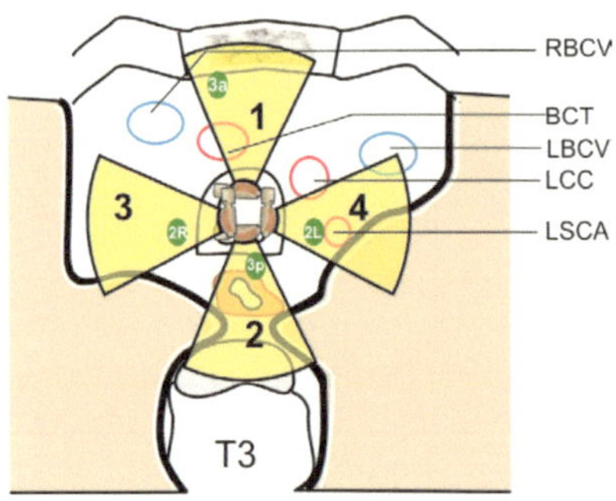

Fig. 11. Imaging from upper trachea - when the scope is positioned in upper trachea the great vessels of neck can be seen. Clock wise rotation of the scope shows the Right Brachiocephalic vein and Brachiocephalic Trunk. The Left common carotid artery and Left Brachiocephalic vein are seen anterior to the trachea and may be more easily seen on anticlockwise rotation. Further anticlockwise rotation may show the Left subclavian artery. A rotation of 180° shows the esophagus lying posterior to trachealis muscle behind the posterior wall of trachea. The yellow beam shows the area of imaging on rotation. 1 = Imaging anterior to trachea, where station 3a (prevascular) lymph nodes are seen, 2 = Imaging posterior to trachea, where station 3b lymph nodes are seen, 3 = Imaging of the right lateral side of trachea, where station 2R lymph nodes, 4 = Imaging of the left lateral side of trachea, where station 2L lymph nodes are seen.

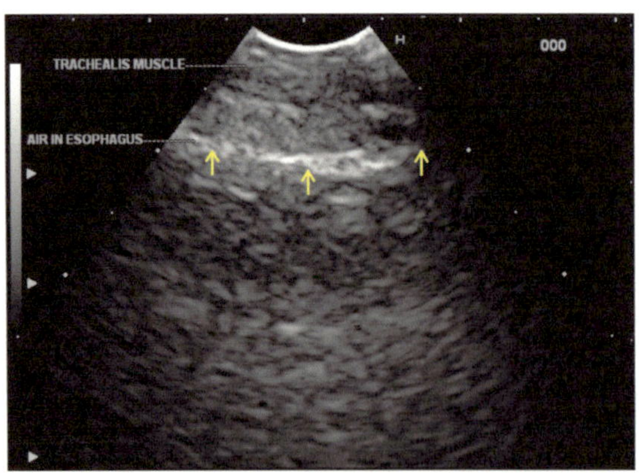

Fig. 12. Imaging of esophagus from trachea -180° rotation from the anterior wall of trachea shows membranous posterior wall of trachea made of trachealis muscle and the multilayered esophagus with air, forming a hyper-echogeneic line in the middle lying behind trachea.

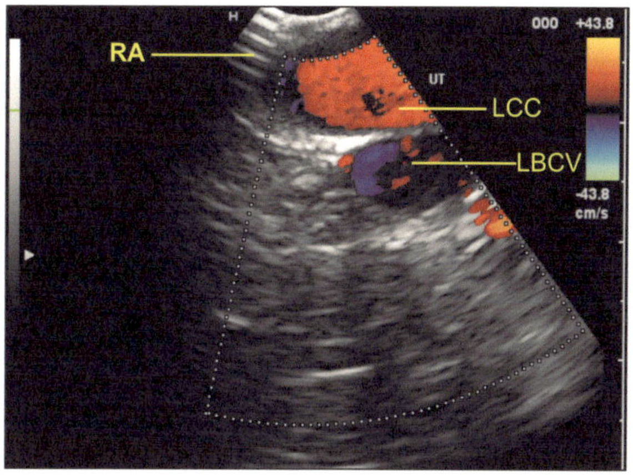

Fig. 13. Imaging of great vessels of neck: Imaging from upper trachea shows reverberation artifact. The trachea has 15 to 20 incomplete horizontally stacked 'C' shaped cartilaginous rings, each of 4 mm vertical diameter, which create alternating zones of reverberation artifact due to cartilage. The breadth of one artifact is likely to match with the breadth of each cartilage (4 mm). Once the arch of aorta is visualized pulling back a little will show the left common carotid coming out from the top of the arch of aorta.

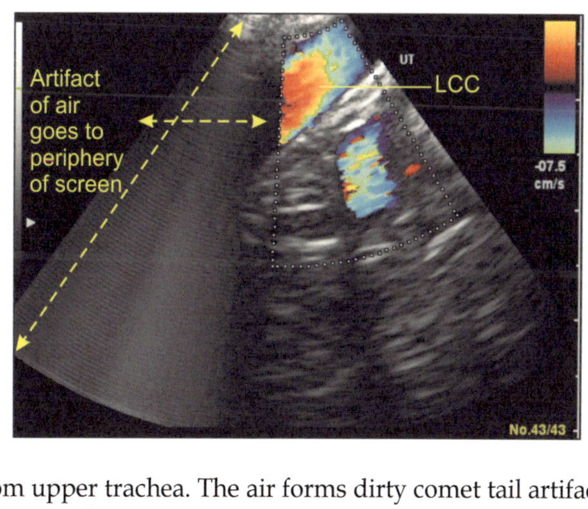

Fig. 14. Imaging from upper trachea. The air forms dirty comet tail artifact which goes to the periphery of the screen in this picture.

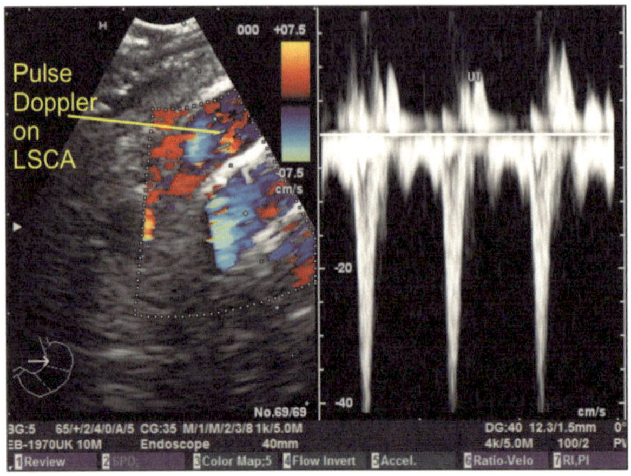

Fig. 15. The left subclavian artery is seen at a little distance away from the trachea with the mirror image artifact due to sharp interface with the left lung (the left common carotid artery generally lies closer to trachea. The application of pulse Doppler confirms the arterial wave form.

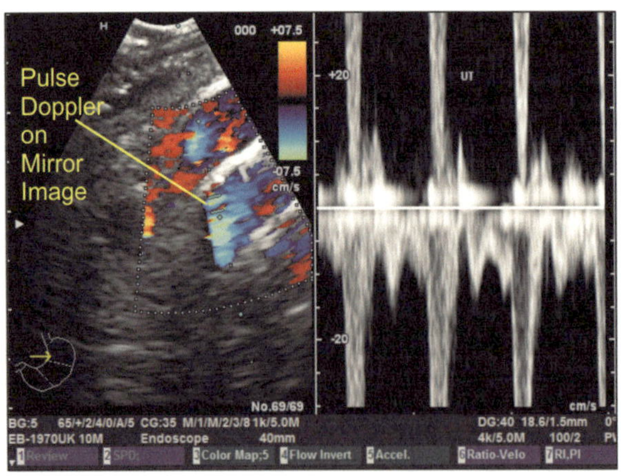

Fig. 16. A 28 year old lady is referred for evaluation of mediastinal lymphadenopathy. Imaging is done from upper trachea. The application of pulse Doppler on the mirror image confirms the arterial wave form on the mirror image also.

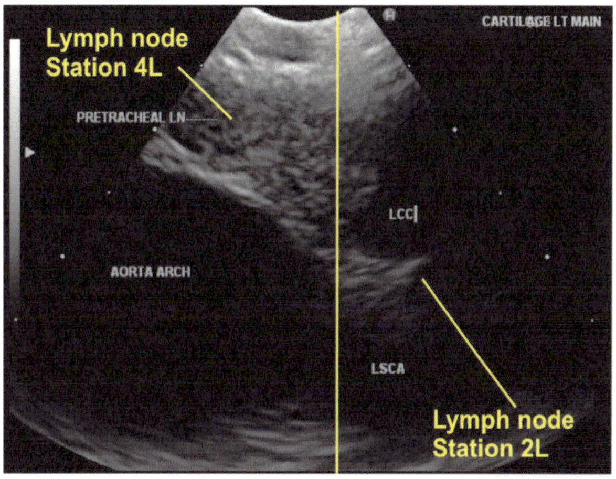

Fig. 17. Imaging is done from upper trachea and reveals a lymph node in front of trachea (Station-4L). The left subclavian artery is seen in the lower part of the screen and one lymph node is seen between the left subclavian artery and left common carotid artery (Station-2L).

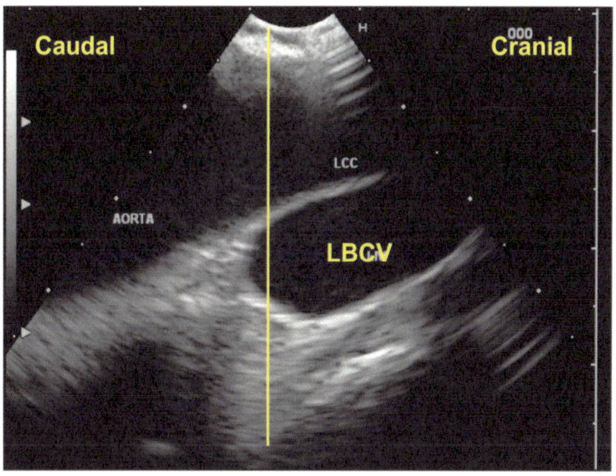

Fig. 18. Imaging is done from upper trachea. Once the arch of aorta is visualized pulling back a little will show the left common carotid coming out from the top of the arch of aorta. The left common carotid artery is seen in this figure and the left brachiocephalic vein is seen crossing in front of left common carotid artery. Vertical yellow line denotes the superior margin of the Aortic arch.

5.2 Station 2: Imaging from lower trachea

A clockwise rotation from above carina shows the right anterolateral wall of the distal one third of trachea where the superior vena cava is seen. If clockwise rotation is continued, the azygos vein can be seen joining the superior vena cava in the right tracheobronchial corner as a kidney-shaped vessel. The inferior border of station 4R is formed by the inferior margin of the azygos vein (Fig. 19, 20 & 21).

An anti-clockwise rotation shows the pulsatile arch of aorta in the left anterolateral wall of distal one third of trachea, the superior margin of which forms the boundary between the station 4L and 2L lymph node stations. Determination of the lower boundary of station 4L and 5 is done from left bronchus after clear visualization of upper rim of left pulmonary artery. Two transverse lines across the upper and lower border of arch are important in determining the area of lymph nodes of station 6 which are better seen by endoscopic ultrasound (Fig. 22).

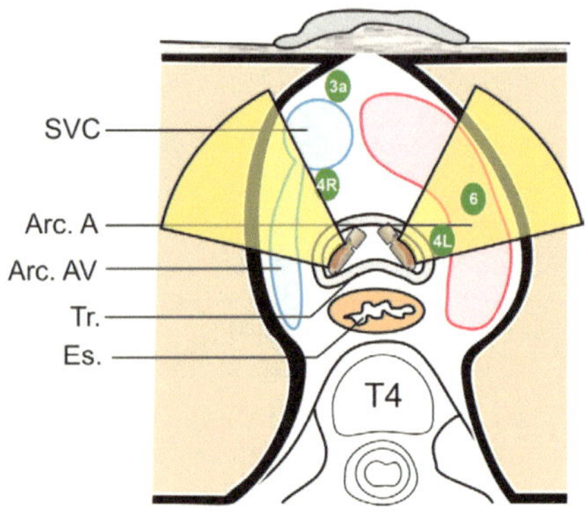

Fig. 19. Cross-sectional illustration from the lower trachea. The arch of the Azygos vein is seen entering the superior vena cava posteriorly on the right lateral side and the arch of aorta is seen in the left lateral side. The illustration shows the station 4R (right para-and pre-tracheal), 4L (lateral to the left lateral margin of trachea), 6 (lateral to the ascending aorta and arch) and 3a (prevascular) lymph nodes.

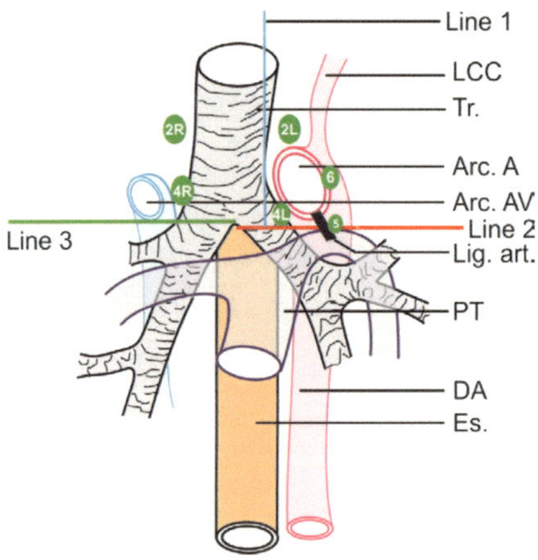

Fig. 20. Illustration of the structures at the lower trachea. The upper level of aortic arch lies anterior and to left of the distal one-third of the trachea. The arch of Azygos vein passes forwards arching over right stem bronchus to open into Superior vena cava, whereas the arch of Aorta passes backwards arching over the left stem bronchus to continue as descending Aorta. Blue line = left lateral border of trachea, the boundary between 2R/4R and 2L/4L, Green line = Inferior margin of Azygos vein = lower boundary of station 4R, Orange line = Superior margin of Left Pulmonary artery, lower boundary of station 4-L and 5. Lymph node stations: 3a = Pretracheal, 4L = Left Paratracheal, 4R = Right Paratracheal & pretracheal, 5= Subaortic nodes lateral to ligamentum arteriosum. 6 = Lateral to ascending Aorta and arch.

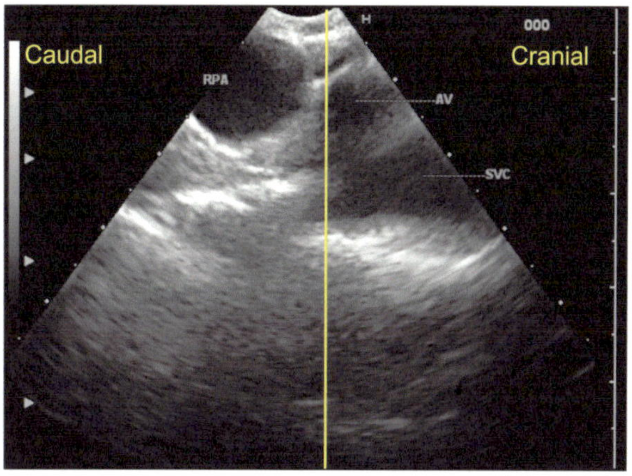

Fig. 21. EBUS image from lower trachea shows the azygos vein joining the superior vena cava posteriorly. The right pulmonary artery is seen just below the union of azygos vein joining the superior vena cava. Vertical yellow line depicts the caudal margin of the azygos vein as it joins superior vena cava.

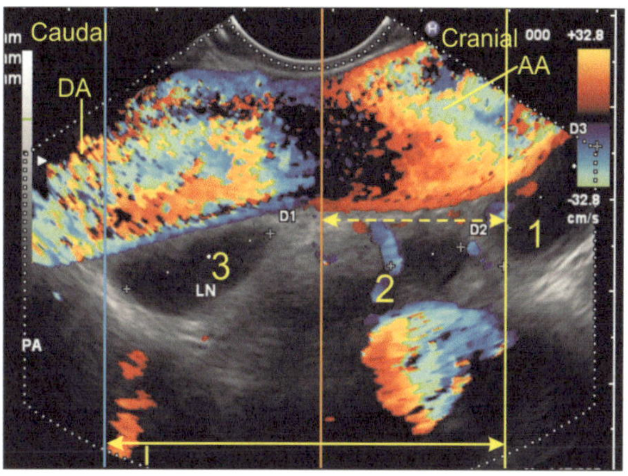

Fig. 22. This is the only EUS image in this article which is given to clarify the borders. EUS image shows the arch of aorta and the left pulmonary artery with lymph nodes (1, 2 & 3). Vertical lines represent-yellow line: upper margin of the arch of aorta, orange line: lower margin of the arch of aorta, blue line: upper margin of the left pulmonary artery. Left right dotted arrow = location of station 6 node. Left right solid arrow = location of station 4L node.). As the ligamentum arteriosum can not be visualized clearly by EBUS, it is often difficult to differentiate the station 4L from the station 5 lymph nodes. Lymph node no. 1= station 2L, No. 2 = station 6 & No. 3= station 5 node.

5.3 Station 3: Imaging from right main bronchus

From the right main bronchus, the subcarinal space, the right pulmonary artery, right pulmonary vein, superior vena cava and ascending aorta are seen close to the anterior wall (Fig. 23, 24, 25 & 26, 27 & 28). Turning the scope anti-clockwise shows station 7 nodes of subcarinal area (Fig 29). Station 10R lymph nodes are seen close to the right main bronchus.

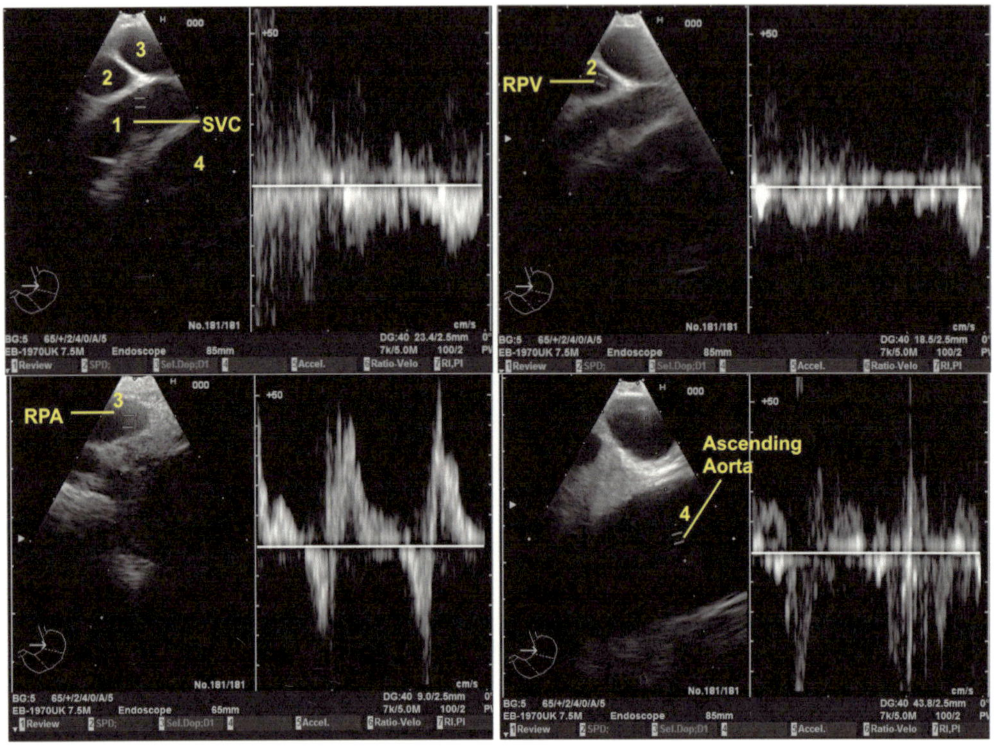

Fig. 23., 24., 25. & 26. Bronchoscopy showed extrinsic compression on the right bronchus. EBUS was done from the right bronchus. Four pulsations are seen. One by one placement of the pulse doppler is done over the pulsations. The pulse Doppler is placed on pulsation 1 in this figure and characterizes it as superior vena cava. The superior vena cava can be followed up by pulling up the scope into right lateral wall of trachea. The rest of the vessels are as follows-2: Right pulmonary vein, 3: Right pulmonary artery, 4: Ascending aorta. SVC = Superior vena cava

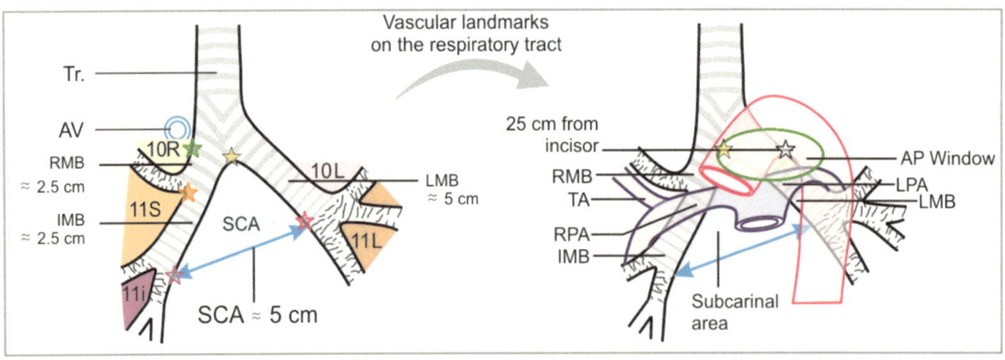

Fig. 27. The 25 cm landmark is an important landmark for EBUS as the trachea divides into right and left bronchus which move towards the respective lungs and opens up a subcarinal window anterior to esophagus. The new IASC classification has redefined the boundaries of subcarinal area (SCA). It is a pyramidal space the tip of which lies at the tracheal bifurcation.

The right boundary (5 cm) is formed by right bronchus (2.5 cm) and intermediate bronchus (2.5 cm). The left boundary is formed by left main bronchus. (5 cm) The lower limit of SCA is formed by an oblique line drawn from the lower border of intermediate bronchus to the lower border of left main bronchus. Just above the origin of apical segment of left lower lobe bronchus (approximately 5 cm long). The upper border of the left atrium is about 3 to 4 cm in breadth and occupies the middle part of this oblique line. More laterally the inferior pulmonary veins form a part of the lower border of subcarinal area which is generally =>1cm for the RIPV and =<, 1cm for LIPV. The dotted blue line shows an axial plane through sub-carinal area which roughly corresponds to the upper border of 10R and 10L. The green line shows the lower border of 10 R. The green bracket shows the area of hilum on the right side which lies opposite sub carinal area on the right side. There is a division between 11s and 11i on the right side. The former indicate the nodes between upper lobe and intermediate bronchus, the latter are situated in between middle and lower lobe. The orange line shows the lower border of 11S on the right side and lies opposite sub carinal area on the right side. The orange arrow shows the inter lobar area on the right side which lies opposite SCA. The blue line with arrows shows the lower limit of SCA. The magenta line shows the lower border of 10 L on the left side and the magenta bracket shows the area of 10 L lymph node which lies opposite SCA on the left side. The 11i lymph node lies above the purple line on the right side and the 11L lie above the brown line on the left side. The hilar nodes of station 10 are situated immediately adjacent to the mainstem bronchus but caudal to the inferior border of azygos vein on the right and superior rim pulmonary veins and artery on the left. Yellow star on 25 cm line = carina, white star on 25 cm line = upper margin of AP window.

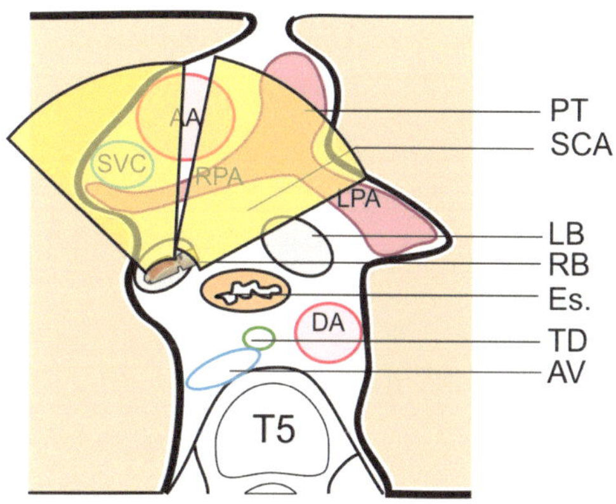

Fig. 28. Imaging from the right main bronchus (Station 3A) – the right main bronchus is Broader, more vertical and about 2.5 cm long. The right pulmonary artery lies immediately anterior to the right main stem bronchus near the origin of the right upper lobe bronchus. The superior vena cava and the ascending aorta lie in front of right pulmonary artery. Imaging from the right bronchus can be done by clockwise and anticlockwise rotation. Clockwise rotation will show the right pulmonary artery superior vena cava and ascending aorta. Anticlockwise rotation will show the subcarinal space. Yellow beam shows the area of imaging.

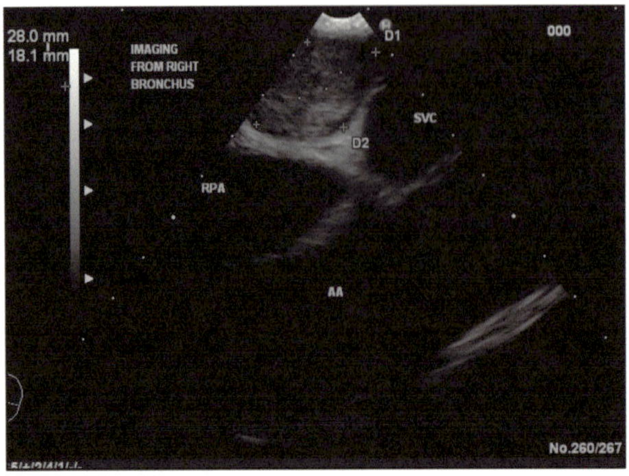

Fig. 29. E-BUS Image from the right main bronchus with anti-clockwise rotation demonstrates station 7 lymph node (subcarinal).

5.4 Station 4: Imaging from intermediate bronchus

Imaging from right intermediate bronchus the subcarinal area (station 7 & 8 nodes) left atrium mitral valve and left ventricle are seen anteriorly (Fig. 30 & 31). On pushing down endoscopic visualization of inferior border of right intermediate bronchus demarcates the lower boundary of station 7 on the right side. Station 11 lymph nodes are seen close to intermediate bronchus.

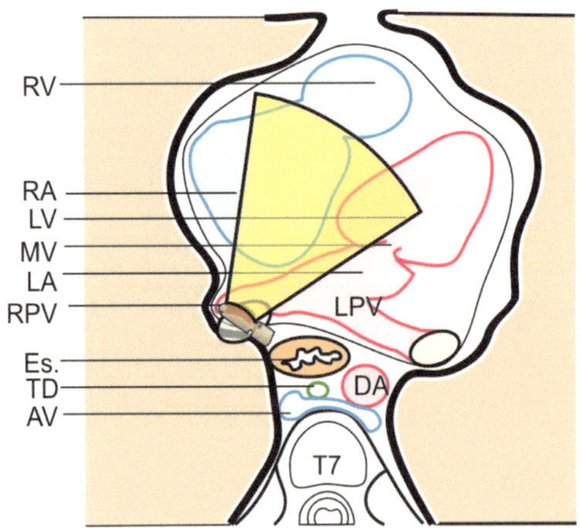

Fig. 30. Imaging from the intermediate bronchus (station 4). The intermediate bronchus lies posterior to the pulmonary veins and the left atrium. On a clockwise rotation the pulmonary veins can be followed into the lung and on anticlockwise rotation they can be followed into the left atrium. From the left atrium the left ventricle and mitral valve can be visualized. Yellow beam shows the area of imaging.

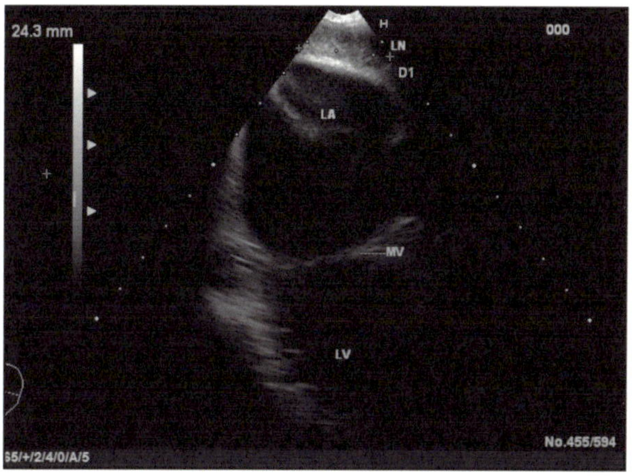

Fig. 31. E-BUS from the lowest part of right intermediate bronchus shows a lymph node between the bronchus and left atrium (Station-8). The left atrium mitral valve and left ventricle are seen in this image.

5.5 Station 5: Imaging from upper part of left main bronchus

The left pulmonary artery is seen in the anterior wall of bronchus. On anticlockwise rotation, the probe faces the posterior wall of left main bronchus where the descending aorta, esophagus and vertebral column are seen (Fig. 32, 33). A clockwise rotation shows station 7 lymph nodes (Fig. 34). Station 10 L lymph nodes are seen near the left main bronchus on anti-clockwise rotation (Fig. 35).

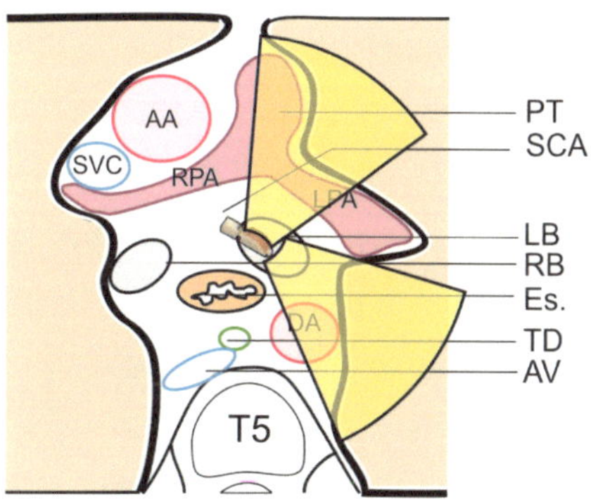

Fig. 32. Imaging from the left main bronchus-The left main pulmonary artery is seen in the anterior wall. The left main bronchus is narrower, less vertical and 5 cm long. It passes to the left inferior to aortic arch through Subaortic Tunnel. From the left main bronchus subcarinal area is identified from the left side by turning the scope in a clockwise direction. It is important to note that in left main bronchus clockwise rotation is required to see the subcarinal area whereas in right main bronchus anticlockwise rotation is required to see the subcarinal area. Identification of the main pulmonary trunk is also possible by clockwise rotation. On anti-clockwise rotation the descending aorta can be visualized and followed up by slow withdrawal along the left wall of bronchus to the aortic arch. Yellow beam shows the area of imaging.

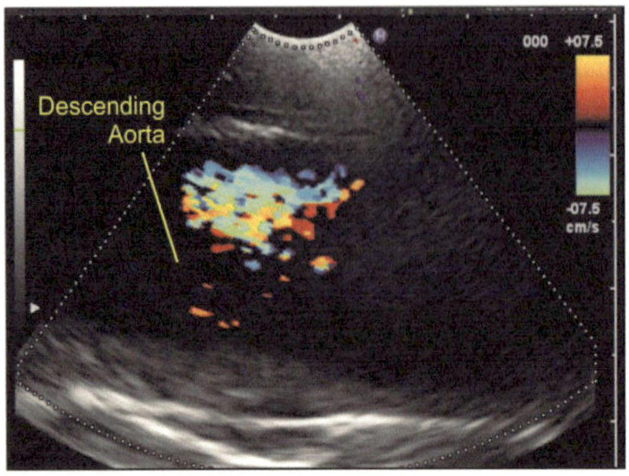

Fig. 33. EBUS Image demonstrates the descending aorta after anticlockwise rotation from the left main bronchus.

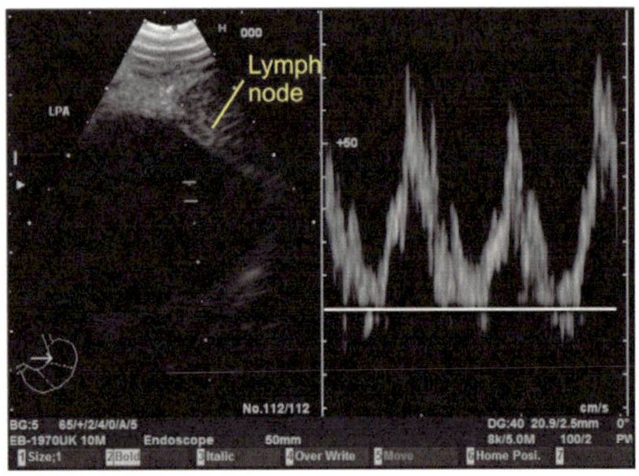

Fig. 34. EBUS image from the left bronchus on clockwise rotation shows station 7 lymph node with the pulmonary trunk lying near the lymph node.

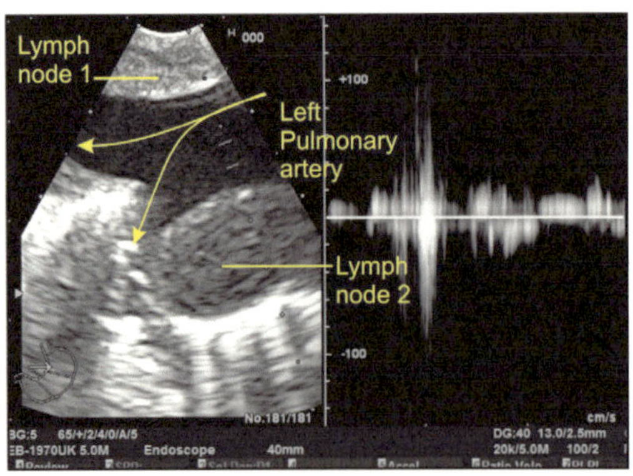

Fig. 35. EBUS from the left bronchus shows the left pulmonary artery anterior to the left bronchus. The lymph node 1 is seen lying close to the bronchus below the upper rim of left pulmonary artery and belongs to station 10-L. The lymph node 2 is lying away from the pulmonary artery after its branching and belongs to station 11-L. Yellow arrow shows the course of pulmonary artery dividing into two branches.

5.6 Station 6: Imaging from lower part of left main bronchus

With the scope in lower part of left bronchus just above the secondary carina the left atrium and station 8 lymph nodes can be identified anteriorly. It is often possible to get a four chambered view of heart with a 75° EBUS scope (Fig. 36). The lymph nodes of station 11L are seen below the secondary carina.

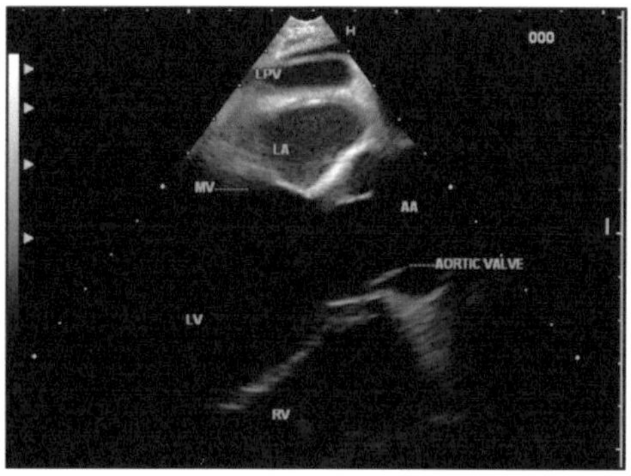

Fig. 36. When the scope is pushed further Down into the left bronchus (Station 6). The left pulmonary vein is seen draining into the left atrium. The mitral valve, the left ventricle, the aortic valve and the ascending aorta are seen in this position. It is important to note that the aortic valve is seen in the root of ascending aorta in front of upper part of left atrium. The lymph node for station 8 is seen at the level of left atrium.

6. Comparison of EBUS and EUS

No standard comparison has been made till now and the choice of procedure (EBUS first or EUS first) is still under debate. The reasons to choose EUS FNA over EBUS FNA for lymph nodes are—

1. EUS scope has a large diameter and it is easier to pass the FNAC needle through the channel of the scope.
2. The field of vision is more with a EUS scope (130° to 180°) as compared to EBUS scope (50 to 70°).
3. The use of elevator allows more angles for the operator to enter the lymph node.
4. The use of right and left knobs allows more angles for entry into the lymph node.
5. The presence of cartilage during entry from trachea may be difficult

7. Abbreviations

GV neck = great vessels of neck, AA = arch of aorta, Arc. AV = Arch of azygos vein,BT = Brachiocephalic Trunk, LCC = Left Common Carotid Artery, LSCA = Left Subclavian Artery, SVC = Superior Vena Cava, RPA = Right Pulmonary Artery, LPA = Left Pulmonary Artery, DA = Descending Aorta, LBCV = Left Brachiocephalic Vein, RBCV = Right Brachiocephalic Vein, AV = Azygos Vein, RPV = Right Pulmonary Vein, LPV = Left Pulmonary Vein, T = Thoracic Vertebra, R = Right, L = Left. Fig. 5 SVC = Superior vena cava, Arc. A = Arch of aorta, AV = Azygos vein, AA = Ascending aorta, RPA = Right pulmonary artery, DA = Descending aorta, LPA = Left pulmonary artery, PT = Pulmonary trunk, LB = Left bronchus, RB = Right bronchus, UT = Upper trachea, LT = Lower trachea,

Es = esophagus. Tr. = Trachea, Es. = Esophagus, PT = Pulmonary trunk, DA = Descending aorta, Es. = Esophagus, Lig. art. = Ligamentum arteri-osum. SCA = Subcarinal area, TD = Thoracic duct, LA = Left atrium, MV = Mitral valve, LV = Left ventricle, RV = Right ventricle, RA = Right atrium, RPV = Right pulmonary vein, LPV = Left pulmonary vein,
RA = Reverberation artifact, SCA = sub carinal area, RMB = right main bronchus, LMB = left main bronchus, TA = Truncus anterior, AP window = aortopulmonary window

8. References

Sharma M., Rameshbabu CS, P. Mohan, Standard Techniques of Imaging of IASLC Borders by Endoscopic Ultrasound Journal of Bronchology & Interventional Pulmonology. 18(1):99-110, January 2011.

Sharma M. Arya CL, Somasundaram A. Rameshbabu CS. Techniques of Linear Endobronchial Ultrasound Imaging Journal of Bronchology & Interventional Pulmonology: April 2010 - Volume 17 - Issue 2 - pp 177-187

Sheski FD, Mathur P. Endobronchial ultrasound. Chest 2008 Jan;133(1):264-70.

Fujita N, Inui K, Kida M, Maguchi H, Yamao K and Yasuda K. S. Standard imaging techniques in the pancreatobiliary region using radial scanning endoscopic ultrasonography. Digestive Endoscopy 2004; 16 (Suppl.), S118-133

Yamao K, Irisawa A, Inoue H et al. Standard imaging techniques of endoscopic ultrasound-guided fine-needle aspiration using a curved linear array echoendoscope. Digestive Endoscopy 2007; 19 (S1), S180 - S205.

Bolliger CT, Herth FJF, Mayo PH, Miyazawa T, Beamis JF; Clinical Chest Ultrasound: from the ICU to the bronchoscopy suite. Prog Respir Res. Basel, Karger, 2009, Vol 37, 153-159

Rusch VW, Asamura H, Watanabe H, Giroux DJ, Rami-Porta R and Goldstraw P. The IASLC Lung Cancer Staging Project. A Proposal for a New International lymph Node Map in the Forthcoming Seventh Edition of the TNM Classification for Lung Cancer. J Thorac Oncol. 2009; 4: 568-577

Ernst A, Herth FJF. Endobronchial ultrasound. An atlas and practical guide. Dordrecht. 2009. Springer. p89-102.

Blank W, Annema JT, Veselic M and Rabe KF. Chest Sonography. Berlin. 2008. Springer.

Agur AMR, Lee MJ. Grant's atlas of anatomy. 10th ed. Philadelphia. 1999. Lippincot-Williams-Wilkins.

Wang KP, Mehta AC, Turner JF. Flexible bronchoscopy. 2nd edition. 2004. Massachusetts. Blackwell science. p36-38

Roose C and Rosse P.G. Hollinshead's Textbook of Anatomy, 5th edition. Philadelphia , Lippincott-Raven, 1997:450-451

Part 3

Clinical Applications of Ultrasonics

9

Ultrasound Imaging of the Fetal Palate

Hong Soo Wong[1,2] and Kevin Craig Pringle[2]
[1]*Australian Women's Ultrasound Centre, Brisbane, Queensland*
[2]*Department of Obstetrics and Gynaecology*
School of Medicine and Health Sciences, University of Otago, Wellington
[1]*Australia*
[2]*New Zealand*

1. Introduction

Ultrasound examination of the fetal palate is known to be problematic. The difficulties identified include shadowing by facial bones, its curved anatomy, and its location deep inside the fetal head especially for the posterior part of palate. The soft tissues in the area, e.g. the fetal tongue, also make it more difficult to delineate the palate. Antenatal detection rate of fetal cleft palate has remained low especially when it is an isolated defect without concomitant cleft lip. The reported detection rate is virtually 0% in these cases (Grandjean et al., 1999; Clementi et.al.. 2000; Shaikh et.al., 2001; Wayne et al., 2002; Hanikeri et al., 2006; Offerdal et al., 2008; Demircioglu et al., 2008). Various methods for examination of the fetal palate have been proposed, including the use of 2-dimensional (2D) and 3-dimensional (3D) ultrasound technology. In this chapter, ultrasound imaging of the fetal palate will be revisited. How these problems may be resolved with ultrasound technology will be discussed.

2. The development of the fetal palate

The fetal palate forms between week 5 to 12 (Moore & Persaud, 2003).
Early in the 6th week, the medial nasal prominences merge to form the median palatine process, or the primary palate, the premaxillary part of the maxilla.
The secondary palate develops early in the 6th week from the lateral palatine processes or the palatal shelves. They are 2 mesenchymal projections that extend from the internal aspects of the maxillary prominences. They elongate and ascent to a horizonatal position superior to the tongue at the 7th to 8th week, fuse with the nasal septum and the posterior part of the primary palate. The primary and secondary palates become ossified. The posterior part of the lateral palatal processes extends beyond the nasal septum forming the soft palate and uvula, and does not become ossified. (Fig. 1)
The fetal palate curves from the premaxilla to the tip of the uvula making almost a 90 degrees turn (Fig. 2). It is like a part of a sphere, with every point on it making a different tangent to any reference plane one may set on this sphere.
Facial clefts could be unilateral, bilateral or midline; anterior, involving the lip with or without the primary palate, or posterior, involving the secondary palate, with or without

involvement of the lip and primary palate, or sometimes involving the uvula only. Overall about a quarter of the facial clefts involve the lip, one half both the lip and palate, and a

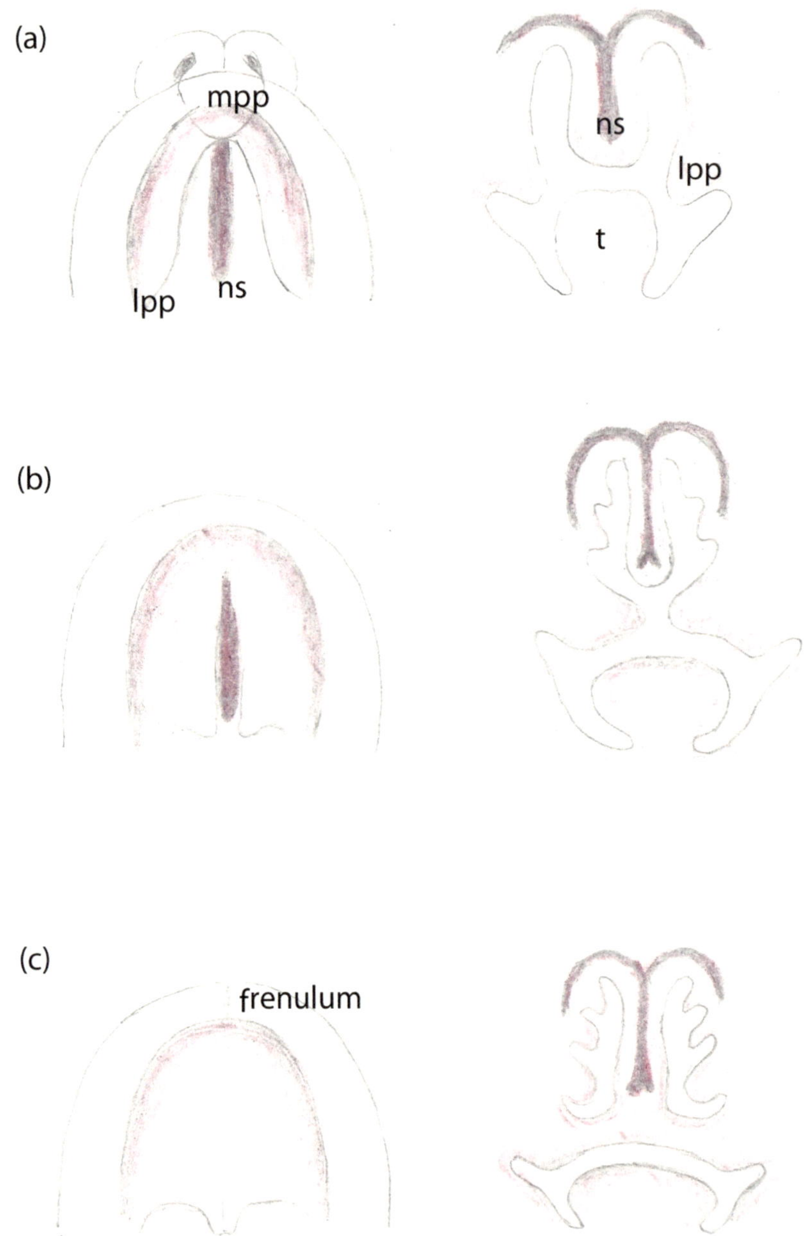

Fig. 1. Development of the fetal palate from the seventh (a), eighth (b) to the tenth (c) week. The images on the left: the palate as seen from below; on the right, coronal plane through the nasal septum and the developing palate; mpp, median palatine process; lpp, lateral palatine process; ns, nasal septum; t, tongue.

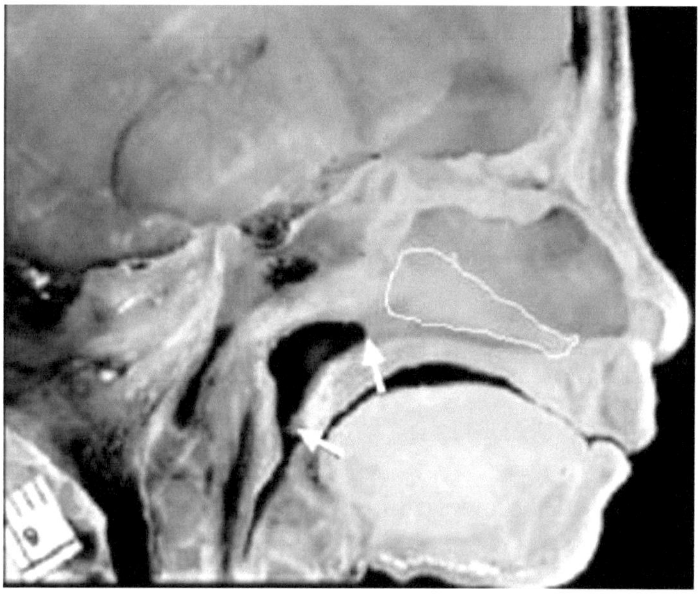

Fig. 2. Sagittal section of a 24 weeks fetus. The soft palate is between the arrows. The vomer bone is outlined. From "Prenatal ultrasound examination of the secondary palate" by Prof. Stuart Campbell, picture courtesy of Dr. Gonzalo Moscoso with thanks, in Ultrasound Obstet Gynecol 2007; 29(2): 124-127. Copyright International Society of Ultrasound in Obstetrics and Gynecology, 2007. Reproduced with permission. Permission is granted by John Wiley & Son Ltd. on behalf of the ISUOG.

quarter the palate only (Offerdal 2008). Therefore assessment of the fetal lip or palate is not complete without the examination of both and the examination of the palate extends from the premaxilla to the tip of the uvula.

3. The use of ultrasound in imaging the fetal palate

3.1 Two-dimensional ultrasound

Before the advent of 3D ultrasound, facial clefts were diagnosed by the 2D oblique face view (Pilu et al., 1986)(Fig. 3). The presence of cleft lip detected in this view leads to further assessment of the fetal palate.

The conventional assessment of the fetal face and anterior part of the palate involves the evaluation of these structures in the axial and coronal planes, which could be obtained in 68-95% of fetuses in the mid-trimester (Pretorius 1995, Babcook 1996). The structures to be assessed in the orthogonal planes are as follows:

Coronal plane	Axial plane	Sagittal view
Soft tissue in the upper lip	Soft tissue of upper lip	Soft tissue of upper lip
-	Alveolar ridge of the maxilla	Any presence of pre-maxillary protrusion

Table 1. The structures to be evaluated on the conventional 2D planes in assessment of fetal lip and palate

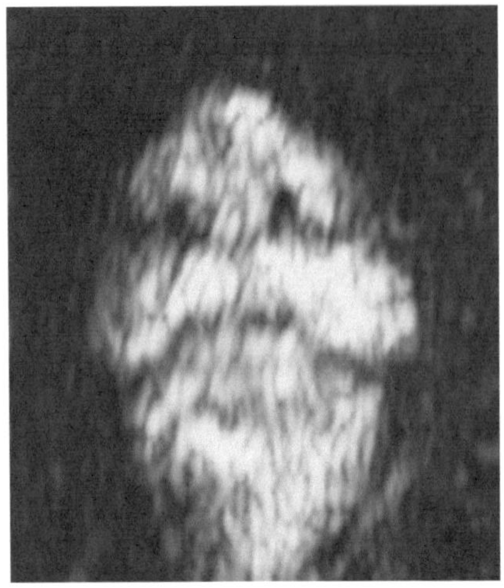

Fig. 3. The 2D view through the lower part of the fetal face showing the nose and the lips.

The sagittal view (or the facial profile) is not always helpful especially in the case of unilateral facial cleft because the view could be very much near normal.

The primary palate and part of the secondary palate are bony. The soft palate including the uvula, is made up of soft tissue. The primary palate is superficial, lying just behind the fetal lip. In contrast, the secondary palate has a dome further inside the head, enclosed by the facial bones (Fig. 2). There are soft tissues present close to the secondary palate in the area e.g. the fetal tongue and the pharynx. The presence of fluid in the oral and pharyngeal cavity and the movement of the tongue may help to define the palate. However, it is known that the hard palate is more difficult to define consistently and the soft palate could not be recognised discretely on 2D ultrasound (Filly & Feldstein, 2000).

3.2 Three-dimensional ultrasound

Ulm et al (1998) used 3D ultrasound to evaluate fetal tooth germs and found it superior to 2D ultrasound with a detection rate of 88-94% versus 56-62%, and noted its usefulness for characterization of facial clefts (Uml et al., 1999).

Fig. 4 and Fig. 5 show the axial plane of the palate in same fetus in 2D and 3D respectively. The application of 3D ultrasound allows the clear visualization of the alveolar ridge in details. The application of 3D ultrasound allows the clear visualization of the alveolar ridge.

Johnson et al. (2000) pointed out the advantages of 3D ultrasound:

a. The fetal face may be viewed in a standard orientation.
b. Interactive display allows the manipulation and scrutinization without the concern for fetal movement
c. Allow artefacts to be detected
d. Allow serial views
e. Allow exact location of the planar images be identified in relation to the rendered image
f. The rendered image allows the family to see the fetal abnormality and the associated abnormality.

Up to this time, shadowing by the alveolar ridge and the facial bones is still an issue for viewing the secondary palate even on 3D ultrasound. Campbell & Lees (2003) introduced the use of three-dimensional reverse face (3D RF) view for the diagnosis of cleft palate (Fig. 6). The usefulness of this technique in the antenatal diagnosis of cleft palate was confirmed

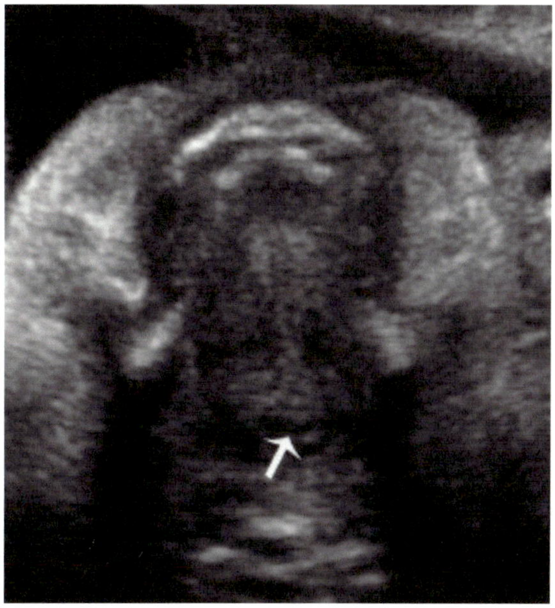

Fig. 4. 2D ultrasound image of the plate. The primary and secondary palate can be seen in this axial plane. The posterior nasal spine is indicated by the arrow. However, due to the anatomy of the palate, the under-surface of the soft palate cannot be seen because it is almost vertical to the insonation beam (Please refer to Fig. 2).

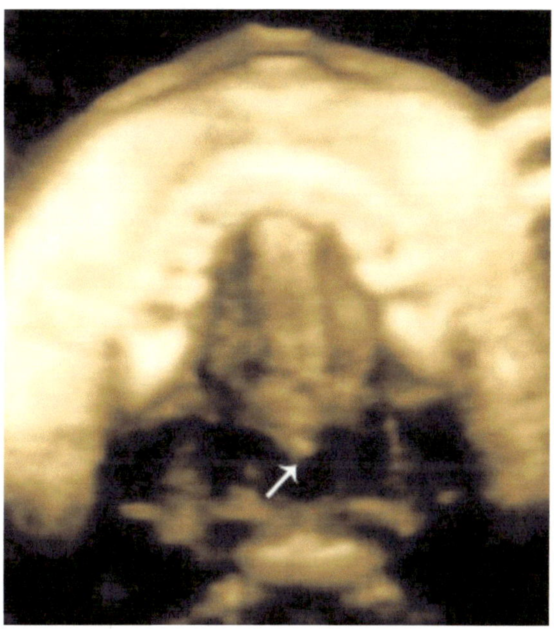

Fig. 5. Axial view on 3D ultrasound. The alveolar ridge is clearly shown in 3D compared with the 2D image in the same fetus in Fig. 4. The arrow points to the tip of the uvula, with the posterior nasal spine in the background.

in 8 cases of suspected craniofacial clefts except in a case of a cleft in the soft palate (Campbell et al., 2005). The face is turned through 180 degrees to be viewed in the reverse direction after a 3D volume is obtained on the fetal face. The shadowing by the alveolar ridge could be largely avoided with clearer demarcation of the edge of the facial cleft with this method.

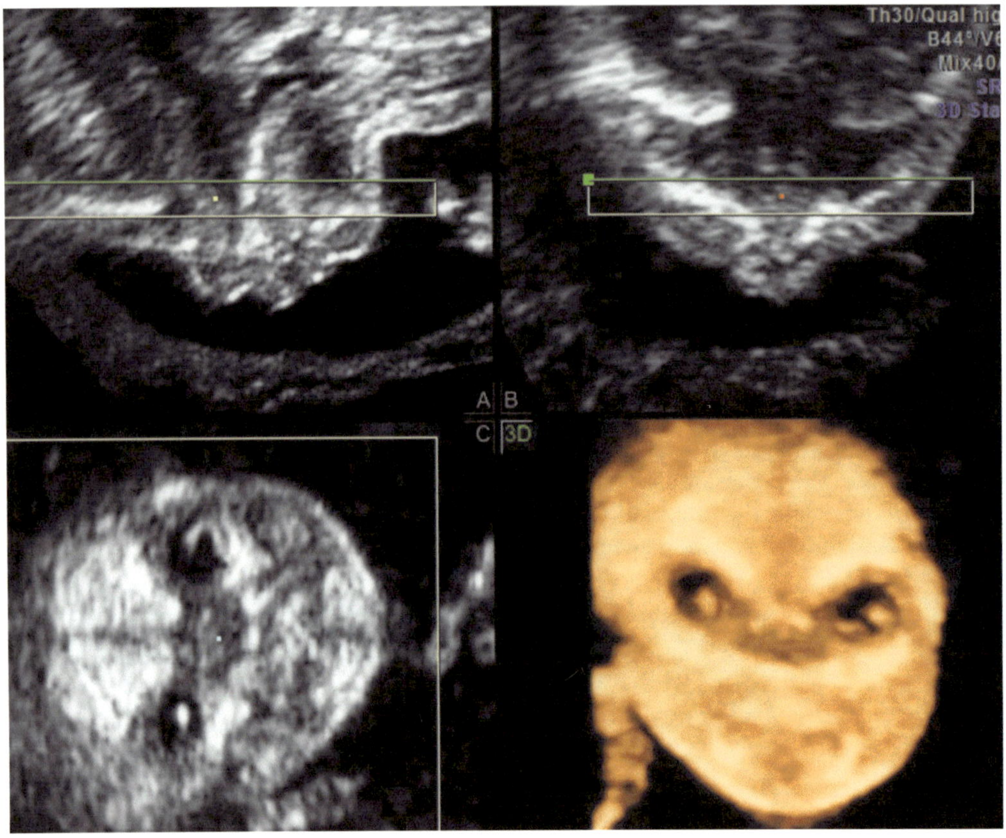

Fig. 6. The reverse face view. The intact palate can be seen as a distinct horizontal line separating the nasal and the oral cavities.

To avoid acoustic shadowing from the alveolar ridge, Pilu & Segata (2006) suggested that the secondary palate to be insonated at a 45 degrees angle in the sagittal plane and 3D ultrasound to be used to construct axial and coronal planes (Fig. 7).
With this method, they were able to obtain satisfactory views of the secondary palate in 10 of 15 cases between 19-28 weeks. They examined the tomographic ultrasound images (TUI) in the orthogonal planes. They confirmed that the axial plane (Fig. 8) allowed the assessment of alveolar ridge defect in cleft lip and palate. However, the tongue might still obscure the edges of the defect in facial cleft. Tomographic ultrasound images of the secondary palate in the coronal plane (Fig. 9) allowed the examination of the secondary palate in serial sections along its length and the edges of the defect appeared to be demarcated. This echoes the finding of Campbell et al. (2003). Although part of the soft palate could be visualized in the sagittal plane, it was not demonstrated in the axial and coronal planes. The limitation with this technique is unfavourable fetal position. (Pilu & Segata 2006)

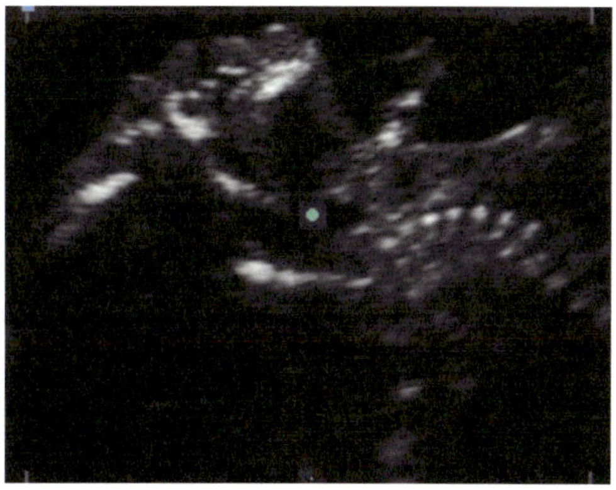

Fig. 7. Insonation of the fetal palate at an angle to avoid acoustic shadowing by the alveolar ridge.

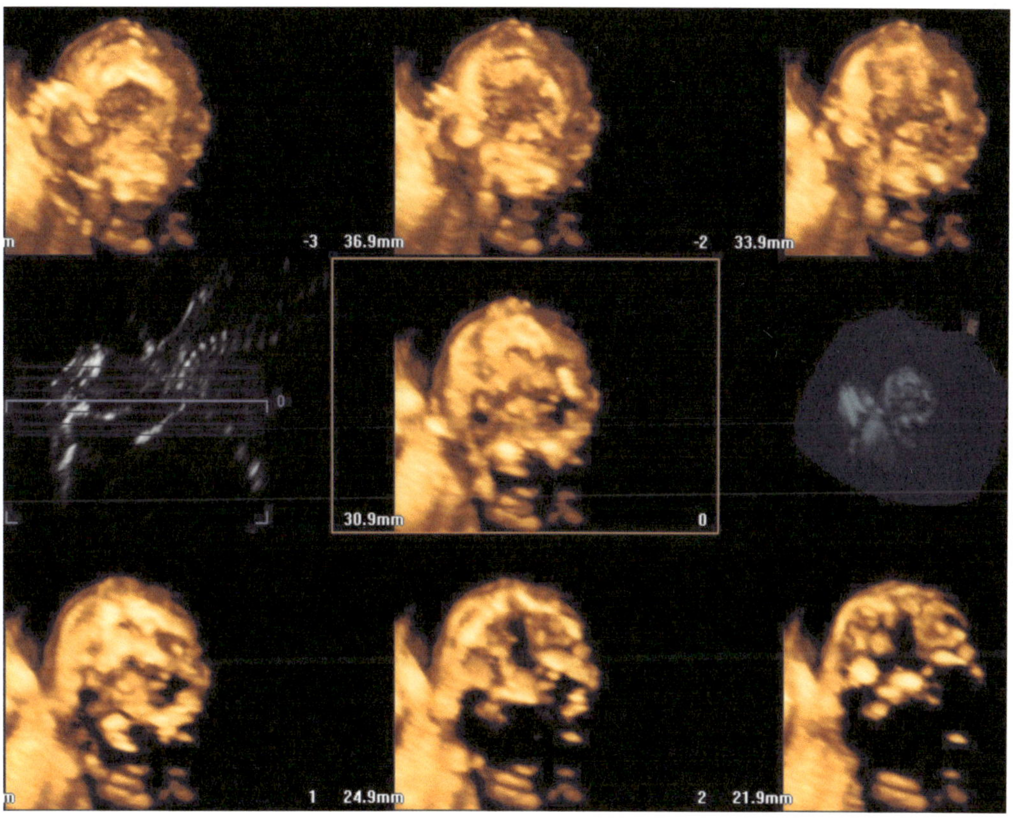

Fig. 8. TUI of the axial view

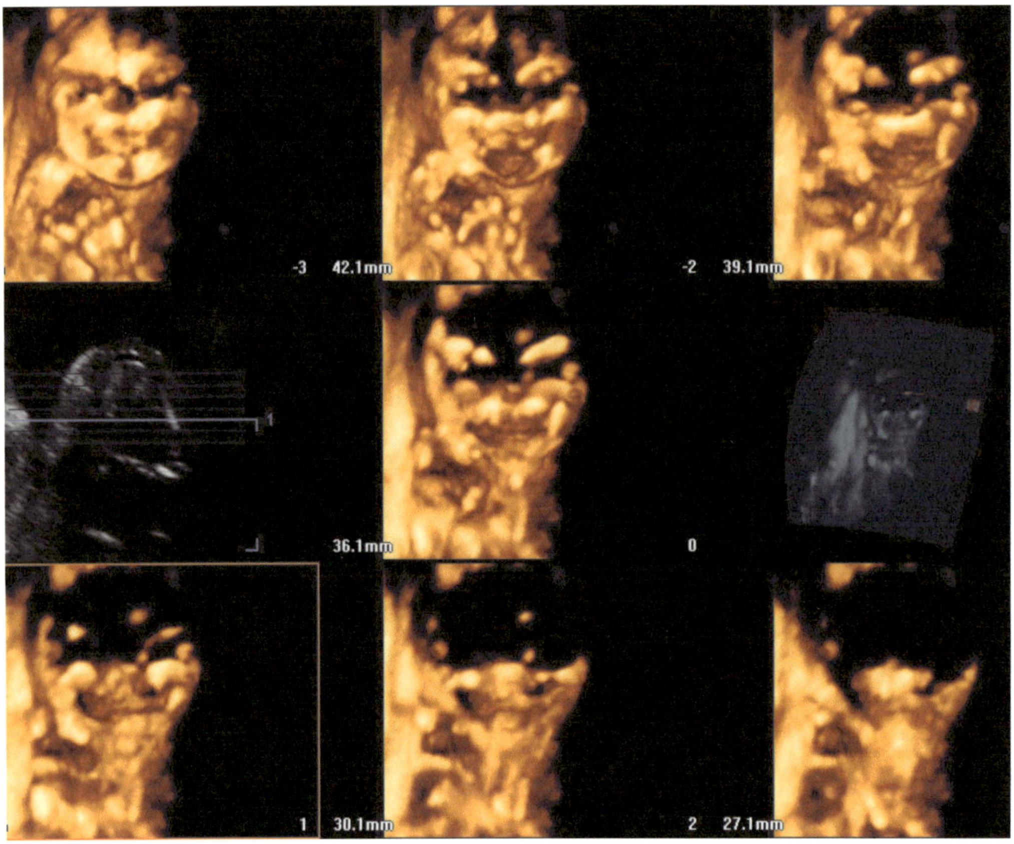

Fig. 9. TUI of the coronal view. The coronal views of the secondary palate could be assessed along the length of the palate in a serial fashion.

Platt et al. (2006) demonstrated the use of the "flipped face" view in antenatal diagnosis of facial clefts. Following acquisition of the 3D volume of the fetal face, the volume is rotated to view the palate from below in a thick slice (Fig. 10). They commented that with this method, the full length and width of the mouth and palate in the axial plane could be examined in 2 minutes.

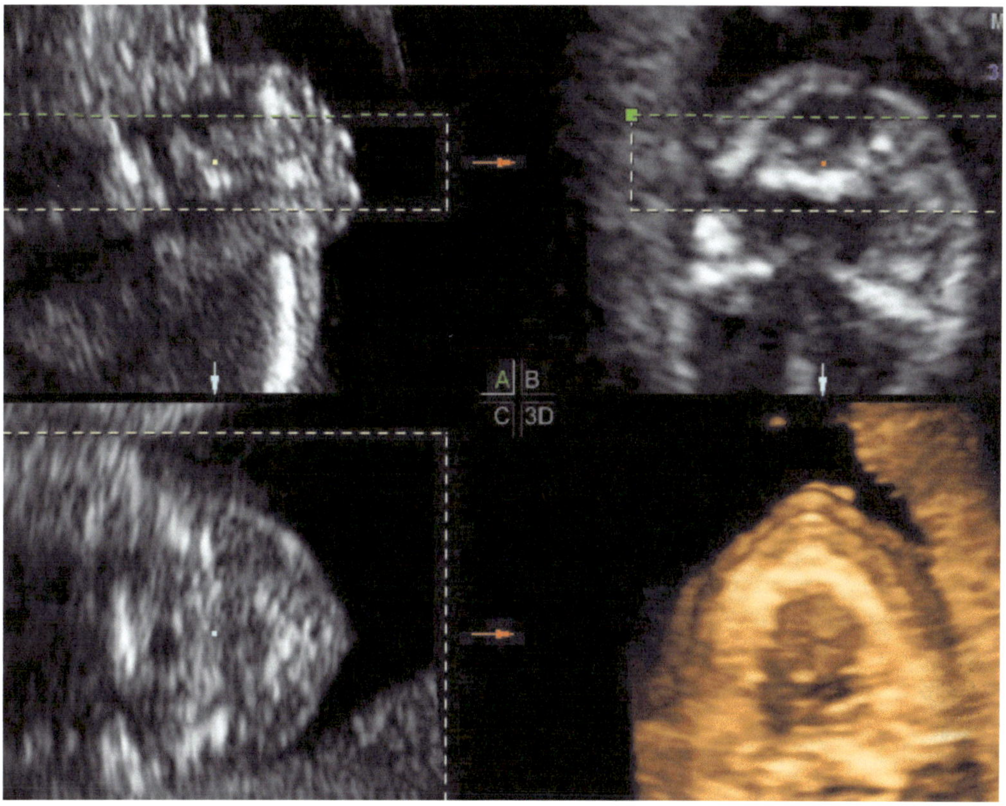

Fig. 10. The "flipped face" view. The alveolar ridge is well seen in this fetus at 18 weeks. The tip of the uvula is visible.

Wong et al (2007, 2008, 2009, and 2010) proposed a rotational method to view the secondary palate especially the soft palate, by rotating the orthogonal planes including the "flipped face" view and the reverse face view to the oblique planes (Fig. 11). With this method, one could view the surfaces of the soft palate at different angles from above or below or from the side with a stored 3D volume of the face. The uvula allows the soft palate to be identified (Fig. 5). The soft tissue around the palate does not appear to affect the view. Similar to the reverse face view, the shadowing by the facial bones and alveolar ridge could largely be avoided because the insonation plane is different from the examination plane.The authors reported the usefulness of this technique in assessing the extent of fetal cleft palate (Wong et al., 2010). However, the application of this method in assessing isolated clefts in the soft palate remains to be tested as this is a less common entity.

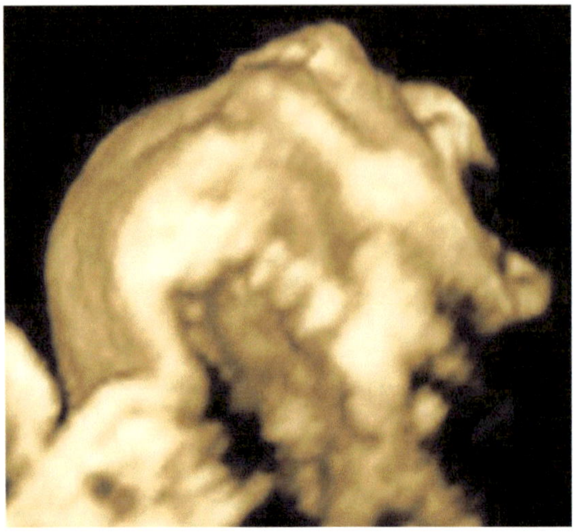

Fig. 11. The oblique axial plane. This is obtained by rotating the axial plane to an oblique plane. The under-surface of the soft palate including the uvula could be seen.

4. Conclusion

We have witnessed the advancement of ultrasound technology in the last few decades, and the increase use of 3D ultrasound in the examination of the fetus in the past 20 years. All the precious experience by previous researchers has contributed to our understand of the issues in the application of ultrasound on examination of the fetal palate and the ways to overcome them. We look forward to see what appears to be a difficult task in the past may possibly be incorporated into routine ultrasound examination of the fetus.

5. References

Grandjean H, Larroque D & Levi S. The performance of routine ultrasonographic screening of pregnancies in the Eurofetus Study. *American Journal of Obstetrics and Gynecology*, Vol 81, No. 2 (August 1999), pp. 446-454., ISSN 0002-9378

Clementi M, Tenconi R, Bianchi F & Stoll C. Evaluation of prenatal diagnosis of cleft lip with or without cleft palate and cleft palate by ultrasound: experience from 20 European registries. EUROSCAN study group. *Prenatal Diagnosis*, Vol. 20, No. 11 (November 2000), pp. 870-875, ISSN 1097-0223

Shaikh D, Mercer NS, Sohan K, Kyle P & Soothill P. Prenatal diagnosis of cleft lip and palate. *British Journal of Plastic Surgery*, Vol. 54, No. 4 (June 2001), pp. 288-289, ISSN 0007-1226

Wayne C, Cook K, Sairam S, Hollis B & Thilaganathan B. Sensitivity and accuracy of routine antenatal ultrasound screening for isolated facial clefts. *British Journal of Radiology*, Vol. 75, No. 895, (July 2002), pp. 584-589, ISSN 1748-880X

Hanikeri M, Savundra J, Gillett D, Walters M & McBain W. Antenatal transabdominal ultrasound detection of cleft lip and palate in Western Australia from 1996 to 2003. *Cleft Palate Craniofacial Journal*, Vol. 43, No. 1, (January 2006), pp. 61-66, ISSN 1545-1569.

Offerdal K, Jebens N, Syvertsen T, Blaas H-GK, Johansen OJ & Eik-Nes SH. Prenatal Ultrasound detection of facial clefts: a prospective study of 49314 deliveries in a non-selected population in Norway. *Ultrasound in Obstetrics and Gynecology*, Vol. 31, No. 6, (June 2008), pp. 639-646, ISSN 0960-7692

Demircioglu M, Kangesu L, Ismail A, Lake E, Hughes J, Wright S & Sommerlad BC. Increasing accuracy of antenatal ultrasound diagnosis of cleft lip with or without cleft palate, in cases referred to the North Thames London Region. *Ultrasound in Obstetrics and Gynecology*, Vol. 31, No. 6, (June 2008), pp. 647-651, ISSN 0960-7692

Moore KL & Persaud TVN (2003). The pharyngeal apparatus. In: *The developing human: clinically oriented embryology*. Moore KL & Persaud TVN (Ed), pp. 201-240, Saunders, ISBN 0-7216-9412-8, Philadelphia, USA.

Pretorius D, House M, Nelson T & Hollenbach, KA. Evaluation of normal and abnormal lips in fetuses: comparison between three- and two-dimensional sonography. *American Journal of Roentgenology*, Vol. 165, No. 5 (November 1995), pp. 165:1233, ISSN 1655-1233

Babcook CJ, McGahan JP, Chong BW, Nemzek WR, Salamat MS. Evaluation of fetal midface anatomy related to facial clefts: Use of US. *Radiology*, Vol. 201, No. 1 (Ocober 1996), pp. 113-118, ISSN 1527-1315

Filly RA & Feldstein VA (2000). Ultrasound evaluation of normal fetal anatomy. In: *Ultrasonography in Obstetrics and Gynecology*, PW Callen (Ed.), 221-276, WB Saunders, ISBN 0-7216-8132-8, Philadelphia, USA.

UlmMR, Kratochwil A, Ulm B, Solar P, Aro G & Bernaschek G. Three-dimensional ultrasound evaluation of fetal tooth germs. *Ultrasound in Obstetrics and Gynecology*, Vol. 12, No. 4, (October 1998), pp. 240-243, ISSN 0960-7692

Ulm MR, Kratochwil A, Ulm B, Lee A, Bettelheim D & Bernaschek G. Three-dimensional ultrasonographic imaging of fetal tooth buds for characterization of facial clefts. *Early fetal development*, Vol. 55, No. 1 (May 1999), pp. 67-75, ISSN 0378-3782

Johnson DD, Pretorius DH, Budorick NE, Jones MC, Lou KV, James GM & Nelson TR. Fetal lip and primary palate: three-dimensional versus two-dimensional US. *Radiology*, Vol. 217, No. 1 (October 2000), pp. 236-239, ISSN 1527-1315

Campbell S and Lees CC. The three-dimenisonal reverse face (3D RF) view for the diagnosis of cleft palate. *Ultrasound in Obstetrics and Gynecology*, Vol. 22, No. 6, (June 2003), pp. 552-554, ISSN 0960-7692

Campbell S, Lees C, Moscoso G and Hall P. Ultrasound antenatal diagnosis of cleft palate by a new technique: the 3D 'reverse face' view. *Ultrasound in Obstetrics and Gynecology*, Vol. 25, No. 1, (January 2005), pp. 12-18, ISSN 0960-7692

Pilu G & Segata M. A novel technique for visualization of the normal and cleft fetal secondary palate: angled insonation and three-dimensional ultrasound. *Ultrasound in Obstetrics and Gynecology*, Vol. 29, No. 2, (February 2007), pp. 166-169, ISSN 0960-7692

Platt LD, DeVore GR & Pretorius DH. Improving cleft palate/cleft lip antenatal diagnosis by 3-dimensional sonography. *Journal of Ultrasound in Medicine*, Vol.25, No. 11 (November 2006), pp.1423-1430, ISSN 1550-9613

Wong HS, Tait J & Pringle KC. The fetal soft palate: not a nowhere land on 3D ultrasound. *Ultrasound in Obstetrics and Gynecology, Vol.* 30, No.4, (October 2007), pp. 484, ISSN 0960-7692

Wong HS, Tait J & Pringle KC. Viewing of the soft and hard palate on routine 3D ultrasound sweep of the fetal face - a feasibility study. *Fetal Diagnosis and Therapy,* Vol. 24, No.2, (August 2008); pp. 146-54., ISSN 1421-9964

Wong HS, Tait J & Pringle KC. Examination of the secondary palate on stored 3D ultrasound volumes of the fetal face. *Ultrasound in Obstetrics and Gynecology,* Vol. 33, No. 4, (April 2009), pp. 407-11, ISSN 0960-7692

Wong HS, Tait J, Pringle KC. The use of oblique planes in assessing fetal cleft palate in stored 3D ultrasound volumes of fetal face. *Ultrasound in Obstetrics and Gynecology,* Vol. 36, Suppl. 1 (October 2010), pp. 249, ISSN 0960-7692

10

Ultrasound Imaging in Vascular Diseases

Mariantina Fragou[1], Andreas Karabinis[2], Eugene Daphnis[3], Nicolaos Labropoulos[4] and Dimitrios Karakitsos[1]
[1]*Department of Intensive Care Unit, General State Hospital of Athens*
[2]*Department of Intensive Care Unit, Onassis Cardiac Surgery Center, Athens*
[3]*Nephrology Department, Heraklion University Hospital, Heraklion, Crete*
[4]*Department of Surgery, Stony Brook University Medical Center, Stony Brook NY*
[1,2,3]*Greece*
[4]*USA*

1. Introduction

Ultrasound scanning has become one of the most important noninvasive investigations used in the assessment of vascular diseases. Duplex ultrasound is currently the main diagnostic modality used in deep venous thrombosis and carotid disease. It enables monitoring of bypasses for patency and neointimal hyperplasia as well as transcranial examination of brain vessels in subarachnoid hemorrhage.

Nowdays, the role of the vascular laboratory is continuously changing with the introduction of new technology. New interventions such as carotid stenting and endovascular aneurysm repair have necessitated the use of duplex ultrasound for detecting in-stent restenosis or endoleaks. Ultrasound is also used intra-operatively in evaluating endovenous procedures such as laser and radiofrequency ablation and the patency of in situ vein bypasses. Arterial mapping of the lower extremity by duplex ultrasound has replaced contrast angiography (CA) and magnetic resonance angiography (MRA) for lower extremity bypass procedures.

Most recently, a variety of new applications for vascular ultrasound has arised. Contrast-enhanced ultrasound imaging allows the assessment of microcirculation and can be used for delivery of drugs and genetic therapies. Physicians use three-dimensional ultrasound to assess carotid plaque volume and monitor its evolution with time and its response to various treatments. In the aera of atherosclerosis, ultrasound has provided a non-invasive way of assessing the elastic properties of an artery and to evaluate the patient's risks of adverse cardiovascular events. Finally, intravascular ultrasound has opened new frontiers in the measuring of intimal thickness and assessing vulnerable plaques.

2. Ultrasound in the era of atherosclerotic disease

2.1 Intravascular ultrasound (IVUS)

Intravascular ultrasound is a promising and rapidly evolving technique that provides high-quality images of the vessel's wall and lumen (Houslay & Uren, 2005) (Fig. 1).

Angiography, the traditionally used "gold-standard" in the imaging of vascular morphology (Liu & Goldberg, 1999) has multiple disadvantages, such as depiction only of contrast agent filled lumen and not the vessel wall, as well as the risk of contrast-induced nenal failure. Moreover, it underestimates the plaque burden, especially for the detection of concentrical lumen narrowing (Liu & Goldberg, 1999).

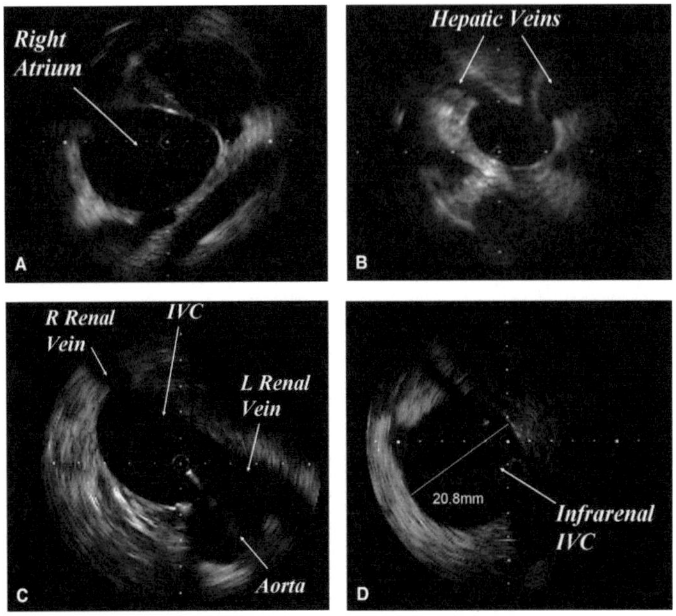

Fig. 1. Intravascular ultrasound (IVUS) advancing via the inferior vena cava (IVC) at various levels depicting the right atrium (A), the hepatic veins (B), the renal veins (C), and the infrarenal IVC (D)

With the use of high-frequency catheter based transducers, all basic components of the vessel are identified: the cross sectional luminal size, shape and vessel wall, as well as the various layers of the wall such as the intima, media, adventitia and perivascular structures (Liu & Goldberg, 1999).

In conventional gray-scale intravascular sonography arteries can be classified as elastic (lying centrally in the arterial tree) or muscular (peripherally distributed). Calcifications are demonstrated as hyperechoic areas, whereas hemorrage or fat deposition inside an atheromatic plaque is hypoechoic. Subsequently, the plaque is subclassified as lipid, calcified and fibrous, according to its differential acoustic properties (Liu & Goldberg, 1999). Furthermore, the concommitant use of colour-flow intravascular sonography allows for a real-time dynamic assessment of plaque morphology and provides a better understanding of the blood flow, the lumen size and the success of endovascular treatment (Zacharatos et al., 2010). Hence, the physician can obtain a realistic virtual histology map of the patient's arteries, visualize the atheroma without the need of true histologic sections of the diseased coronary arteries and tailor his treatments (Fayad & Fuster, 2001; Martin et al., 1997).

The correlation of IVUS plaque characteristics and histopathologic speciments is well validated in literature (Potkin et al., 1990).The CAPITAL study showed a strong correlation of IVUS findings with histologic speciments from endarterectomy (Diethrich et al., 2007) while Potkin et al compared IVUS with coronary histopathologic speciments, to show that fibrous and calcified plaques were identified with good precision (Potkin et al., 1990).

In patients with coronal artery stenosis IVUS can act as a prognostication tool, as vulnerable plaques, heavy in fat deposition are considered at higher risk for cardiovascular events and might need more aggressive treatment. In addition, plaque regression in respond to lipid lower therapies with statins has been successfully monitored by the use of serial IVUS (Crouse et al., 2007; Nissen, 2005; Nissen et al., 2008). Many dynamic phenomena in the setting of an atheroma, such as positive and negative remodeling or restenosis after angioplasty and stenting are timely demonstrated and treated accordingly (Liu & Goldberg, 1999).
The concommitant use of intravascular elastography(Fayad & Fuster, 2001) (images obtained from cardiac IVUS images associated with intraluminar pressures during the cardiac circle) expands the frontiers of the IVUS technique, as it illustrates the mechanical properties of the vessel wall and provides strain information. IVUS allows a direct visualization of the processes associated with lumen expansion by ballon dilation. It is believed that about 80% of the post-dilation increase in the lumen area is due to an increase in vessel size, and 20% is due to a reduction in plaque area, due to axial plaque redistribution (Liu & Goldberg, 1999).
IVUS can be utilized as a means of planning and evaluating the effects of vascular brachytherapy in the treatment of post-stent restenosis (Carlier et al., 2000). Apart from coronal artery disease, it is a safe method of choosing the appropriate intervention procedure in peripheral vascular disease (Fig. 2) and carotid stenting (Liu & Goldberg, 1999). It's only risk, the disruption of a plaque and release of embolic material, seems minor compared to it's numerous advantages.

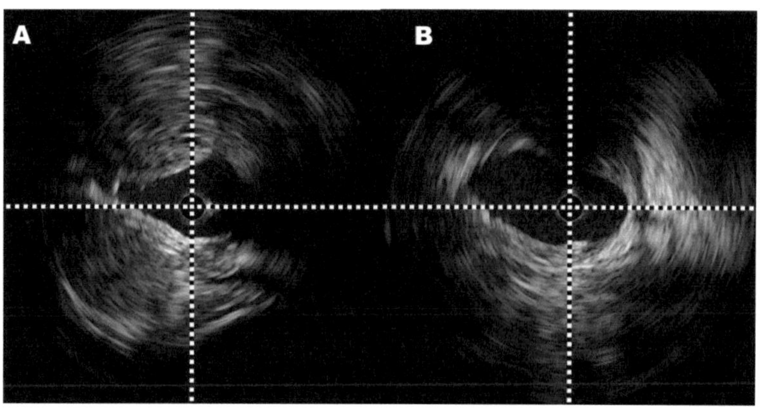

Fig. 2. Obstruction of the iliac vein: pre-intervention imaging (A) and post-intervention result (B) by intravascular ultrasound (IVUS)

2.2 3D ultrasound

Three-dimentional ultrasound is a recent development that came as an answer to the multiple problems inherent to 2D ultrasound images, leading to incorrect quantification of plaque morphology, difficult localization and significant operator dependence (Fenster et al., 2004) (Fig. 3).
3D imaging of atherosclerotic plaques can allow reproducible quantitative monitoring of plaque progression and regression and provide important information regarding the plaques' response to therapy, as its morphology and geometry is accessed (Weyman, 2009). With this technique vascular branches, accessory vessels and their intimate relationships can

be easily demonstrated (Liu & Goldberg, 1999). Arterial dissections, aneurysms and aortic dissections and flaps are depicted with 3D IVUS much better than conventional angiography.

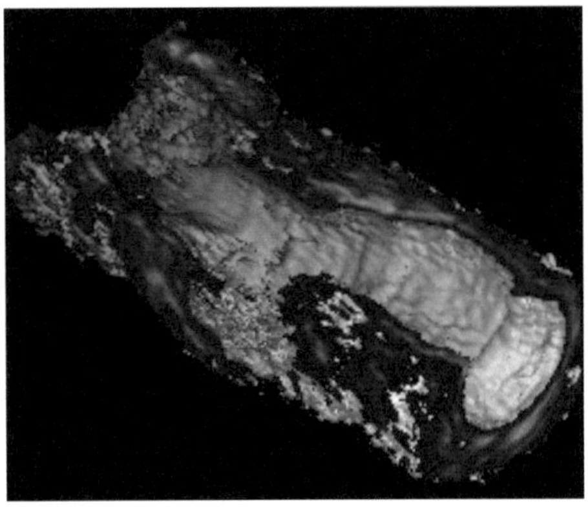

Fig. 3. 3D IVUS of an iliac artery

Although the importance of 3D imaging has been demonstrated in several studies, the widespread use of this technique has been prevented by inherent disadvantages, such as the slow frame rate, the lengthy analysis time and the limited spacial resolutions (Weyman, 2009). The combination of contrast with 3D ultrasound will likely compensate for the latter and should enhance its value in areas such as stress echocardiography (Liu & Goldberg, 1999).

2.3 Flow mediated dilatation (FMD) and carotid intima-media thickness

Endothelial dysfunction and its effect on modulation of vascular tone is considered to play an important role in the pathogenesis of the atherosclerotic process (Ghiadoni et al., 2008). The degree of vasodilation is a measure of endothelial function; the greater the vasodilation, the higher the endothelial function.

A novel non invasive technique called the "flow-mediated dilation" (FMD) of the brachial artery is nowdays widely used in current clinical practice to assess the function of the endothelium and its relationship to coronary artery disease. Ischemia of the brachial artery is induced by the inflation of an arterial cuff for five minutes. After cuff deflation brachial artery flow increases and this also increases shear stress of the artery resulting in vasodilation. It is believed that the endothelium locally produces NO in response to stress induced phosphorylation of the endothelial NO synthase (Ghiadoni et al., 2008). In arteries with impaired NO production, due to decreased endothelial function the above response is diminished.

Decreased brachial artery FMD has been associated with all the major risk factors for cardiovascular disease, such as smoking, diabetes, advanced age and hypercholesterolemia. Faulx et al have demonstrated that FMD was almost as sensitive and more specific in detecting coronary artery disease in comparison to stress electrocardiography (Faulx et al., 2003). Lerman et al showed that FMD significantly predicted cardiovascular events, independently of traditionally used cardiovascular risk factors (Lerman & Zeiher, 2005).

Limitations of this promising technique are the potential small vessel size of the brachial artery that often renders the measurement erroneous and the ambiguity in image timing after cuff deflation (Faulx et al., 2003).

Another marker used to quantify atherosclerosis by B-mode ultrasound is the measurement of carotid intima-media thickness (CIMT) (de Groot et al., 2008; Labropoulos et al., Dec 2005). A simple distance measurement between the leading edges of the lumen-intima and media-adventitia ultrasound interfaces is performed and this measurement can be used to measure the degree of existing atherosclerosis and future cardiovascular disease risk (de Groot et al., 2008; Bots et al., 1997; Chambless et al., 1997). Futhermore, several studies in literature have proved the efficacy of CIMT in monitoring the patient's response to lipid lowering therapies (Blankenhorn et al., 1993; de Groot et al., 1998; Furberg et al., 1994; Smilde et al., 2001).

3. Pre-operative ultrasound use

In patients with lower extremity ischemia, angiography has traditionally been considered the "gold standard" of arterial mapping. However, in recent years, duplex ultrasonography (DA) has gained a major role in the pre-operative evaluation of patients undergoing lower extremity bypass (Ascher et al., 1999; Grassbaugh et al., 2003; Ligush et al., 1998; Pemberton et al., 1996; Proia et al., 2001). Mazzariol et al reported that the use of dupplex ultrasonography can provide enough information for surgery in more than 83% of patients with arterial stenosis and that an abnornal femoral artery waveform was 100% predictive for detecting stenosis greater than 80% (Mazzariol et al., 2000) Proia et al have also confirmed these results (Proia et al., 2001).

In comparison with conventional angiography or MRA, DA has a lower sensitivity for detecting arterial disease of the lower extremity. Moreover, it is often cumbersome and time-consuming to scan the entire arterial tree from the aorta to the pedal vessels. Imaging can also be obscured in obese patients or heavily calcified vessels. Nevertheless, the simplicity and safety of this technique underlines its importance as a first-line examination before planning a bypass surgery (Pearce & Astleford, 2004).

4. Intra-operative and post-operative ultrasound

Completion angiography has been traditionally used as an adjunctive technique after bypass procedures to scan the graft for anatomic and flow abnormalities. Nowdays, duplex scanning is used as a safer alternative to visualize these abnormalities (Johnson et al., 2000). Defective grafts are identified by direct measurement of PSV and ratio at the lesion devided by proximal velocity (Johnson et al., 2000).

Moreover, surveillance Duplex ultrasound has acquired an important role in the post-operative assessment of patients following lower extremity revascularization. It enables prompt detection of hemodynamically significant lesions and early intervention (Bandyk, 2002, Mills et al., 2001). Patients undergoing EVAR (endovascular aneurysm repair) are also monitored by serial ultrasound examinations (Bendick et al., 2003; Carter et al., 2000; McWilliams et al., 1999; Pearce & Astleford, 2004). The value of duplex ultrasound scanning in this group of patients is that repeated studies can be performed frequently to detect an endoleak or a restenosis, without the risk of contrast-induced nephropathy or the presence of adjuscent metal artifacts.

Carotid artery stenting (CAS) is currently being clinically evaluated as an alternative to conventional carotid endarterectomy (CEA). Dupplex ultrasound is commonly used to monitor restenosis in patients following CEA. Several authors in literature begin to report their experience in the use of ultrasonography as a follow-up tool in CAS too (Lal et al., 2004).

5. Ultrasound in venous disease

In the field of deep venous thrombosis ultrasound is nowdays the sole diagnostic modality in most centers and has contibuted extensively in our understanding of the natural history and the pathophysiology of the disease (Labropoulos et al., Feb 2005; Labropoulos et al., Jan 2010; Apr 2010) (Figures 4, 5).

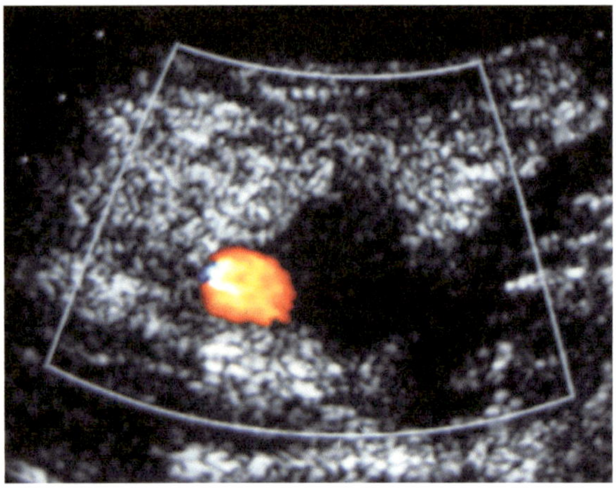

Fig. 4. Acute thrombosis in the common femoral vein. There is absence of color, the vein is dilated (twice the size of the adjacent common femoral artery in red) with homogenous echolucent texture

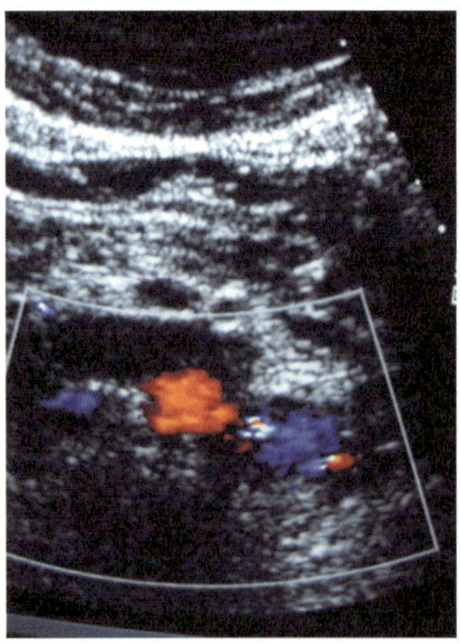

Fig. 5. Chronic inferior vana cava (IVC) obstruction with partial recanalization. The lumen of IVC is smaller compared to the adjacent aorta. The azygos vein is dilated and larger than the aorta.

Duplex ultrasound is also used as a follow-up tool to detect venous reflux up to six months after treatment (Labropoulos et al., Feb 2005) (Fig. 6) and to investigate conditions such as thrombus neovascularization (Labropoulos et al., Sep 2005).

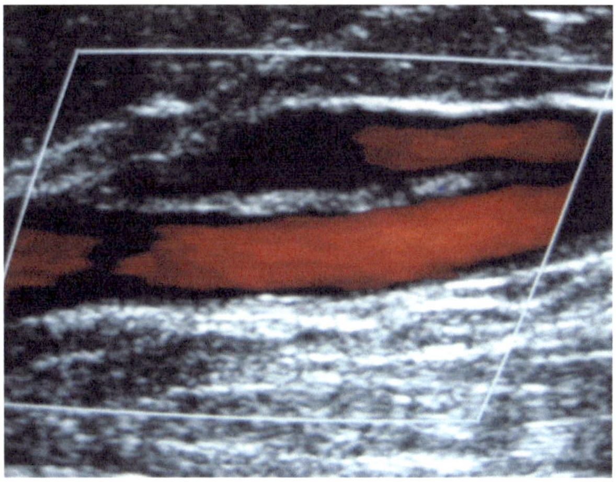

Fig. 6. Chronic thrombus with partial recanalization in great saphenous vein. Flow channels with reflux are seen over the old thrombus that is seen as an echogenic band in the lumen

Patients undergoing varicose vein stripping and venous ablative surgery routinely undergo preoperative ultrasound scanning to assure that the deep venous system is clot-free and to identify the location of perforators and accessory veins as well as the presence of lesser saphenous reflux. Intraoperatively, the use of ultrasound allows for placement of a catheter under direct guidance close to the sapheno-femoral junction, and then the anesthesia agent is injected (Min et al., 2001; Pichot et al., 2004). Successful ablation is then established by monitoring venous occlusion by means of ultrasonography.

6. Contrast-enhanced ultrasound

Gramiak was the first to describe contrast enhanced ultrasound in 1969, using air bubbles in the aorta (Gramiak et al., 1969). In modern clinical practice contrast agents for ultrasound use are microbubbles of different gases, 1-7μm in diameter (Cosgrove, 2006). The gas can be air, which unfortunately dissolves quickly in water or blood, or newer agents such as sulphur hexafloride, perfluocarbons or heavy gases, which minimally dissolve in water (Cosgrove, 2006). In order to reach and persist in systemic circulation the microbubbles are stabilized with albumin, simple phospholipids micelles, bilayered membranes and biocompatible polymers (Cosgrove, 2006). Inside the vessels microbubbles expand and contract in the alternating pressure waves of the ultrasound beam, while tissues are almost incompressible. Special software using multiple pulse sequences enhances this blood-tisue border detection (Weyman, 2009). Adverse effects of contrast agents are headache, bruising, injection site pain, paresthesias and burning.

Microbubbles are currently used to improve Doppler studies especially when flow information makes conventional imaging difficult, a technique called "Doppler rescue" (Cosgrove, 2006). Common applications include imaging of the basilar and vertebral arteries, transcranial ultrasound examinations in patients with severe hyperostosis of the skull, measurement of internal carotid stenosis in calcified arteries (Cosgrove, 2006) and differentiation of subtotal stenosis from occlusion in acute stroke (Seidel & Meairs, 2009). Moreover, contrast enhanced ultrasound has been used in renal artery stenosis, portal and hepatic artery examinations (e.g. in cirrhosis, tips shunts or after liver transplantation) (Furlow, 2009) and in liver oncology (Wilson & Burns, 2006) (Fig. 7).

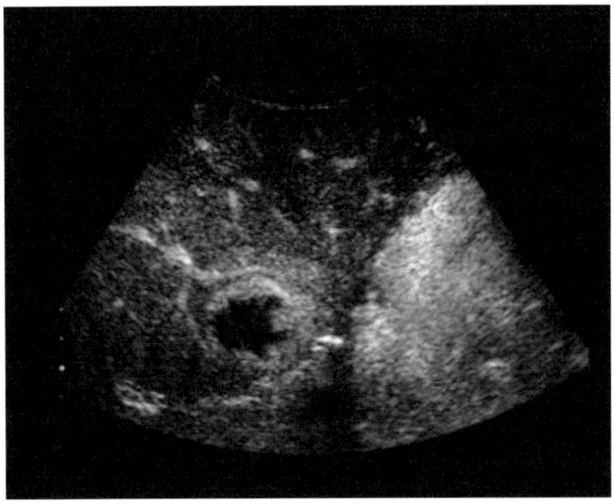

Fig. 7. Contrast-enhanced ultrasound of an hepatic hemangioma

Neurosurgeons can intra-operatively assess vascular pathologies such as middle cerebral artery aneurysms and arteriovenous malformations in real time and make appropriate surgical planning (Hölscher et al., 2007).

The microbubbles used in contrast-enhanced ultrasound techniques after attachment of antibodies or other ligants to their shell can bind to specific cell receptors in areas of disease (Voigt, 2009), thus provide information about the stage of the disease (Lindner, 2009). Several promising studies have targeted pathologic processes with contrast-enhanced ultrasound (Lindner, 2009; Voigt, 2009), such as angiogenesis (by targeting endothelial integrins) (Lerman & Zeiher, 2005), thrombus (by targeting IIbIIIa receptors or fibrinogen) (Alonso et al., 2007), inflammation (by targeting ICAM-1, VCAM-1 P- and L- selectin) and plaque (by targeting ICAM-1, VCAM-1 and several angiogenesis markers) (Voigt, 2009). In fact, it is believed that by targeting plaque inflammation and neovascularization we could identify patients at high risk for cardiovascular events well before angiography (Lindner, 2009; Voigt, 2009) or even recognise "vulnerable plaques" and begin early treatment (Vicenzini et al., 2009).

Several future promising therapeutic applications of microbubbles are under research. Therapeutic agents, genes, siRNAs, drugs and molecules can be attached to or dissolved within the surface shell or deposited within the bubbles themselves (Hernot & Klibanov, 2008; Hynynen, 2008; Weyman, 2009).

Local cavitation due to microbubble destruction can produce clot fragmentation and enhance thrombolysis (Medel et al., 2009; Trübestein et al., 1976). Continuous transcranial Doppler has been shown to augment the t-PA induced arterial recanalization in stroke victims (Alexandrov et al., 2004). Future studies need to be performed in order to improve the safety profile and therapeutic indexes of these challenging techniques.

7. Conclusion

Ultrasound imaging in vascular diseases has evolved during the past years due to new challenging technologies. Virtually all peripheral arterial and venous structures can be visualized with color duplex ultrasound. In the era of atherosclerosis, the use of intravascular ultrasound, contrast-enhanced ultrasound, 3D ultrasound, flow mediated dilatation and carotid intima media thickness techniques allow for more precise and localized diagnosis, treatment and follow-up. Ultrasound techniques routinely performed before, during or after surgical procedures are nowdays commonplace. The low cost and noninvasive aspect of most ultrasound methods make it the technique of choice in studying the human vasculature.

8. References

Alexandrov AV, Molina CA, Grotta JC, Garami Z, Ford SR, Alvarez-Sabin J, Montaner J, Saqqur M, Demchuk AM, Moyé LA, Hill MD & Wojner AW. Ultrasound-enhanced systemic thrombolysis for acute ischemic stroke. *N Engl J Med,* Vol. 351, No. 21, (Nov 2004), pp. 2170-2178

Alonso A, Della Martina A, Stroick M, Fatar M, Griebe M, Pochon S, Schneider M, Hennerici M, Allémann E, Meairs S. Molecular imaging of human thrombus with novel abciximab immunobubbles and ultrasound. *Stroke,* Vol. 38, No. 5, (May 2007), pp. 1508-1514

Ascher E, Mazzariol F, Hingorani A, Salles-Cunha S & Gade P. The use of Duplex ultrasound arterial mapping as an alternative to conventional arteriography for primary and secondary infrapopliteal bypasses. *Am J Surg,* Vol. 178, No. 2, (Aug 1999), pp. 162–165

Bandyk DF. Infrainguinal vein bypass graft surveillance: how to do it, when to intervene, and is it cost effective? *J Am Coll Surg,* Vol. 194, No. 1 suppl, (Jan 2002), pp. 540-552 Bendick PJ, Bove PG, Long GW, Zelenock GB, Brown OW & Shanley CJ. Efficacy of ultrasound scan contrast agents in the noninvasive follow-up of aortic stent grafts. *J Vasc Surg,* Vol. 37, No. 2, (Feb 2003), pp. 381–385

Blankenhorn DH, Selzer RH, Crawford DW, Barth JD, Liu CR, Liu CH, Mack WJ & Alaupovic P. Beneficial effects of colestipol niacin therapy on the common carotid artery. Two- and four-year reduction of intima-media thickness measured by ultrasound. *Circulation,* Vol. 88, No. 1, (Jul 1993), pp. 20-28

Bots ML, Hoes AW, Koudstaal PJ, Hofman A & Grobbee DE. Common carotid ntima-media thickness and risk of stroke and myocardial infarction: the Rotterdam Study. *Circulation,* Vol. 96, No. 5, (Sep 1997), pp. 1432-1437

Carlier SG, Coen VL, Sabaté M, Kay IP, Ligthart JM, Van Der Giessen WJ, Levendag PC, Bom K & Serruys PW. The role of intravascular ultrasound imaging in vascular brachytherapy. *Int J Cardiovasc Intervent,* Vol. 3, No. 1, (Mar 2000), pp. 3-12

Carter KA, Nelms CR, Bloch PHS, Gregory RT, Parent EN & DeMasi RJ. Doppler waveform assessment of endoleak following endovascular repair of abdominal aortic aneurysm: predictors of endoleak thrombosis. *J Vasc Technol,* Vol. 24, No. 2, (2000), pp. 119 122

Chambless LE, Heiss G, Folsom AR, Rosamond W, Szklo M, Sharrett AR & Clegg LX. Association of coronary heart disease incidence with carotid arterial wall thickness and major risk factors: the Atherosclerosis Risk in Communities (ARIC) Study, 1987-1993. *Am J Epidemiol,* Vol. 146, No. 6, (Sep 1997), pp. 483-494

Cosgrove D. Ultrasound contrast agents: an overview. *Eur J Radiol*, Vol. 60, No. 3, (Dec 2006), pp. 324-330

Crouse JRr, Raichlen JS, Riley WA, Evans GW, Palmer MK, O'Leary DH Grobbee DE & Bots ML. Effect of rosuvastatin on progression of carotid Intima media thickness in low-risk individuals with

subclinical atherosclerosis: the METEOR Trial. *JAMA*, Vol. 297, No. 12, (Mar 2007), pp. 1344-1353

de Groot E, Jukema JW, Montauban van Swijndregt AD, Zwinderman AH, Ackerstaff RG, van der Steen AF, Bom N, Lie KI & Bruschke AV. B-mode ultrasound assessment of pravastatin treatment effect on carotid and femoral artery walls and its correlations with coronary arteriographic findings: a report of the Regression Growth Evaluation Statin Study (REGRESS). *J Am Coll Cardiol*, Vol. 31, No. 7, (Jun 1998), pp. 1561-1567

de Groot E, van Leuven SI, Duivenvoorden R, Meuwese MC, Akdim F, Bots ML & Kastelein JJ. Measurement of carotid intima-media thickness to assess progression and regression of atherosclerosis. *Nat Clin Pract Cardiovasc Med*, Vol. 5, No. 5, (May 2008), pp. 280 288

Diethrich EB, Pauliina Margolis M, Reid DB, Burke A, Ramaiah V, Rodriguez - Lopez JA, Wheatley G, Olsen D & Virmani R. Virtual histology intravascular ultrasound assessment of carotid artery disease: the Carotid Artery Plaque Virtual Histology Evaluation (CAPITAL) study. *J Endovasc Ther*, Vol. 14, No. 5, (Oct 2007), pp. 676-86

Faulx MD, Wright AT & Hoit BD. Detection of endothelial dysfunction with brachial artery ultrasound scanning. *Am Heart J*, Vol. 145, No. 6, (Jun 2003), pp. 943-951

Fayad ZA & Fuster V. Clinical imaging of the high-risk or vulnerable atherosclerotic plaque. *Circ Res*, Vol. 89, No. 4, (Aug 2001), pp. 305-316

Fenster A, Landry A, Downey DB, Hegele RA & Spence JD. 3D ultrasound imaging of the carotid arteries. *Curr Drug Targets Cardiovasc Haematol Disord*, Vol. 4, No. 2, (Jun 2004), pp. 161-175

Furberg CD, Adams HPJ, Applegate WB, Byington RP, Espeland MA, Hartwell T, Hunninghake DB, Lefkowitz DS, Probstfield J & Riley WA. Effect of lovastatin on early carotid atherosclerosis and cardiovascular events. Asymptomatic Carotid Artery Progression Study (ACAPS) Research Group. *Circulation*, Vol. 90, No. 4, (Oct 1994), pp. 1679-1687

Furlow B. Contrast-enhanced ultrasound. *Radiol Technol*, Vol. 80, No. 6, (Jul Aug 2009), pp. 547S-561S

Ghiadoni L, Versari D, Giannarelli C, Faita F & Taddei S. Non-invasive diagnostic tools for investigating endothelial dysfunction. *Curr Pharm*, Vol. 14, No. 35, (Dec 2008), pp. 3715-3722

Gramiak R, Shah PM & Kramer DH: Ultrasound cardiography: contrast studies in anatomy and function. *Radiology*, Vol. 92, No. 5, (Apr 1969), pp. 939-948

Grassbaugh JA, Nelson PR, Rzucidlo EM, Schermerhorn ML, Fillinger MF, Powell RJ, Zwolak RM, Cronenwett JL & Walsh DB. Blinded comparison of preoperative duplex ultrasound scanning and contrast arteriography for planning revascularization at the level of the tibia. *J Vasc Surg*, Vol. 37, No 6, (Jun 2003), pp. 1186-1190

Hernot S & Klibanov AL. Microbubbles in ultrasound-triggered drug and gene delivery. *Adv Drug Deliv Rev*, Vol. 60, No. 10, (Jun 2008), pp. 1153-1166

Hölscher T, Ozgur B, Singel S, Wilkening WG, Mattrey RF & Sang H. Intraoperative ultrasound using phase inversion harmonic imaging: first experiences.

Neurosurgery, Vol. 60, No. 4, Suppl. 2, (Apr 2007), pp. 382-386, discussion 386-387
Houslay ES & Uren NG. Intravascular ultrasound: defining plaque regression. *Hosp Med*, Vol. 66, No. 1, (Jan 2005), pp. 27-31

Hynynen K. Ultrasound for drug and gene delivery to the brain. *Adv Drug Deliv Rev*, Vol. 60, No. 10, (Jun 2008), pp. 1209-1217

Johnson BL, Bandyk DF, Back MR, Avino AJ & Roth SM. Intraoperative duplex monitoring of infrainguinal vein bypass procedures. *J Vasc Surg*, Vol. 31, No. 4, (Apr 2000), pp. 678-690

Labropoulos N, Bhatti AF, Amaral S, Leon L, Borge M, Rodriguez H & Kalman P. Neovascularization in acute venous thrombosis. *J Vasc Surg*, Vol. 42, No. 3, (Sep 2005), pp. 515-518

Labropoulos N, Kokkosis AA, Spentzouris G, Gasparis AP & Tassiopoulos AK. The distribution and significance of varicosities in the saphenous trunks. *J Vasc Surg*, Vol. 51, No 1, (Jan 2010), pp. 96

Labropoulos N, Leon L, Kwon S, Tassiopoulos A, Gonzalez-Fajardo JA, Kang SS, Mansour MA & Littooy FN. Study of the venous reflux progression. *J Vasc Surg*, Vol. 41, No. 2, (Feb 2005), pp. 291-295

Labropoulos N, Leon LRJ, Brewster LP, Pryor L, Tiongson J, Kang SS, Mansour MA & Kalman P. Are your arteries older than your age?. *Eur J Vasc Endovasc Surg*, Vol. 30, No. 6, (Dec 2005), pp. 588-596

Labropoulos N, Jen J, Jen H, Gasparis AP & Tassiopoulos AK: Recurrent deep vein thrombosis: long-term incidence and natural history. *Ann Surg*, Vol. 251, No. 4, (Apr 2010), pp. 749-753

Lal BK, Hobson RW 2nd, Goldstein J, Chakhtoura EY & Duran WN. Carotid artery stenting: is there a need to revise ultrasound velocity criteria? *J Vasc Surg*, Vol. 39, No.1, (Jan 2004), pp. 58–66

Lerman A & Zeiher AM. Endothelial function: cardiac events. *Circulation*, Vol. 111, No. 3, (Jan 2005), pp. 363-368

Ligush J Jr, Reavis SW, Preisser JS & Hansen KJ. Duplex ultrasound scanning Defines operative strategies for patients with limb-threatening ischemia. *J Vasc Surg*, Vol. 28, No. 3, (Sep 1998), pp. 482–490

Lindner JR. Contrast ultrasound molecular imaging of inflammation in cardiovascular disease. *Cardiovasc Res*, Vol. 84, No. 2, (Nov 2009), pp. 182-189

Liu JB & Goldberg BB. 2-D and 3-D endoluminal ultrasound: vascular and nonvascular applications. *Ultrasound Med Biol*, Vol. 5, No. 2, (Feb 1999), pp. 159-173

Martin AJ, Ryan LK, Gotlieb AI, Henkelman RM & Foster FS . Arterial imaging: comparison of high-resolution US and MR imaging with histologic correlation. *Radiographics*, Vol. 17, No. 1, (Jan- Feb 1997), pp. 189-202

Mazzariol F, Ascher E, Hingorani A, Gunduz Y, Yorkovich W & Salles-Cunha S. Lower-extremity revascularisation without preoperative contrast arteriography in 185 cases: lessons learned with duplex ultrasound arterial mapping. *Eur J Vasc Endovasc Surg*, Vol. 19, No. 5, (May 2000), pp. 509-515

McWilliams RG, Martin J, White D, Gould DA, Harris PL, Fear SC, Brennan J, Gilling-Smith GL, Bakran A & Rowlands PC. Use of contrast-enhanced ultrasound in follow-up after endovascular aortic aneurysm repair. *J Vasc Interven Radiol* , Vol. 10, No. 8, (Sep 1999), pp. 1107–1114

Medel R, Crowley RW, McKisic MS, Dumont AS & Kassell NF. Sonothrombolysis: an emerging modality for the management of stroke. *Neurosurgery*, Vol. 65, No. 5, (Nov 2009), pp. 979-993, discussion 993

Mills JL Sr, Wixon CL, James DC, Devine J, Westerband A & Hughes JD. The natural history of intermediate and critical vein graft stenosis: recommendations for continued surveillance or repair. *J Vasc Surg*, Vol. 33, No. 2, (Feb 2001), pp. 273–278 [discussion 278–280]

Min RJ, Zimmet SE, Isaacs MN & Forrestal MD. Endovenous laser treatment of the incompetent greater saphenous vein. *J Vasc Interven Radiol,* Vol. 12, No. 10, (Oct 2001), pp. 1167–1171

Nissen SE. Effect of intensive lipid lowering on progression of coronary atherosclerosis: evidence for an early benefit from the Reversal of Atherosclerosis with Aggressive Lipid Lowering (REVERSAL) trial. *Am J Cardiol,* Vol. 96, No. 5A, (Sep 2005), pp. 61F-68F

Nissen SE, Nicholls SJ, Wolski K, Rodés-Cabau J, Cannon CP, Deanfield JE, Després JP, Kastelein JJ, Steinhubl SR, Kapadia S, Yasin M, Ruzyllo W, Gaudin C, Job B, Hu B, Bhatt DL, Lincoff AM & Tuzcu EM. Effect of rimonabant on progression of atherosclerosis in patients with abdominal obesity and coronary artery disease: the STRADIVARIUS randomized controlled trial. *JAMA*, Vol. 299, No. 13, (Apr 2008), pp. 1547-1560

Pearce WH & Astleford P: What's new in vascular ultrasound. *Surg Clin North Am,* Vol. 84, No. 4, (Aug 2004), pp. 1113-1126

Pemberton M, Nydahl S, Hartshorne T, Naylor AR, Bell PR & London NJ. Colour-coded duplex imaging can safely replace diagnostic arteriography in patients with lower-limb arterial disease. *Br J Surg*, Vol. 83, No. 12, (Dec 1996), pp. 1725–1728

Pichot O, Kabnick LS, Creton D, Merchant RF, Schuller-Petroviae S & Chandler JG. Duplex ultrasound scan findings two years after great saphenous vein radiofrequency endovenous obliteration. *J Vasc Surg*, Vol. 39, No. 1, (Jan 2004), pp. 189–195

Potkin BN, Bartorelli AL, Gessert JM, Neville RF, Almagor Y, Roberts WC, & Leon MB. Coronary artery imaging with intravascular high frequency ultrasound. *Circulation,* Vol. 81, No. 5, (May 1990), pp. 1575-1585

Proia RR, Walsh DB, Nelson PR, Powell RJ, Zwolak RM, Fillinger MF & Cronenwett JL. Early results of infragenicular revascularization based solely on duplex arteriography. *J Vasc Surg*, Vol. 33, No. 6, (Jun 2001), pp. 1165–1170

Seidel G & Meairs S. Ultrasound contrast agents in ischemic stroke. *Cerebrovasc Dis,* Vol. 27, No. Suppl 2 (2009), pp. 25-39

Smilde TJ, van Wissen S, Wollersheim H, Trip MD, Kastelein JJ & Stalenhoef AF. Effect of aggressive versus conventional lipid lowering on atherosclerosis progression in familial hypercholesterolaemia (ASAP): a prospective, randomised, double-blind trial. *Lancet,* Vol. 357, No. 9256, (Feb 2001), pp. 577-581

Trübestein G, Engel C, Etzel F, Sobbe A, Cremer H & Stumpff U. Thrombolysis by ultrasound. *Clin Sci Mol Med,* Vol. Suppl 3, (Dec 1976), pp. 697s-698s

Vicenzini E, Giannoni MF, Benedetti-Valentini F & Lenzi GL. Imaging of carotid plaque angiogenesis. *Cerebrovasc Dis*, Vol. 27, No. Suppl 2, (2009), pp.48-54

Voigt JU. Ultrasound molecular imaging. *Methods,* Vol. 48, No. 2, (Jun 2009), pp. 92-97

Weyman AE. Future directions in echocardiography. *Rev Cardiovasc Med,* Vol. 10, No. 1, (Winter 2009), pp. 4-13

Wilson SR & Burns PN. Microbubble contrast for radiological imaging: 2. Applications. *Ultrasound Q,* Vol. 22, No. 1, (Mar 2006), pp: 15-18

Zacharatos H, Hassan AE & Qureshi A. (2010). Intravascular ultrasound: principles and cerebrovascular applications. *AJNR Am J Neuroradiol*, Vol. 31, No. 4, (Apr 2010), pp. 586-597

11

The Role of Obstetric Ultrasound in Reducing Maternal and Perinatal Mortality

Yaw Amo Wiafe, Alexander T. Odoi and Edward T. Dassah
Komfo Anokye Teaching Hospital
Ghana

1. Introduction

The joy that every expectant couple, family, or community has when a woman gets pregnant is suddenly turned into sorrow and mourning when the woman dies during pregnancy or child birth, or when the baby dies. According to the World Health Organization (WHO), the five major causes of maternal mortality are hemorrhage, sepsis, complications of abortion, eclampsia, and obstructed labour (Bale et al, 2003).

The WHO similarly lists the most common causes of neonatal mortality as infections, birth asphyxia, birth injuries, preterm births, and birth defects (Bale et al., 2003). It is worth noting that these mortality causes are conditions for which timely ultrasound imaging could be of immense help in early diagnosis and hence intervention, leading to the reduction of mortality rates among mothers and their babies.

It is also notable that most of these avoidable deaths (99%) occur in developing countries, where ultrasound imaging is currently underutilized, and financial constraints have been cited as the main reason. However, the usefulness of ultrasound imaging in preventing these needless deaths has not been fully exploited. It is anticipated that low resource settings could benefit by prudent application of this modern technology which is a relatively affordable and safe imaging modality. In recent times technology has made this modality so affordable and widely available, that it is unacceptable to watch such needless deaths occur when ultrasound application could help improve survival rates.

This chapter discusses the usefulness of ultrasound imaging at various stages of pregnancy, whether in apparently normal or high risk situations. Current advances in obstetric ultrasound application and imaging techniques that are helpful for improving pregnancy outcome are discussed. The chapter also addresses the availability of more affordable but high quality ultrasound equipment that can improve obstetric healthcare, accentuating the need to implement sustainable ultrasound practice standards in developing countries where the current rate of maternal and perinatal mortalities is unacceptably high.

It must be emphasised that the objective and focus of this chapter is the role ultrasound plays in the diagnosis and in some cases follow-up or interventionary guidance, not the management of the various conditions. Readers may consult other literature for the specific management of these conditions.

2. Reducing mortality rates by ultrasound imaging in the first trimester

Ectopic pregnancy, abortion, and gestational trophoblastic diseases (GTDs) are the commonest conditions of the first-trimester that can cause maternal mortality, due to the possibility of severe haemorrhage, shock or sepsis. Patients usually present with bleeding and/or pain but can also remain asymptomatic for a long time. In some cases patients don't even realize that they are pregnant, particularly in some cases of ectopic pregnancy and missed abortion. Ultrasound imaging is extremely useful for obtaining accurate diagnosis for these first trimester conditions. It is therefore important to exclude early pregnancy pathology in every woman of reproductive age who presents with amenorrhoea, abnormal bleeding and/or pain, using diagnostic ultrasound imaging in combination with beta human chorionic gonadotropin (β-HCG). This approach to medical care can potentially reduce maternal mortality rates.

In terms of perinatal mortality the role of ultrasound imaging in detecting markers for chromosomal anomalies and structural defects in the fetus to enable early intervention or close monitoring is very important.

2.1.1 Ectopic pregnancy

Ectopic pregnancy accounts for 9% of all pregnancy-related deaths (Uzelac and Garmel, 2007). However, because of improved diagnostic capabilities, notably in ultrasound imaging, the incidence of mortality has relatively declined in the US and other developed countries since the 1970s, despite the increasing number of ectopic pregnancies (Lawson et al, 1988; Levine, 2000). This implies that improving on the use of ultrasound imaging in developing countries could equally improve survival rates of deaths caused by ectopic gestation.

In the evaluation of suspected ectopic pregnancy β-HCG and ultrasound complement each other. Transvaginal sonography (TVS) is able to reliably identify an intrauterine gestational sac when the serum β-HCG is 1000mIU/ml and transabdominal sonography (TAS) when the β-HCG level is 1800-3600mIU/ml. Thus TVS detects either a normal or an abnormal intrauterine gestational sac earlier than TAS. With TVS the transducer is closer to the uterus and adnexae allowing higher frequencies to be used, since there are fewer tissue interfaces with less beam scatter and the effect of abdominal wall fat is avoided, (details of the TVS technique are described in another section of this chapter).

In sonographic diagnosis of ectopic pregnancy, TVS may reveal only a thickened decidualised endometrium. With more advanced ectopic pregnancies, decidual sloughing with resultant fluid or blood in the cavity may lead to the formation of a small and irregular intrauterine structure, the so-called pseudogestational sac. Diagnostic accuracy is further enhanced by the use of transvaginal colour Doppler sonography (TV-CDS) compared with the use of TVS alone, which will detect an increased peritrophoblastic flow on colour Doppler at the site of implantation.

In a patient with a positive β-HCG who has no sonographic evidence of an intrauterine pregnancy, the presence of an adnexal mass is suggestive of ectopic pregnancy with a positive predictive value of 70% to 75% (Nyberg et al, 1991).

In some cases, an echogenic adnexal ring will be seen separate from the ovary, known as tubal ring. Tubal ring has been detected in 68% of unruptured tubal pregnancies using TVS, with a positive predictive value of 100% (Fleischer et al, 1990; Nyberg et al, 1991)

The specific diagnosis of ectopic pregnancy however, is the demonstration of a gestational sac with an embryo in the adnexa (Nyberg et al, 1991) (Figure 1). A live extrauterine fetus can be detected with TVS in 17% to 28% of patients with ectopic pregnancies (Thorsen et al, 1990; Fleischer et al, 1990) compared with approximately 10% with TAS (Mahony et al, 1985), implying that an examiner should progress to TVS if TAS findings are suboptimal.

With TV-CDS an adnexal peritrophoblastic flow with a high-velocity and low-resistance spectral pattern may be demonstrated, separate from the ovary (Pellerito et al, 1992).
Also the presence of free fluid in the pouch of Douglas is a nonspecific finding that suggests the presence of an ectopic pregnancy in the appropriate clinical setting. The amount of fluid and the echogenicity of the fluid are important clues in predicting the presence of a ruptured ectopic pregnancy. Large amounts of fluid and increased echogenicity of the fluid are both more indicative of a ruptured ectopic pregnancy (Frates et al, 1994). In patients with suspected ectopic pregnancy, the combination of an adnexal mass and echogenic free fluid is associated with a 97% positive predictive value for ruptured ectopic pregnancy (Nyberg et al, 1991). Detecting the ectopic pregnancy before rupture will avoid blood loss and consequent morbidity and mortality (Dassah et al, 2009). Even when rupture has occurred early detection by ultrasound imaging will obviously help to prevent further blood loss.

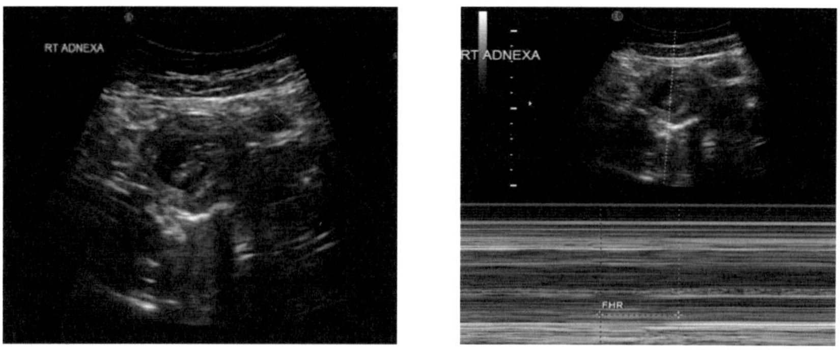

(a) (b)

Fig. 1. (a)&(b) shows a right adnexal ectopic gestation with a live embryo demonstrated by M mode assessment of fetal heart rate (FHR).

2.1.2 Abortion

Unsafe abortion is known to account for 13% of maternal mortality (WHO 2005). Regardless of whether an abortion is spontaneous or induced, subsequent events and the care received determine whether the abortion is safe or unsafe. If an incomplete abortion is not appropriately treated, it can lead to haemorrhage, shock, sepsis and death. Ultrasound imaging is useful for obtaining definitive diagnosis, as the symptoms of incomplete abortion and ectopic pregnancy may be similar. Moreover if a miscarriage is assumed to have occurred, or termination of pregnancy is carried out without an initial ultrasound imaging, one may not know whether subsequent complaints of bleeding and pain are caused by retained products of conception, ectopic pregnancy or even a haemorrhagic corpus luteum. Additionally, early ultrasound imaging may prevent uterine perforation which can occur during evacuation of an incomplete abortion or termination of pregnancy as a result of retroverted/retroflexed uterus. Ultrasound is also useful in determining which pregnancies are viable and which are most likely to miscarry. Ultrasound findings of incomplete abortion may vary depending on the amount of products expelled; it may appear as a reduced sac-size with irregular shape, and/or an echogenic material representing placental tissue within the uterus. An irregular gestational sac without a yolk sac or embryo is consistent with a blighted ovum (Figures 2A and 2B), whereas a foetus without a cardiac activity is consistent with a missed abortion (Figure 2c).

Where available it is important to use TAS or TVS with colour and spectral Doppler application when excluding retained products of conception from a tissue that is no longer viable and is likely to be expelled spontaneously. Colour Doppler will usually demonstrate a focally increased colour Doppler flow in the region of retained products, if present.

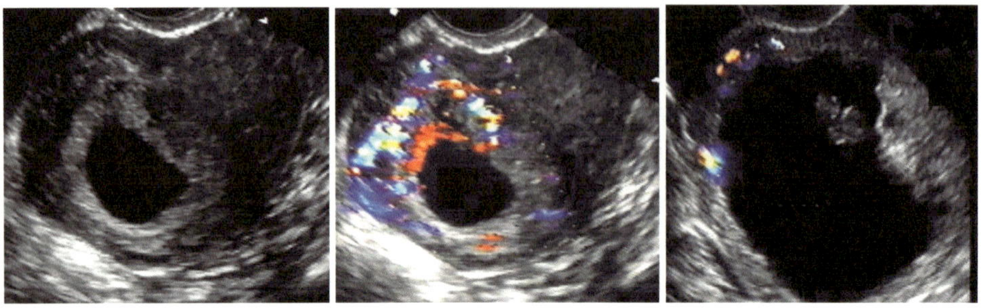

(a) (b) (c)

Fig. 2. (a),(b) and (c) A&B: Blighted Ovum; C: Missed Abortion- Note the non-viable embryo. In B there is increased vascularity on colour Doppler at implantation site.

2.1.3 Gestational trophoblastic diseases

Gestational trophoblastic diseases are a spectrum of benign and malignant conditions of the trophoblast comprising hydatidiform mole, invasive mole, choriocarcinoma, placental site trophoblastic tumour, and epithelioid trophoblastic tumour. Aside vaginal bleeding or brownish spotting which is common with early pregnancy conditions, molar pregnancies may present with a larger-than-date uterus, hyperemesis, passage of grape-like vesicles per vaginum, preeclampsia and hyperthyroidism. Complications of molar pregnancy can be life-threatening and include: (1) Haemorrhage from an existing mole or local invasion; (2) Anaemia due to maternal blood loss; (3) Rupture of, or haemorrhage into theca lutein cysts; (4)Pulmonary embolism or pulmonary oedema due to the migration of trophoblastic tissue through the uterine veins, and (4) Progression to malignancy.

The role of ultrasound imaging in GTDs is based on providing evidence for the diagnosis of hydatiform mole. Once diagnosed, tumor response to therapy can also be monitored, and the presence of metastatic sites can be ascertained.

The characteristic sonographic appearance in most molar pregnancies is the demonstration of hydropic villi. The typical sonographic appearance of a complete mole is that of a complex and echogenic intrauterine mass containing many small cystic spaces, which correspond to the hydropic villi on gross pathology (Benson et al, 2000) (Figure 3a). One may also see a large, central fluid collection that mimics an anembryonic gestation or abortion (Figure3c -& d). Occasionally, there is merely a central mass of variable echogenicity. Colour Doppler sonography is used to detect areas of increased blood flow within the myometrium(Kawano, et al, 1996) (Figure 3b) and can be used as a means of monitoring the effectiveness of chemotherapy (Bidzinski et al, 1999). Even though best practice requires that all products of conception from non-viable pregnancies should be examined histologically, irrespective of ultrasonographic findings, ultrasound will in the first place determine whether the pregnancy is viable or not. This does not downplay the importance of ultrasound in this condition. Secondly in rural settings access to histological report may delay, or may not be available at all. Ultrasound imaging will therefore assist in the initial diagnoses and in carefully selecting those patients at higher risk for malignancy for histological evaluation, especially where the laboratory facilities for histology are not available.

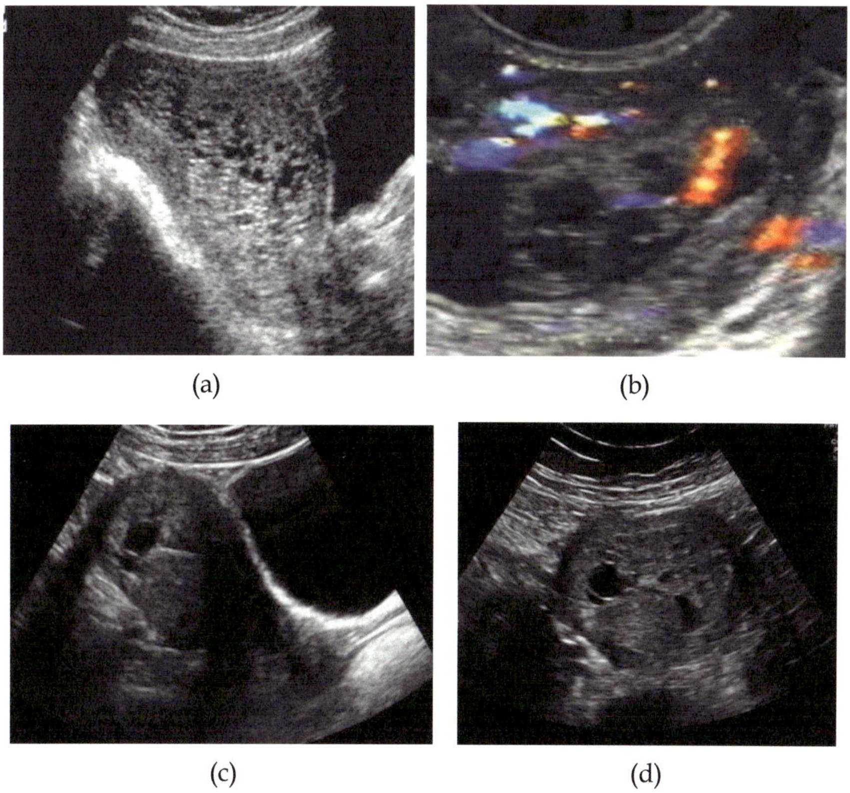

Fig. 3. (a) is a typical appearance of complete mole as described in the text
(b) shows increased flow within myometrium in regions of invasion of a mole
(c) & (d) are sagittal and transverse views of the same case respectively, showing atypical appearance of molar pregnancy

2.2 Gestational age estimation

In the first trimester a patient can benefit from ultrasound imaging in the estimation of gestational age (GA), particularly those who cannot recall their last menstrual period (LMP), or those who do not have regular 28 day menstrual cycle. Gestational age has emerged as one of the most important predictors of perinatal mortality (Markestad et al, 2005). The outcome of pregnancy is more closely related to gestational age as determined by ultrasound imaging. Accurate GA enables future detection of intrauterine growth restriction (IUGR), large for gestational age (LGA), and also essential in decision making for delivery or conditions such as premature rupture of membrane (PROM), postdates, placenta previa, hypertensive disorders, etc. The most accurate estimation of GA therefore, is done in the first trimester (7-13weeks gestation) using the crown-rump length (CRL), and is even more reliable than using clinical date (Eik-Nes et al, 2000). A CRL is determined by measuring the maximal straight line distance from the fetal head to the rump (Figure 4a & b).

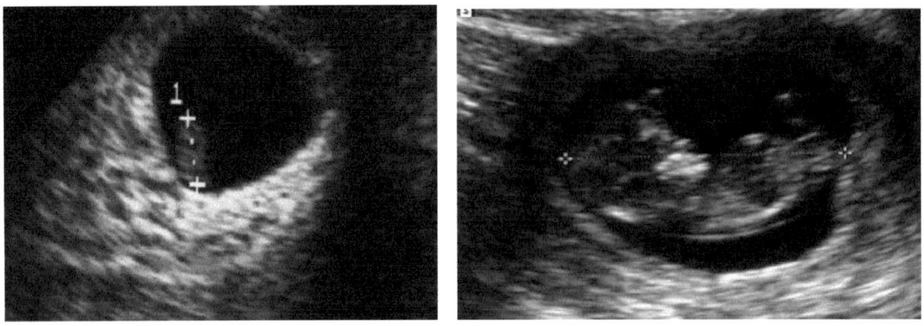

(a) (b)

Fig. 4. CRL measurement can be used for pregnancy dating in early first trimester as figure 4a, and late first trimester as figure 4b. This is the most accurate way to date a pregnancy

2.3 Multiple pregnancy

Ultrasonography is the diagnostic tool of choice for detecting a multiple pregnancy (as early as five weeks gestation) using TVS. The perinatal mortality rate in twins is about 5-times higher than in singletons, with higher incidence in monochorionic (5%) than dichorionic (2%) twin pregnancies (Sebire et al 1997). Again, the prevalence of pre-eclampsia is about 4-times greater in twin than in singleton pregnancies (Savvidou et al 2001). Other complications include increased risk of miscarriage and pre-term delivery. There is increased risk of placenta previa, malpresentation, and abruptio placenta. Anaemia is three times more common compared to singletons. The risk of atonic postpartum haemorrhage is also far higher in twins. Also,there is increased risk of operative intervention to the mother. Increased surveillance in the antepartum period is therefore required, making early detection by ultrasound imaging an appropriate practice.

In the first trimester, dichorionic twins can easily be distinguished by the presence of a thick septum between the chorionic sacs; the septum forms the chorionic component of the inter-twin membrane. This septum becomes thinner as the pregnancy progresses, but remains thicker and easier to identify at the base of the membrane as a triangular tissue projection, the so-called lambda sign (Sepulveda et al 1996). Sonographic examination of the base of the inter-twin membrane for the presence or absence of the lambda sign (Figure 5) provides reliable distinction between dichorionic and monochorionic pregnancies. This definitive diagnosis of chorionicity may not be possible with second and third trimester scans; hence the importance of first trimester scans.

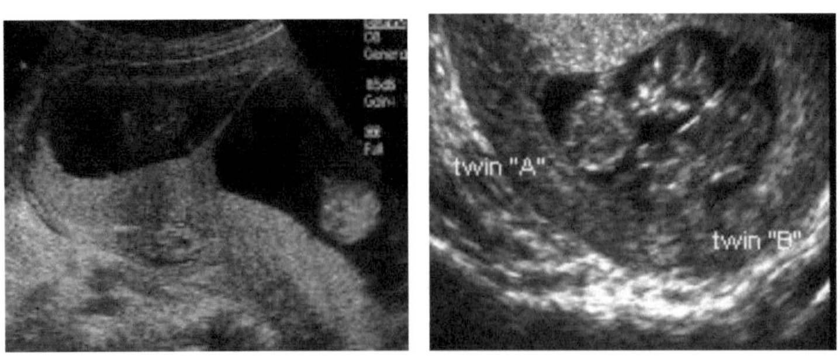

(a) (b)

Fig. 5. (a) shows the triangular tissue projection (lambda sign). This is absent in figure 5b

2.4 Early detection of chromosomal and structural anomalies (11-14weeks'-scan)

Late first trimester ultrasound imaging for anomaly detection is typically performed at 11-14 weeks primarily for measuring nuchal translucency (NT). The NT is ultrasound description of a subcutaneous physiologic fluid collection between the skin and the cervical spine of the foetus which can be used for obtaining diagnostic information when the CRL of the foetus is 45 - 84mm (figure 6a & b) NT increases with GA hence accurate CRL is needed for interpretation of NT measurement.

Measurement of the NT is useful for determining aneuploidy, a major cause of perinatal mortality. At 11 - 14 weeks, all major chromosomal defects are associated with increased NT thickness (Nicolaides et al 1992). In a chromosomally normal fetus, increased NT thickness is also associated with major abnormalities of the heart and great vessels, diaphragmatic hernia, exomphalos and asphyxiating thoracic atrophy (Souka et al, 2004). Further sonographic evaluation with echocardiography and/or 3D imaging may therefore be requested to rule out these anomalies. Other defects detectable at this gestational age are: acrania, anencephaly, encephalocele, gastroschisis, cleft palate, etc.

The role of ultrasound imaging in early prediction of aneuploidy and structural defects reduces the number of perinatal deaths resulting from birth defects, as it offers the couple an opportunity to decide whether or not to terminate the chromosomally abnormal fetus. Termination of pregnancy at this early gestation is associated with less maternal morbidity and mortality.

In developed countries, the practice of early termination of chromosomally abnormal foetus has significantly reduced perinatal mortality (Briker et al, 2000), and may become useful in developing countries; since with increasing education, women in these countries are now giving birth later in life, putting them at greater risk of having chromosomally abnormal babies.

Invasive prenatal testing by amniocentesis or chorionic villous sampling, which is needed for a definitive diagnosis, also requires ultrasound guidance. This invasive procedure can unfortunately result in the miscarriage of a normal pregnancy.

The important role of ultrasound, therefore, is based on the fact that most foetuses with chromosomal abnormalities have either major structural malformations or minor abnormalities (markers) that can be sonographically detected at this early stage of pregnancy (Nicolaides, 1993), and enable termination of pregnancy with less morbidity and mortality.

Even if the couple decides to keep the pregnancy, the knowledge of structural defects enables referral to a tertiary centre to improve post-delivery care.

Table 1 show first trimester anomalies (markers) associated with aneuploidy, based on the reported findings of Nicolaides (2004).

Even though NT can be accurately measured with TAS in about 95% of cases, whereTAS assessment of NT and structural abnormalities are inclusive, a combination of TAS and TVS is required. The advantage of TAS is that it allows flexibility of probe manipulation. However, TVS offers better resolution and visualisation.

In a study by Braithwaite et al, which compared foetal anatomy at 12 to 13 weeks using TVS and TAS, they found that a complete survey of the anatomy was possible in 72% of women using TAS, 82% with TVS, and 95% by combining the two (Braithwaite et al. 1996).

Additional sonographic findings by M-mode assessment of fetal heart rate is also useful for predicting aneuploidy in the late first trimester ultrasound imaging. The normal fetal heart rate (FHR) increases from about 100 bpm at 5 weeks of gestation to 170 bpm at 10 weeks, and then decreases to 155 bpm by 14 weeks (Nicolaides et al, 2004). At 10–14 weeks, trisomy

13 and Turner's syndrome are associated with tachycardia, whereas in trisomy 18 and triploidy there is fetal bradycardia (Liao et al 2001). In trisomy 21, there is a mild increase in FHR (Nicolaides et al 2004).

The detection rate of the additional structural abnormalities, some of which are listed in table 1, depends very much on the skill and experience of the sonographer, and to a lesser extent on the machine. With state of the art ultrasound machine many structural abnormalities have been detected in recent years. In five separate studies of screening an unselected population in the first trimester, the detection rates of fetal abnormality ranged from 33%-64.7% (Peregrine and Pandya, 2005).

The importance of 3-D ultrasound imaging especially in high-risk families further enhances detection of abnormality (Pretorius et al, 1995). Some investigators have suggested that 3-D ultrasound imaging is the tool of choice in evaluating the skeletal structures and the thorax, especially the long bones, due to capability of rotating the volumes (Ploeckinger-Ulm et al, 1996). However, fast movement of the foetus, and the positioning of the extremities adjacent to the uterine wall, can potentially be an obstacle in their evaluation. Although 4-D imaging may prove to be more useful, the primary stumbling blocks remain the same.

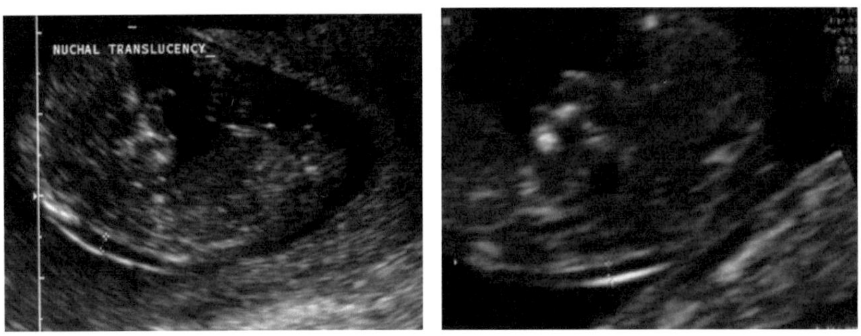

(a) (b)

Fig. 6. (a)-(b) shows the NT region; zoom the image closer as in 6b for a clear visualization of the NT space.

Aneuploidy	Ultrasound findings
Trisomy 21	Absent nasal bone(60-70% of cases), short maxilla (25% of cases), Abnormal ductus venosus waveform (80% of cases)
Trisomy 18	Absent nasal bone (55% of cases), Single umbilical artery (75% of cases), exomphalos (30% of cases), bradycardia and early onset of fetal growth restriction
Trisomy 13	Holoprosencephaly, tachycardia (70% of cases), exomphalos (40% of cases), megacyst, and early onset of fetal growth restriction
Turner's syndrome	Tachycardia (50% of cases), and early onset of fetal growth restriction
Triploidy	Holoprosencephaly, exomphalos, bradycardia (30% of cases), posterior fossa cyst (40% of cases), molar changes in placenta (30% of cases), and early onset of fetal growth restriction

Table 1. Sonographic markers for aneuploidy in first trimester

3. Reducing mortality rates by ultrasound imaging in the second trimester

Second trimester ultrasound imaging is typically performed between 18 and 24 weeks of gestation. Ultrasound imaging is performed to evaluate fetal and maternal structures for abnormalities that could lead to maternal and/or perinatal mortality. The structures evaluated are fetal anatomy, fetal biometry, amniotic fluid volume, placenta, maternal cervix and Doppler velocimetry of uterine and umbilical arteries . The purpose is to exclude findings associated with fetal chromosomal abnormalities, pre-term delivery, IUGR and pre-eclampsia.
Pre-eclampsia and intrauterine growth restriction remain the two most important causes of maternal and neonatal death that need to be detected as early as possible (Sibai, Dekker , Kupferminc, 2005; Walker, 2000).These 2 conditions are thought to be the result of abnormal placentation in which there is failure of trophoblastic invasion of the spiral artries resulting in increased vascular resistance in the uteroplacental circulation (Pijnenborg et al, 1991).
Pre-eclampsia can cause serious maternal complications including the HELLP syndrome (microangiopathic Hemolysis, Elevated Liver enzymes, Low Platelet count), eclampsia, coagulopathy, stroke and death (Wen et al, 2005; Roberts JM and Cooper DW, 2001).
Early prediction of pre-eclampsia and intrauterine growth restriction by ultrasound imaging in the second trimester is therefore paramount to providing appropriate antenatal surveillance and therapy in an effort to improve pregnancy outcomes. It must be pointed out, however, that prediction of these conditions in the second trimester is only possible if accurate dating from either early ultrasound examination or known conception dates has been previously established.

3.1 Assessment of fetal anatomy in the second trimester

The use of ultrasound imaging to exclude fetal structural defect in the second trimester has been a common practice in most developed countries for sometime. Over the past decade researchers have identified specific structural defects/markers and their specific syndromal pattern of abnormalities, most of which have been listed in table 2. The overall risk of chromosomal abnormalities increases with the total number of defects that are identified (Nicolaides et al, 1992). Considering that birth defects are among the list of common causes of perinatal mortality, detection of these defects by ultrasound imaging assists mothers to know their risk of chromosomal abnormalities. Based on the ultrasound findings they can consider termination, particularly if the mother's conditions such as age, medical history, and previous pregnancies, puts her at risk of losing her own life. In resource-poor countries where expensive invasive procedures such as amniocentesis may not be cost-effective or readily available, ultrasound imaging may be the only affordable modality for determining a woman's risk of delivering a chromosomally abnormal baby who is more likely to die in the perinatal period than a chromosomally normal baby, so that they might consider termination. Even in pregnant women with high risk factors who can afford invasive procedures, ultrasound imaging is still indicated, as the initial less expensive and non-invasive procedure before ultrasound-guided amniocentesis is considered. If no defect is detected on ultrasound imaging, the mother's risk of chromosomal abnormality is reduced, and she may decide not to proceed with an amniocentesis proecudure with its associated risk of miscarriage.

3.2 Assessment of fetal size (biometry)

Second trimester clinical determination of gestational age/fetal size using LMP and uterine size are rather subjective. This is because clinical dating can be negatively affected by wrong information on LMP, maternal body habitus, fibroids and multiple pregnancy.

The indication for ultrasound imaging, however, may be requested, not just for estimating gestational age (and date of delivery), but more importantly, to exclude intra-uterine growth restriction (IUGR).

SYNDROME	COMMON ULTRASOUND FINDINGS
Trisomy 21	Brachycephaly, mild ventriculomegaly, flattening of the face, nuchal edema, atrioventricular septal defects, duodenal atresia and echogenic bowel, mild hydronephrosis, shortening of the limbs, sandal gap and clinodactyly or mid-phalanx hypoplasia of the fifth finger.
Trisomy 18	strawberry-shaped head, choroid plexus cyst, absent corpus callosum, Dandy-Walker complex, facial cleft, micrognathia, nuchal edema, heart defects, diaphragmatic hernia, esophageal atresia, exomphalos, renal defects, myelomeningocele, growth retardation and shortening of the limbs, radial aplasia, overlapping fingers, and talipes or rocker bottom feet
Trisomy 13	Holoprosencephaly, microcephaly, cardiac abnormalities, enlarged and echogenic kidneys, exomphalos and postaxial polydactyly
Triploidy	IUGR, molar placenta, mild ventriculomegaly, micrognathia, cardiac abnormalities, myelomeningocoele, syndactyly, and 'hitch-hiker' toe deformity.
Turner syndrome	cystic hygromata, generalized edema, mild pleural effusion and ascites, and cardiac abnormalities

Table 2. Sonographic markers for aneuploidy in second trimester

Many sonographic parameters have been used for estimating gestational age in the second and third trimesters. The commonly used parameters are: fetal head circumference (HC) and biparietal diameter (BPD), abdominal circumference (AC) and femur length (FL).

The measurements obtained from these parameters are used in conjuction with other sonographic findings including oligohydramnios (subjectively assessed) and the placental size and echotexture. In twin pregnancy, twin-to-twin transfustion can also be determined by measuring the size of the fetuses using the same parameters stated for assessing each fetus.

3.3 Assessment of placenta

Evaluation of the placental size, location and the retroplacental area should be part of every antenatal ultrasound examination performed in the second trimester. Placental size is a reflection of the health and size of the fetus and correlates with pregnancy outcome (Dawn, 1995; Theam et al, 2001). Also, there is positive correlation between placental volume and neonatal birth weight and babies length (Sivaro et al, 2002).

The size is estimated by either measuring the placental thickness or its volume (Geirsson et al., 1985). A thin placenta (<10mm) may be due to IUGR, placental infarction, or pre-clampsia (Chase and Cayea, 1991). In recent times, the development of 3D ultrasound has improved the clinical ability to obtain a placental volume measurement (Jurkovie et al., 1994).

Secondly, placental previa must be excluded. Placental previa refers to a placenta that is close to the maternal internal cervical os, or covers the os either partially or completely.
It is a dangerous and sometimes fatal condition for mother and/or baby due to the possibility of severe haemorrhage. Accurate and timely diagnosis of placenta previa is therefore indispensable. Fortunately, major degrees of placenta previa are easily recognised by ultrasound imaging around 18-20 weeks gestation. Although TAS imaging may be unable to see the precise relationship between the lower placental edge and the internal os in cases of suspected minor previa, further TAS evaluation in the third trimester will usually delineate the placental site, and should be performed first with a partially filled bladder and then with an empty bladder, to avoid false positive diagnoses. Where concerns persists, a TVS in the third trimester will accurately define the relationship between the lower edge of the placenta and the internal cervical os (Figure 8b). As a general guide, a placenta-internal os distance of >2cm is required for safe vaginal delivery.
Another important concept in ultrasound imaging of the placenta is observation of the retroplacental hypoechoic complex which is composed of uteroplacental vessels, myometrium and decidua. Absence of the hypoechoic space may be seen in placenta percreta, a condition where the placenta has invaded the whole myometrial thickness. It is therefore logical to exclude placental percreta in pregnant women at high risk, as it could result in severe hemorrhage and maternal death.

3.4 Assessment of maternal cervix

Assessment of the cervix can assist in management decisions by predicting those patients who are at risk of preterm birth. Shortening of the cervix (Iams et al, 1996; Welsh A, Nicolaides, 2002) or dilatation/funneling of the internal os (Guzman et al, 2001) is associated with increased risk of premature delivery. Early prediction is important because premature birth is responsible for 75% of neonatal mortality and morbidity (Iams JD, 2003). In the past, clinical examination was the only method available for evaluation of the cervix.
However, clinical examination is subjective. This is especially true when it comes to estimation of the length of the cervix. Furthermore, detection of changes in the internal cervical os or cervical canal is impossible with a closed external os. When cervical dilatation or shortening of the cervix is noted by ultrasound imaging, cervical cerclage (and sometimes conservative management with bed rest) can help reduce the likelihood of premature births that are caused by cervical incompetence, thereby reducing perinatal mortality.
There are three approaches to scanning the cervix: TAS, TVS and transperineal (translabial). TVS approach is the gold-standard technique for optimal imaging, and should be employed when imaging by the TAS approach is suboptimal. Generally in our practice TAS approach has been accurate in the second trimester, but difficulty may occur in the third trimester as the pregnancy advances which may require the use of TVS. In assessing the cervix with TVS, scan gel is applied to the tip of the transvaginal transducer, which is then covered with a clean or sterile condom or glove to avoid cross infection. Lubricating gel is applied over the cover and the transducer tip is introduced into the vagina, about 2-3cm depth and away from the cervix. Sonographic visualization starts as soon as the transducer is introduced. Inserting the transducer tip too far can cause the examiner to miss seeing the cervix and lower uterine segment as the transducer tip reaches the posterior or anterior fornix. The cervical length is measured by orienting the transducer in the sagittal plane (figure 8a). The transducer is then oriented in the coronal plane to assess the internal os

and the canal for further evaluation of any dilatation, funneling of the internal os, or ballooning of the lower uterine segment which may appear as a bulging of amniotic fluid sac into the cervical canal.

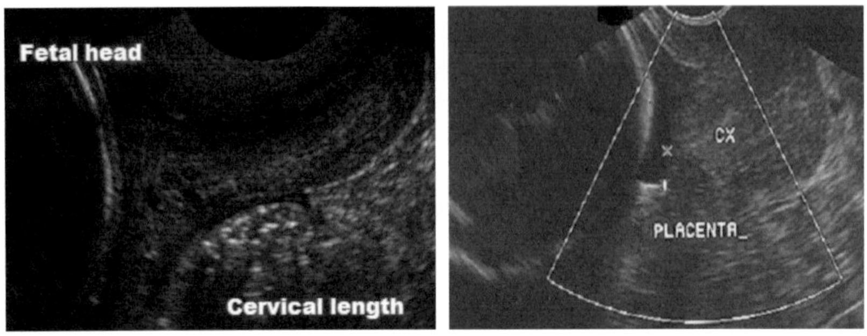

(a) (b)

Fig. 8. (a) and (b) - TVS demonstration of cervical length. Measurement of the distance of the placenta from the internal os can be made

3.5 Doppler velocimetry of the second trimester

Doppler assessment of uterine and umbilical arteries is a reliable technique for predicting the level of risk for preeclampsia and intrauterine growth restriction, preterm delivery, gestational diabetes and fetal asphyxia (Martin et al, 2001, Reese et al, 1994; Bromley et al, 1994). Uterine artery assessment may be performed via the TVS or TAS route in the second trimester (18-22weeks) for high risk population. A high resistance waveform in uterine artery, or a waveform with a notch (Figure 9), implies inadequate trophoblastic invasion of the endometrial and myometrial spiral vessels.

Umbilical artery assessment is performed via the TAS route. Increased umbilical artery systolic/diastolic (S/D) ratio, or reduced diastolic flow, is also an indication of a rising placental vascular insufficiency. The diastolic flow may eventually disappear (figure 10a) or may even reverse in direction (Figure 10b), indicating that events may lead to intra-uterine death. These are clinically significant findings for uteroplacental vascular resistance associated with risk of hypertensive disorders, small for gestational age, preterm delivery, and gestational diabetes. Early detection improves management leading to improved survival.

4. Reducing mortality rates by ultrasound imaging in the third trimester

Maternal death may occur in the third trimester of pregnancy due to conditions such as antepartum hemorrhage, hypertensive disorders ,thromboembolism, chorioamnionitis, cardiac disease, anaemia (sickle cell disease), rupture of uterine scar, etc.

Perinatal mortality may also be caused by conditions such as prematurity, macrosomia, IUGR, infections, maternal diabetes, and maternal isoimmunisation. Additionally, all the major causes of maternal death may also lead to perinatal death.

Ultrasound imaging plays a role in the assessment of fetal growth and well being, fetal presention, placental location, ultrasound-guided procedures; all of which are useful for management decisions if an intervention should be carried out to improve survival rates.

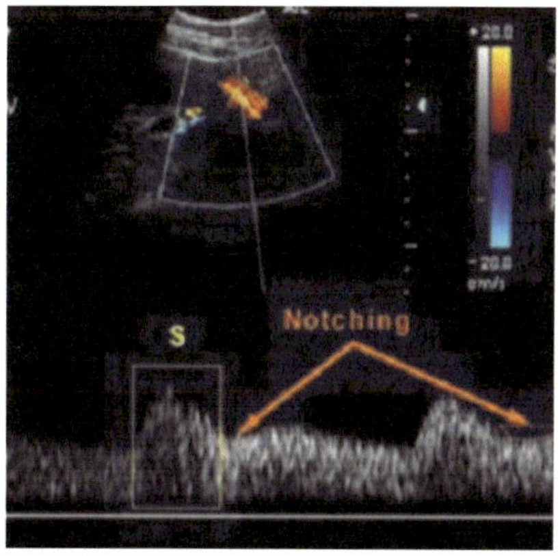

Fig. 9. Uterine artery waveform with a notch.

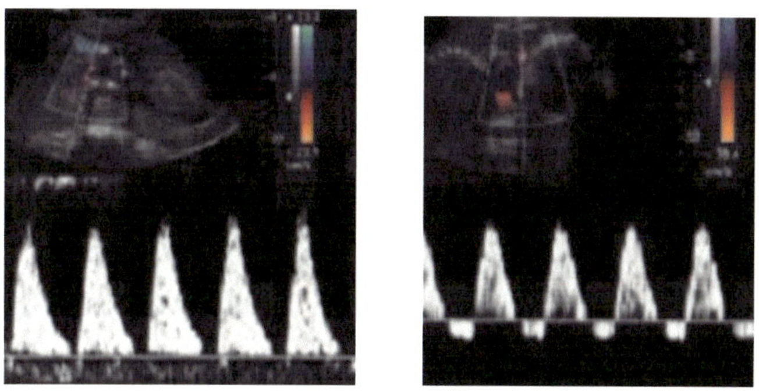

(a) (b)

Fig. 10. (a)-(b) Umbilical artery waveform; a (absent diastole) and b (reversed diastole)

4.1 Disproportionate fetal growth (IUGR and LGA)

Perinatal death may occur in cases of IUGR due to increased risk of fetal hypoxia and acidosis, neonatal hypoglycemia, meconium aspiration syndrome, etc.

Serial ultrasound examinations are important in documenting growth and excluding structural anomalies. Accurate early dating of the pregnancy is very important for comparison purposes. It must be emphasized again that the establishment of conditions such as IUGR later in a pregnancy is only possible if accurate dating from either early ultrasound examination or known conception dates has been previously established.

Once true dating of the pregnancy has been established, measurements of the fetal head (BPD and HC), abdomen (AC) and femur (FL)may be obtained for comparison purposes. From these measurements, the estimated fetal weight (EFW) can be calculated using one of several published formulae on EFW. This is then plotted on a percentile growth chart, showing the estimated fetal weight versus gestational age. IUGR is suspected if the estimated weight is below the 10th percentile. Antenatal diagnosis of IUGR is however not precise because the EFW cannot be directly measured, but calculated from a combination of measured parameters with a prediction error rate 10-20% (Degani, 2001). Abdominal circumference measurement is the most useful measurement for evaluating fetal growth, as

it reflects the volume of fetal subcutaneous fat and the size of the liver which in turn correlate with the degree of fetal nutrition. Moreover, fetal hypoxia is more common when the abdominal circumference is below the 5th percentile (Degani, 2001).
Decreased amniotic fluid volume is clinically associated with IUGR and may be the earliest sign detected on ultrasound. Therefore liquor volume measurement should be carried out in cases of suspected IUGR. In the third trimester, amniotic fluid index (AFI) is the most commonly used method of amniotic fluid volume assessment, as it is easy to perform and is reproducible. This is the sum of the largest vertical pocket of amniotic fluid measured in centimetres in each of the four quadrants of the uterus. The deepest (largest) vertical pocket is used for the assessment, particularly in multiple pregnancies. In twin pregnancies measurement of the deepest vertical pocket of each individual fetus is taken. An AFI of less than 5cm, or a largest single vertical pocket of less than 2cm is considered oligohydramnios.
In addition, umbilical artery (UA) Doppler velocimetry can estimate the likelihood of adverse perinatal outcome in IUGR fetuses, and may be useful in determining the intensity of fetal surveillance. In the early phase of fetal hypoxia retrograde diastolic flow in the UA is a sign of severe hypoxemia and acidemia (Baschat and Weiner, 2000). Doppler flow study is therefore helpful in terms of reducing intervention and improving the overall fetal outcome.
In addition, abnormal middle cerebral artery (MCA) and UA S/D ratio are strongly associated with low birth weight and low umbilical artery pH in fetuses with suspected IUGR, and occurrence of fetal distress. An abnormal Doppler cerebro-placental ratio, (i.e. MCA pulsatile index divided by UA pulsatile index) also has been associated with a statistically significant increase in perinatal mortality (Sterne et al, 2001). In addition to the AU and MCA, the descending aorta has an altered perfusion in fetuses with both IUGR.
A careful and targeted ultrasound examination is therefore necessary to determine the degree of fetal well being using these sonographic parameters.
On the other hand, LGA fetuses, defined as fetuses above the 90th percentile of weight for any specific gestational age, are also associated with increased perinatal mortality. Generally macrosomia is when the fetus has an EFW of 4.5kg or more. The risk of perinatal morbidity and mortality is greater for babies with birth weight of 4kg or more. Causes of macrosmia include diabetes, obesity, postdatism and previous macrosomic babies. Complications include stillbirth, shoulder dystocia (during delivery), birth trauma, etc.

4.2 Hypertensive disorders in pregnancy

Hypertensive disorders are among the 5 most common causes of maternal mortality in the world, and the leading cause in the authors' center. This disorder comprise gestational hypertension, pregnancy induced hypertension that may progress to preeclampsia (mild or severe) and eclampsia, chronic hypertension, chronic hypertension with superimposed preeclampsia and/or superimposed eclampsia.
Ultrasound imaging is useful in preventing maternal and perinatal mortality due to accurate dating of gestational age, especially when obtained in the first trimester. Ultrasound is also used for monitoring fetal growth and well being to enable early intervention when necessary.
Moreover, with an accurate gestational age of 32-34 weeks, delivery can be effected if any maternal or fetal complication sets in, once there is very high chance of neonatal survival.
The role of ultrasound in antenatal fetal monitoring therefore, is through biometric measurement to detect IUGR, EFW, biophysical profile (BPP) and Doppler velocimetry to evaluate uteroplacental blood flow and fetal circulation.

The biophysical profile (BPP) is a useful method of predicting antepartum fetal acidemia. Studies in centers at 4 different geographic locations demonstrated reduction in perinatal mortality in high risk patients who were managed on the basis of BPP (Harman, 2005). Although the BPP test can be used as a primary method of fetal surveillance, it can be especially helpful in cases where the non-stress test (NST) is not reactive. There is some evidence that the BPP may even be useful during labour as an adjunct to fetal heart rate monitoring (Kim et al, 2003).The five components of a BPP integrate fetal cardiac activity, amniotic fluid assessment, fetal breathing, fetal movement and tone. Each component is scored 2 if present or reassuring and 0 if abnormal. Fetal breathing is the first parameter affected, and is probably as reliable as the NST in predicting early fetal acidosis. As the insult becomes more profound and chronic, fetal breathing, then body movement, then tone are compromised. The amount of amniotic fluid reflects the placental health as well as fetal well being, and is a marker for chronic hypoxia when reduced. The fetal health can therefore be accurately predicted, allowing the pregnancy to continue with low risk of fetal loss and long term morbidity if the score is normal. Timely intervention can be executed when fetal compromise is detected, to lower perinatal mortality. A BPP test can be completed in as little as five minutes if the fetus is active and awake, or can take as long as 30 minutes. Stimulation of the fetus by shaking the probe is appropriate for shortening the time of the study.

4.3 Antepartum haemorrhage (placenta previa, abruption and vasa previa)

Placenta previa can lead to severe hemorrhage and profound shock in the antenatal period, during delivery and immediately after delivery.

Perinata death may occur in cases of placental previa due to the likelihood of preterm delivery, severe malformations in central nervous, cardiovascular, or gastrointestinal systems which may occur in the process of labour and delivery, and stillbirth from maternal shock.

Ultrasound diagnosis of placenta previa was described in the section on second trimester ultrasound imaging. In the third trimester, repeat scan is recommended for all patients who were diagnosed of placenta previa in the second trimester, and new patients reporting for the first time in the third trimester with antepartum hemorrhage must be scanned.

Abruptio placenta refers to premature separation of a normally situated placenta.

After the separation bleeding may be concealed beneath the placenta with seeping into the myometrium or track down per vaginum (revealed). Concealed abruptio placentae have more severe complications. Maternal death may occur due to the likelihood of severe hemorrhage (ante- and postpartum), shock, disseminated intravascular coagulation and renal failure. Perinatal mortality is mainly due to fetal hypoxia from the premature separation of the placenta, IUGR, low birth weight, congenital malformation, and fetal anemia.

The diagnosis of abruptio placenta is usually clinical, but ultrasound can be helpful in some concealed cases with large retroplacental clot. This appears as hyperechoic, isoechoic, or sonolucent in comparison with the placenta, depending on the age of the clot. Resolving clot appears hyperchoic within one week and sonolucent within 2 weeks. Abruptio placenta may also present as an abnormal thickening or rounding of the placental edge.

However ultrasound is not an accurate tool in the diagnosis of abruption. Its main usefulness is in excluding placenta previa, as a number of placenta previa cases may also have abruption. The size of the clot, and the fetal growth and liquor volume are closely

monitored in such cases. This is useful during conservative management to achieve fetal maturity. Intervention is carried out if clot enlarges, fetal distress sets in, or severe growth restriction sets in. If IUGR sets in, ultrasound plays further role in monitoring fetal well being through BPP and Doppler velocimetry.
Vasa previa is a condition in which the umbilical vessels divide within the amniotic membrane before they reach the placenta (velamentous cord insertion). These vessels may cross the internal os below the fetal presenting part, which is called vasa previa. The vessels may rupture spontaneously and cause rapid fetal exsanguination. This condition can easily be detected by ultrasound imaging with colour Doppler application. Appropriate intervention can then be executed before rupture occurs.

4.4 Deep vein thrombosis and thrombo embolism

Pregnancy significantly increases the risk of venous thromboembolism (VTE) due to increased concentration of clotting factors (fibrinogen, factors VII, VIII, X, XII) and venous stasis. Pulmonary embolism is a common cause of death. Fatal pulmonary thromboembolism (PTE) usually occurs after delivery, more commonly following caesarean section. Majority occurs within 2 days of delivery but may occur as late as 42 days. Antenatal PTE can occur at any trimester but more common in third trimester. Clinical diagnosis of the condition is inaccurate and unreliable, and the most reliable diagnostic modality of venography (considered previously to be the gold standard) is not suitable in pregnancy due to small risk of radiation and contrast agents.
The use of duplex ultrasound imaging with compression is therefore recommended, as it is non-invasive and has a high degree of accuracy for detecting thrombus in femoropopliteal and calf veins. The iliac veins may however not be well seen during pregnancy, and may require magnetic resonance imaging. The details of the scanning techniques and the diagnostic features of thrombosed vein, are described in a separate chapter of this book.

4.5 Rh Isoimunisation

The Rhesus (Rh) antigens are lipoproteins on the red blood cell membrane. The mother may be isoimmunized through incompatible blood transfusion or following feto-maternal hemorrhage between a fetus with incompatible rhesus status and the mother. Rh- positive fetal red cells entering into the maternal circulation will provoke antibody formation against the fetal red blood cells leading to fetal hemolysis and fetal anemia. Severe fetal anemia may result in hydropic fetus with ascites, pericardial effusion and heart failure.
To determine the severity of the anemia, duplex ultrasound imaging of the proximal third of the MCA can be estimated. High peak velocity blood flow of the MCA correlates well with severe fetal anemia (Mari et al, 2000). This test may be performed at two weeks interval in these patients, thus avoiding more invasive diagnostic interventions until there is evidence of severe anemia. If severe anemia is suspected, ultrasound-guided cordoscentesis is helpful in detecting the degree of fetal anemia. Ultrasound-guided amnioscentesis is also helpful, in detecting the level of bilirubin in the amniotic fluid as a measure of fetal hemolysis using spectrophotometry.
Furthermore, ultrasound plays an important role in monitoring the iso-immunized patient for hydrops through evaluation of fetal heart size, detection of pericardial effusion and fetal ascites, and measurement of amniotic fluid volume (Roman and Martin, 2007).
In terms of treatment, if the fetus is preterm, ultrasound-guided intrauterine transfusion can be performed directly into the umbilical veins (Roman and Martin, 2007). Other

interventions aided by ultrasound include aspiration of pericardial effusion and ascites, and ultrasound-guided amniocentesis to test for fetal lung maturity before expediting delivery.

4.6 Abnormal lie and malpresentation

Malpresentation can cause, birth injury and umbilical cord compression and prolapse during delivery, which can lead to perinatal death.

Ultrasound is used to confirm abnormal lie and malpresentation of the fetus, so that a decision on the route of delivery can be made. If there is no contraindication external cephalic version can be done under ultrasound guidance at 37 weeks gestation to achieve vaginal delivery.

4.7 Cesarean scar rupture

Uterine rupture carries with it a high rate of maternal and perinatal mortality and is estimated to occur in up to 4% of pregnancies with history of caesarean delivery ( ). This rupture may occur silently (asymptomatically) in the antenatal period, commonly in the third trimester. Ultrasound has been found to be useful in diagnosing silent rupture or scar dehiscence in the antenatal period.

5. Labour, delivery and post-delivery issues

Most maternal deaths occur during labour and delivery, and most perinatal deaths are due to events that occur during labour and delivery. Causes of maternal death at this stage include: prolonged labour with its sequel of water and electrolyte imbalance, obstructed labour with sequel of water and electrolyte imbalance and uterine rupture, eclampsia, hemorrhage and thromboembolism, and complications of anesthesia for cesarean section; all of which may lead to perinatal death as well.

During delivery, perinatal death may also result from vacuum delivery complications, which include subgaleal hemorrhage, subdural hematoma, cerebral infaction, skull fracture, and neonatal jaundice (Odoi and Opare Addo, 2002). Birth injuries sustained during shoulder dystocia and breech delivery can all result in perinatal death. Almost all of these could be prevented by proper case selection, and good labour management including use of partograph.

Ultrasound imaging is helpful in the delivery process, including assessing cervical length during induction, knowing the head position and descent during labour, case selection for vagina birth after caesarean section (VBAC), detection of uterine rupture, preventing obstructed labour, identifying cause of intrapartum hemorrhage and monitoring fetal heart.

5.1 Induction delivery interval: cervical length and dilatation

The success of labour induction is directly related to the favourability of the cervix shown by the Bishop score. Ultrasound accurately measures the cervical length and dilatation to help determine the score to avoid prolonged labour [Rane et al, 2005].

The assessment of the cervical length was described in the second trimester.

Secondly, TVS measurement of fetal head to perineum distance and, TAS measurement of fetal head position, offers the most accurate prediction of successful induction of labour [Eggebø et al, 2008].

5.1.1 Progress of labour in terms of head descent and position

Studies have shown that sonographic measurement of head position and descent is more accurate than digital examination. More recently, it has been suggested that the angle formed by a line connecting the lowest point of the fetal head to the inferior edge of the pubic symphysis provides an objective, accurate and reproducible means of assessing descent, using the translabial sonography approach. At angle of progression of about 120 degrees or more, there is a high probability of either spontaneous vaginal delivery or an easy and successful vacuum extraction [Kalache et al, 2009]. Also, the gold standard technique for assessing fetal head position during labour is transabdominal suprapubic transverse ultrasound [Sherer et al, 2002]. Therefore lack of progress as shown by partographic presentation of this sonographic finding prompts intervention.

5.1.2 Selection of cases for vaginal birth after Caesarean section (VBAC)

The main concern about VBAC is the uterine scar rupture. Predisposing factors to uterine rupture include fetal size and scar thickness. The estimation of fetal size and weight aids selection of cases. Studies have found that the antepartum uterine scar thickness inversely correlates with the risk of intrapartum uterine rupture, and that intrapartum assessment of uterine scar can predict uterine rupture with a high degree of accuracy. There is evidence that ultrasound imaging may be useful in determining the uterine scar thickness [Asakura, 2000] and aid in case selection for VBAC.

5.1.3 Detection of uterine rupture

Uterine rupture during labour and delivery is mostly diagnosed clinically; hence if clinical diagnosis is clear, precious time should not be wasted on ultrasound imaging [Yeboah et al, 2010].

However where the clinical features are not obvious, as may occur in pre-labour silent rupture, or occasionally in labour especially with epidural, ultrasound imaging may show the rent in the uterine wall [Ogbole et al, 2008], with herniated membrane as a cystic structure through the defect [Acton et al, 2004].

5.1.4 Head position for vacuum

The success of vacuum delivery depends, among other conditions, on where the cap is positioned. Wrong placement may deflex the fetal head and lead to failure of the procedure. The cap must be placed at or close to the flexion point on the vertex. Ultrasound aided examination has been shown to detect this flexion point better than digital examination alone [Wong, 2007; Molina and Nicholides, 2010]

5.1.5 Cord presentation

This condition, if not detected will lead to umbilical cord prolapse when the fetal membranes rupture. It may be difficult to feel a presenting cord. Colour Doppler sonography can clearly detect this cord to direct appropriate intervention to avert fetal or neonatal death.

5.1.6 Preventing obstructed labour

Fetal macrosomia, malpresentation and abnormal lie are all causes of obstructed labour. Apart from macrosomia, all the other conditions also predispose to cord prolapse.

Ultrasound is useful in detecting all these for appropriate intervention to prevent the obstruction or cord prolapse by assessing fetal biometry and EFW, and presentation / lie.

5.1.7 Fetal heart rate detection

Occasionally the fetal heart rate may not be heard with the Pinard fetal stethoscope.
As ultrasound is becoming more and more available than sonicaid (audio Doppler) or cardiotocography (CTG) machine, especially in low-income countries, ultrasound is used to check the fetal condition and if fetus is alive and in distress, prompt delivery by caesarean section or vacuum will prevent perinatal death.

5.1.8 Version in the second stage of labour for second twin

There is increased perinatal mortality associated with the second twin compared to the first twin due to cord accidents, premature separation of the placenta and other factors after delivery of the first twin. There is therefore the need to expedite delivery of the second twin as early as possible. After delivery of the first twin, if the second twin is not cephalic, external cephalic version (if membranes are intact) or internal podalic version (if membranes are intact or just ruptured) may be done under ultrasound guidance to achieve vaginal delivery

5.2 Post-partum complications

Uterine inversion leading to hemorrhage and shock, retained products of conception leading to hemorrhage and infection, puerperal sepsis, postpartum eclampsia, and thromboembolism are major causes of maternal death after delivery.
The usefulness of ultrasound imaging in detecting thromboembolism and the imaging technique has been discussed earlier.
In some cases of uterine inversion where clinical diagnosis is not obvious, ultrasound has been used to elicit the diagnosis [Momin et al, 2009] to enable appropriate management.
In cases of retained products of conception ultrasound can differentiate between retained products and endometritis [Zuckerman et al 1997] Even tiny retained products of conception as occurs in first trimester miscarriage is accurately detected by TVS with Doppler application [Ustunyurt et al., 2007]

5.2.1 Postpartum detection of uterine rupture

Sometimes the suspicion of uterine rupture does not arise until after delivery, especially if it occurs in the second stage of labour. There is evidence that ultrasound can detect caesarean section scar rupture after delivery (Henrich et al, 2005) and even scar defect after the puerperium (Amstrong et al, 2003). Others have suggested that a combined anterior uterine wall and bladder thickness (<3mm) associated with ballooning of the lower segment indicates a defect in the myometrium (Champmank, 1994).

5.2.2 Postpartum detection of broad ligament hematoma

Broad ligament hematoma may occur when there is uterine rupture or cervical tear with upper extension, and can cause shock in the post-partum period that may be out of proportion. Ultrasound imaging can aid the detection of the hematoma.

5.2.3 Puerperal sepsis

Apart from aiding in the diagnosis of postpartum endometritis, ultrasound accurately detects pelvic abscess, which may appear as a focal collection, either hypoechoic or complex.

6. Routine obstetric ultrasound- would it improve survival rates in the developing world?

Routine obstetric scanning refers to regular ultrasound imaging for each and every pregnancy conducted either at the first, second or third trimester to separate specific pregnancy abnormalities from normally progressing pregnancies. In many developed countries, such as Great Britain, Germany, France and those of Scandinavia, routine obstetric ultrasound imaging at about 18 weeks' has become standard of care. In United States routine ultrasound was not endorsed untle recently when the American College of Obstetricians and Gynecologists (2007) recommended routine aneuploidy screening for pregnant women. One published large-scale observational study in Sweden concluded that a significant benefit could be obtained from even a single routine obstetric ultrasound at approximately 15 weeks 'gestation (Waldenstrom et al, 1988). Among the important benefits of routine ultrasound are the accuracy in gestational age determination, and detection of multiple pregnancies (Neilson et al 1998). In most developing countries, accurate estimation of gestational age by ultrasound imaging is likely to be more beneficial and significant than developed countries, as the majority of pregnant women in those areas cannot recall their LMP (van Dyk et al, 2008) probably due to the high illiteracy rates among the pregnant women. This makes them far more vulnerable to unrecognized preterm delivery (a major cause of perinatal mortality), and post-maturity syndromes associated with fetal distress and long-term development disorders.

However, the impact of routine ultrasound imaging in terms of significantly improving the over-all pregnancy outcome has been disputed by many observational studies conducted mostly in developed countries. But considering the fact that there are no sufficient studies conducted in developing countries, it is still unclear whether the impact as described in developed countries will produce similar results in developing countries. Until then, one cannot rule out the possible impact routine ultrasound imaging can have in developing countries, as most of the victims of maternal and perinatal mortality live in these areas.

The major challenge for routine ultrasound however, has been cost effectiveness.

In England routine antenatal ultrasound screening has been estimated to cost the National Health Service (NHS) £14 to £16 per scan, while the family contribute between £9 and £15 per scan, giving an indication of how expensive routine ultrasound can be for developing coutries (Henderson et al 2002). But the Canadian and most European health policy-makers support the view that the benefits of routine ultrasound outweigh the cost, and in those countries routine ultrasound screening is either a national policy or a recommendation (Saari-Kemppainen et al., 1990; Public Health Agency of Canada, 2006). Moreover, maternal and newborn deaths is said to be representing an estimated annual global financial loss of $15 billion in potential productivity (USAID, 2001). So that if observational studies on the significant impact of routine obstetric ultrasound in developing countries should show a positive impact, there may be the need for international support to assist in financing routine ultrasound imaging in antenatal care for developing countries, as part of efforts to reach the Millennium Development Goals on reducing maternal and neonatal deaths.

Secondly, routine ultrasound has also been critisized for prompting unncessary intevention, creating anxiety related to false-positive diagnoses and giving false assurances to women who may be dissuaded from undergoing further examination because of a normal ultrasound. Therefore we recommend that if some form of routine ultrasound imaging will ever be considered for developing countries, then standardized guidelines will have to be in place in terms of training qualified personnel, quality assurance of ultrasound machine and regulating ultrasound practice to minimize such problems.

7. Sustainability of ultrasound imaging for the developing world

WHO has recommended ultrasound for dissemination to developing nations during the second phase of its earlier basic radiology system initiative (WHO, 1998). Ultrasound was described as a "sustainable technology" for developing and low-resource countries, because of its relatively low cost of purchase, low cost for maintenance and supplies, portability, and durability in comparison with all other imaging modalities (Goldberg, 2003). Currently the increasing availability of affordable and smaller ultrasound scanners is a clear indication of the sustainability of ultrasound for the developing world and its potential role in reducing maternal and perinatal mortality(Harris and Mark, 2009). A market survey we conducted (unpublished) revealed that a new ultrasound machine could cost as low as $5000, and can be used for basic obstetric assessment such as gestational age, foetal viability, placental position, and may even be used for foetal anatomical survey. Further evaluation with more sophisticated and relatively expensive machines can then be arranged for selected cases with suspected anomalies, as a form of 'level 2' or 'level 3' scanning conducted by an advanced practitioner or specialist. Moreover the practice of donating slightly used but good quality machines continues to be helpful and should be encouraged.

Manufacturers of ultrasound systems must support developing countries by providing offices, sales representatives, and applications personnel in these regions, so that they can assist with the dissemination of equipment, initial installation and instruction on equipment usage, and equipment maintenance.

Lack of adequately trained physicians and sonographers, and limited means of equipment maintenance in developing countries has been a major challenge (Munjanja, 1993). Even though some developed countries around the world have made a concerted effort to provide education, it continues to be provided in a random fashion and has never been able to keep up with the need for adequate training for physicians and sonographers. One proposal at using a low cost system for training ultrasound imaging techniques has been via use of a PC platform that uses interface components from the Nintendo Wii games console (as a simulator) to aid remote mentoring by experienced ultrasound professionals. The proposers cited their experience with this technique in Ghana as an example (Ap Cenydd et al, 2009).

Another recommendation has been to incorporate a diploma in clinical ultrasound for medical graduates of local universities (Mindel, 1997). The use of existing allied health professionals such as nurses/midwives or radiographers who have received additional training in ultrasound has been valuable in some developed countries, and may be cost-effective in developing countries. A new model in developing countries is the creation of Bachelor degree programs in Sonography in existing university settings. Graduates of these university sonography programss may be utilized as sonographers, or professionals in ultrasound imaging and may help to ease the pressure on doctors in developing countries. It is the belief of the authors that a three-pronged approach must be utilized for the sustainability of ultrasound in developing countries: First, the development of a new career path through the university setting for sonographers; Second, the creation of long-term comprehensive sonography education programs for physicians; and Thirdly, involvement of government agencies and institutions for regulatory policy setting. Clearly, creative and novel approaches that serve the unique situations of developing countries and address the need for both trained operators of ultrasound equipment and people with biotechnical skills for ongoing maintenance would be highly beneficial (Spencer and Adler, 2008).

8. Conclusion

In spite of increasing technological advancement, including ultrasound imaging, maternal and perinatal mortality globally have not decreased and indeed in some developing countries there is increase.

The major causes of maternal mortality include abortion related complications, hemorrhage from various conditions, hypertensive disorders, thrombo-embolism, obstructed labour, prolonged labour, ruptured uterus and puerperal infection. Causes of perinatal mortality include prematurity, birth asphyxia, congenital malformations, IUGR, traumatic delivery, and cord prolapsed. A significant number of these conditions that lead to maternal death also lead to perinatal death.

Fortunately, ultrasound is a non-invasive and safe tool that can aid in the diagnosis of most of these conditions, prevent the effects of these complications and in some cases guide in treatment. Thus wider use of ultrasound is advocated in obstetric practice. It is important for every medical doctor in the obstetric unit and indeed midwives to be trained in basic use of ultrasound in obstetrics. The need for advanced practice training for specialist obstetricians as sonologists, and professional sonographers as advanced ultrasound practitioners is recommended for the future in developing countries as currently practiced in some developed countries.

Governments should be committed to the purchase and maintenance of ultrasound machines for healthcare facilities, especially in obstetric units. A more widespread use of ultrasound imaging and improvement in treatment approach should lead to reduction in maternal and perinatal mortality.

9. References

Acton C, King V, Whitehead J.(2004).Sonographic diagnosis of uterine rupture with successful out. *Australian and New Zealand journal of Obstetric and Gynecology.* Vol 44(5), pp 473-474

AMERICAN COLLEGE OF OBSTETRICIANS AND GYNECOLOGISTS 2007: Screening for fetal chromosomal abnormalities. ACOG Practice Bulletin No. 77. Obstetrics and Gynecology, 109:27. BAKKETEIG, LS; EIK-NES, SH; JACOBSEN, G; ULSTEIN, MK; BRODTKORB, CJ; BALSTAD, P; ERIKSEN, BC & JORGENSEN, NP 1984: Randomised controlled trial of ultrasonographic screening in pregnancy. Lancet; 2:207-211

Amstrong V, Hansen WF, Voorhis BJV, Syrop CH. (2003). Detection of ceasarian scars by transvaginal ultrasound, *Obstet Gynecol* Vol 101(1), pp 61-65

Ap Cenydd L, John NW, Vidal FP, Gould DA, Joekes E, Littler P. (2009). Cost effective ultrasound imaging training mentor for use in developing countries. *Stud Health Technol Inform.* Vol 142, pp 49-54.

Asakura H, Nakai A, Ishikawa G. (2000). Predicting of uterine dehiscence by measuring lower segment thickness prior to the onset of labour: Evaluation by transvaginal sonogragraphy. *J Nippon Med Sci*, Vol 67,No.5 pp 352-6 ISSN:1345-4676

Bale JR, Lucas AO, Stoll BJ (eds). (2003). Improving Birth Outcomes. Washington, DC: Institute of Medicine of theNational Academies, National Academies Press

Baschat A, Weiner CP. (2000). Umbilical artery Doppler screening for detection of small fetus need of antepartum surveillance. *Am J Obstet Gynecol* vol 182 p154 PMID: 10649171

Benson C, Benson CB, Genest DR, Bernstein MR, Soto-Wright V, Goldstein DP, Berkowitz RS. (2000). Sonographic appearance of first trimester complete hydatidiform moles. *Ultrasound in Obstetrics and Gynecology*. Vol.16, pp. 188–191

Bidzinski M, Sobiczewski P, Derlatka P, Pietrzak K, Wierzba W. (1999). Clinical usefulness of color doppler flow examination during treatment of gestational trophoblastic disease. *Ginekol Pol.* Vol.70, No. 2 pp 88-92

Brace RA, Wolf EJ. (1989). Normal amniotic fluid volume changes throughout pregnancy. *Am J Obstet Gynecol* Vol. 161, pp 382-388

Bricker L, Garcia J, Henderson J, Mugford M, Neilson J, Roberts T, et al. (2000). Ultrasound screening in pregnancy: a systematic review of the clinical effectiveness, cost effectiveness and women's views. *Health Technol Assess* Vol. 4, No. 16, pp

Bromley B, Frigoletto FD, Harlow BL, Pauker S, Benacerraf B. (1994). The role of Doppler velocimetry in the structurally normal second-trimester fetus with elevated levels of maternal serum α-fetoprotein. *Ultrasound Obstet Gynecol.*Vol. 4, pp377-380

Champmank MH, Champtman R. (1994). The value of serial ultrasounds in the management of recurrent uterine scar rupture. *BrJObstet Gynaecol* Vol.101, pp549-551.

Chase, L.M. and Cayea, P.D. (1991) : The placenta and umbilical cord. IN Berman, M.C. (ed). *Diagnostic Medical Sonography. A Guide to Clinical Practice.* 1st ed. Philadelphia, J.B. Lippincott Company, p. 301-330.

Dassah ET, Odoi AT, Opoku BK. (2009) Advanced twin abdominal pregnancy: diagnostic and therapeutic challenges. *Acta Obstet Gynecol Scand.* Vol.88, No.11, pp 1291-3

Dawn, C.S. (1995) : Hypertensive disorders in pregnancy. Int. Dawn, C.S. (ed). Textbook of Obstetrics.

Degani S. (2001). Fetal biometry: Clinical, pathological, and techinical considerations. *Obstet Gynecol Surv* Vol. 56. p159

Eggebø TM, Heien C, Økland I, Gjessing LK, Romundstad P, Salvesen KA. (2008) Ultrasound assessment of fetal head-perineum distance before induction of labor. *Ultrasound Obstet Gynecol.* Vol.32, No.2, pp199-204.

Eik-Nes SH, Salvesen KA, Okland O, Vatten LJ. (2000). Routine ultrasound fetal examination in pregnancy: the "Alesund" randomized, controlled trial. *Ultrasound Obstet Gyneco* Vol.15, pp473- 8

Fleischer AC, Pennell RG, McKee MS, et al. (1990). Ectopic pregnancy: features at transvaginal sonography. *Radiology* Vol.174, pp375.

Frates MC, Brown DL, Doubilet PM, et al. (1994). Tubal rupture in patients with ectopic pregnancy: diagnosis with transvaginal US. *Radiology* Vol.191, p769.

Geirsson, R.T.; Ogston, S.A.; Patel, N.B.; Christie, A.D. (1985) : Growth of total intrauterine, intra-amniotic and placental volume in normal singleton pregnancy measured by ultrasound. *Br. J. Obstet. Gynaecol.* Vol.92, pp46-53.

Goldberg BB. (2003).International arena of ultrasound education. *J Ultrasound Med* Vol.22, pp549–551

Guzman ER, Walters C, Ananth CV, et al(2001): A comparison of sonographic cervical parameters in predicting spontaneous preterm birth singleton gestations. *Ultrasound Obstet Gynecol* Vol. 18, No.3, pp204-210

Harman CR. Biophysical Profile Scoring, In: *Diagnostic Ultrasound,* Rumack CM, Wilson RS, Charboneau JW(eds),p1521, Elsevier MOSBY ISBN-9997629523 St.Louis Missouri

Harris RD, Cho C, Wells WA. (1996) Sonography of the placenta with emphasis on pathological correlation. *Semin Ultrasound CT MRI* Vol.17, pp66-89.

Harris RD, Marks WM. (2009). Compact ultrasound for improving maternal and perinatal care in low-resource settings: review of the potential benefits, implementation challenges, and public health issues. *J Ultrasound Med.* Vol.28, No.8 pp1067-76.

Henderson J, Bricker L, Roberts T, Mugford M, Garcia J, Neilson J.(2002) British National Health Service's and women's costs of antenatal ultrasound screening and follow-up tests. *Ultrasound Obstet Gynecol.* Vol.20, No.2, (Aug 2002) pp154-62. [PubMed]

Henrich W, Dudenhausen J, Fuchs I, Kamena A, Tutschek B (2006). Intrapartum translabial ultrasound (ITU): sonographic landmarks and correlation with successful vacuum extraction. *Ultrasound Obstet Gynecol.* Vol.28, pp753–760.

Iams JD. (2003). Prediction and early detection of preterm labor. *Obstet Gynecol* Vol.2, pp402-412

Iams JD, Goldenberg RL. Meis PJ, et al. (1996). The length of the cervix and the risk of spontaneous premature delivery. *N Engl J Med* Vol.334, pp567-572

Johnson DD, Pretorius DH, Riccabona M, et al. (1997). Three-dimensional ultrasound of the fetal spine.*Obstet Gynecol* Vol.89, No.3, pp434–8.

Jurkovic, D.; Jauniaux, E. and Cobnpbell, S. (1994) : Three dimensional ultrasound in obstetrics and gynecology. In Kurjak, A. and Chervenak, F.A (eds.). *The fetus as patient*, pp. 135-40. (Carnlortl, U.K : The Parthenon Publishing Group).

Kalache KD, Dückelmann AM, Michaelis SAM, Lange J, Cichon G, Dudenhausen JW. (2009). Transperineal ultrasound imaging in prolonged second stage of labor with occipitoanterior presenting fetuses: how well does the 'angle of progression' predict the mode of delivery? *Ultrasound Obstet Gynecol* Vol.33, pp326–330.

Kawano M, et al. (1996)Transvaginal color Doppler studies in gestational trophoblastic disease. *Ultrasound Obstet Gynecol*. Vol.7, No.3,(March 1996) pp197-200

Kim SY, Khandelwal M, Ganghan JP, et al. (2003). Is the intrapartum biophysical profile useful? *Obstet Gynecol* Vol.102. pp471-6

Lawson HW, Atrash HK, Saftlas AF, et al. (1988). Ectopic pregnancy surveillance, United States, 1970-1985. MMWR CDC *Surveill Summ* Vol.37, p9.

Levine D: Ectopic Pregnancy, In: *Ultrasonography in Obstetrics and Gynecology,* Callen PW(ed), Saunders ISBN: 0-7216-8132-8, Philadelphia

Lin CC, Santolaya-Forgas J. (1998). Current concepts of fetal growth restriction: Part I. Causes, classification, and pathophysiology. *Obstet Gynecol* Vol.92, pp1044-1055

Lockwood CJ, Weiner S. (1986). Assessment of fetal growth. *Clin Perinatol* Vol.13, pp3-35

Mahony BS, Filly, RA, Nyberg DA, et al. (1985). Sonographic evaluation of ectopic pregnancy. *J Ultrasound Med* Vol.4, p221.

Magann EF, Perry KG, Jr., Chauhan SP, et al. (1997).The accuracy of ultrasound evaluation of amniotic fluid volume in singleton pregnancies: the effect of operator experience and ultrasound interpretative technique. *J Clin Ultrasound* Vol.25, pp249-253.

Mari G et al. (2000). Noninvasive diagnosis by doppler ultrasonography of fetal anemia due to maternal red-cell alloimmunization. Collaborative Group for Doppler Assessment of the Blood Velocity in Anemia. *N Engl J Med* Vol.342, p9

Markestad T, Kaaresen PI, Ronnestad A, Reigstad H, Lossius K, Medbo S, Zanussi G, Engelund IE, Skjaerven R, Irgens LM. (2005). Early death, morbidity, and need of treatment among extremely premature infants. *Pediatrics*. Vol.115, pp1289–1298. doi: 10.1542/peds.2004-1482. [PubMed] [Cross Ref]

Martin AM, Bindra R, Curcio P, et al. (2001) Screening for pre-eclampsia and fetal growth restriction by uterine artery Doppler at 11-14 weeks of gestation. *Ultrasound Obstet Gynecol* Vol.18, pp583-586

Mindel S. (1997). Role of imager in developing world. *Lancet* Vol.350, pp426–429

Molina FS, Nicholaides KH. (2010) Ultrasound in Labour and Delivery. *Fetal Diagn Ther* Vol.27 No.2, pp61-7

Momin AA, Saiffi SG, Pethani NR, Mitha SH. (2009). Sonography of postpartum uterine inversion from acute to chronic stage.*Jclinica ultrasound*. Vol.37, No.1, pp53-56

Munjanja SP. Ultrasound in developing world: appropriate technology?, In: *Obstetric Ultrasound*, Neilson JP, Chambers SE (eds), pp 191-194, Oxford University Press, ISBN 0192622242, Oxford

Nicolaides KH, Azar G, Byrne D, Mansur C, Marks K. (1992).Fetal nuchal translucency:ultrasound screening for chromosomal defects in first trimester of pregnancy. *BMJ* Vol.304, pp867–869.

Nicolaides KH, Snijders RJM, Gosden RJM, et al. (1993). Sonographically detectable markers of fetal chromosomal abnormalities. *Lancet* Vol.340. pp704-707.

Nicolaides KH. (2004). Nuchal translucency and other first-trimester sonographic markers of chromosomal abnormalities. *Am J Obstet Gynecol* Vol.191, pp45-67

North RA, Ferrier C, Long D, Townend K, Kincaid-Smith P. (1994)Uterine artery Doppler flow velocity waveforms in the second trimester for the prediction of pre-eclampsia and fetal growth retardation. *Obstet Gynecol.* Vol.83, pp378-386.

Nyberg DA, Hughes MP, Mack LA, et al. (1991). Extrauterine findings of ectopic pregnancy at transvaginal US: importance of echogenic fluid. *Radiology* Vol.178, p823.

Odoi AT, Opare-Addo HS, Operative vaginal delivery: Forceps delivery and vacuum extraction. In Comprehensive obstetrics in the Tropics.2002 Kwawukume EY, Emuveyan E (eds), 340-51

Ogbole GI, Ogunseyinde OA, Akinwuntan. (2008).Intrapartum rupture of the uterus diagnosed by ultrasound. *Afri Health Sci* Vol.8, No.1, pp 57-59

Pellerito JS, Taylor KJW, Quedens-Case C, et al. (1992) Ectopic pregnancy: evaluation with endovaginal colour flow imaging. *Radiology* Vol.183, p407.

Peregrine E, Pandya P: Structural Anomalies in the First Trimester, In: *Diagnostic Ultrasound,* Rumack CM, Wilson RS, Charboneau JW(eds),p1152, Elsevier MOSBY ISBN-9997629523 St.Louis Missouri

Pijnenborg R, Anthony J, Davey DA, et al. (1991). Placental bed spiral arteries in the hypertensive disorders of pregnancy. *Br J Obstet Gynaecol* Vol.98, pp648-655.

Roman AS, Martin LP. Late Pregnancy Complications, In: *Current diagnosis &Treatment OBSTETRICS & GYNECOLOGY,* Decherney AH, Nathan L, Goodwin TM, Laufer N (eds), p285 McGraw-Hill, ISBN-13:978-0-07-110509-5, New York

Rane SM, Guirgis RR, Hggin B, Nicholaides KH. Models for successful induction of labour based on pre-induction sonographic measurement of of cervical length

Reese EA, Homko CJ, Wiznitzer A. (1994). Doppler velocimetry and the assessment of fetal well-being in normal and diabetic pregnancies. *Ultrasound Obstet Gynecol.* Vol.4, pp508-514.

Rembouskos G, Cicero S, Longo D, Vandecruys H, Nicolaides KH. (2004). Assessment of the fetal nasal bone at 11-14 weeks of gestation by three-dimensional ultrasound.*Ultrasound Obstet Gynecol* Vol.23, pp232-236

Roberts JM, Cooper DW. (2001). Pathogenesis and genetics of pre-eclampsia. *Lancet* Vol.357, pp53-56

Saari-Kemppainen A, Karjalainen O, Ylostalo P, Heinonen OP (1990). Ultrasound screening and perinatal mortality: Controlled trial of systematic one-stage screening in pregnancy. The Helsinki Ultrasound Trial. *Lancet,* Vol.336, No.8712, pp387-391.

Savvidou MD, Karanastasi E, Skentou C, Geerts L, Nicolaides KH. (2001). Twin chorionicity and pre-eclampsia. *Ultrasound Obstet Gynecol* Vol.18, pp228–231.

Sebire NJ, Snijders RJM, Hughes K, Sepulveda W, Nicolaides KH. (1997). The hidden mortality of monochorionic twin pregnancies. *BJOG* Vol.104, pp1203–1207

Sepulveda W, Sebire NJ, Hughes K, Odibo A, Nicolaides KH. (1996).The lambda sign at 10–14 weeks of gestation as a predictor of chorionicity in twin pregnancies. *Ultrasound Obstet Gynecol* Vol.7, pp421–423.

Sherer D, Miodovnik M, Bradley K, Langer O. (2002).Intrapartum fetal head position II: comparison between transvaginal digital examination and transabdominal ultrasound assessment during the second stage of labor. *Ultrasound Obstet Gynecol.* Vol.19, pp264–8

Sibai B, Dekker G, Kupferminc M. (2005). Pre-eclampsia. *Lancet* Vol.365, pp785-99.

Sickler GK, Nyberg DA, Sohaey R, et al. (1997). Polyhydramnios and fetal intrauterine growth restriction: ominous combination. *J Ultrasound Med* Vol.16, pp609-614.

Sivaro, S.; Vidyadaran, M.K.; Jammal, A.B.; Zinab, S. and Ramesh, K.N. (2002) : Weight, volume and surface area of placenta of normal pregnant women and their relation to maternal and neonatal parameters in Malay, Chinese, and Indian ethnic group. *Placenta* Vol.23, No.8-9, pp691-6.

Souka AP, von Kaisenberg CS, Hyett JA, Sonek JD, Nicolaides KH. (2004). Increased nuchal translucency with normal karyotype. *Am J Obstet Gynecol*

Spencer JK, Adler RS.(2008). Utility of portable ultrasound in a community in Ghana. *J Ultrasound Med* Vol.27, pp1735–1743.

Sterne G et al. (2001). Abnormal fetal cerebral and umbilical doppler measurements in fetuses with intrauterine growth restriction predicts the severity of perinatal morbidity. *J clin Ultrasound* Vol. 29:146

Theam M,Osmond C, Wilks R, Benett FI and Forrester, TE (2001). Second trimester placental volume and infant size at birth. *Obstet Gynecol* Vol.98, No.2, pp279-283.

Thorsen MK, Lawson TL, Aiman EJ, et al. (1990). Diagnosis of ectopic pregnancy: endovaginal vs transabdominal sonography. *Am J Roentgenol* Vol.155, p307.

USAID. 2001. USAID Congressional Budget Justification FY2002: Program, Performance and Prospects - The Global Health Pillar.

Ustunyurt E, Kaymak O, Iskendar C, Ustunyurt OB, Celik C, Danisman N. (2007). Role of Transvaginal ultrasound in the diagnosis of retained products of conception. *Archives of Gynae Obstet*, Vol.277, No.2, pp 151-4

Uzelac PS,Garmel SH: Early Pregnancy Risks, In: *Current diagnosis &Treatment OBSTETRICS & GYNECOLOGY*, Decherney AH, Nathan L, Goodwin TM, Laufer N (eds), pp259-272 McGraw-Hill, ISBN-13:978-0-07-110509-5, New York

Van den Elzen HL, Cohen-Overbeek TE, Grobbee DE, et al. (1995). Early uterine artery Doppler velocimetry and outcome of pregnancy in women aged 35 years and older. *Ultrasound Obstet Gynecol.* Vol.5, pp328-333

Van Dyk B, Motto JA, Buchmann EJ. (2008). The value of routine mid-trimester ultrasound in low-risk pregnancies at primary care level. *The Free Library.com .Health SA Gesondheid*

Walker JJ. (2000). Pre-eclampsia. *Lancet* Vol.356, pp1260-1265.

Wen SW, Huang L, Liston R, et al. (2005). Maternal Health Study Group, Canadian Perinatal Surveillance System. Severe maternal morbidity in Canada, 1991-2001. *CMAJ* Vol.173, pp759-64.

Welsh A, Nicolaides K. (2002). Cervical screening for preterm delivery. *Curr Opin Obstet Gynecol 2002*, Vol.14, No.2, pp195-202.

Wong GY, Mok YM, Wong SF. (2007).Transabdominal ultrasound assessment of the fetal head and the accuracy of vacuum cup application. *Int J Gynecol Obstet* Vol.98, pp 120-123.

World Health Organization. (1998). Training in Diagnostic Ultrasound: Essentials, Principles and Standards. Report of a WHO Study Group. Geneva, Switzerland, World Health Organization. Technical report series 875.

World Health Organization. Making pregnancy safer. In: *The World Health Report 2005: Making Every Mother and Child Count.* Geneva, Switzerland: World Health Organization; 2005:41–52

Yeboah MY, Dassah ET, Odoi AT, Manu AA. (2010). The appropriateness of healthcare provider requests for obstetric and gynecologic ultrasound in a low resource setting. *Int J Gynecol Obstet* Vol.111, pp271-3

Zuckerman J, Levine D, McNicholas MM, Kanopka S, et al. (1997). Imaging of pelvic postpartum complications. *Amj Roentgenolog* Vol.168, pp663-668

12

Role of the Endoscopic Ultrasonography in the Management of Gastric Lymphomas: Our Experience and Review of Literature

Calogero Vetro, Alessandra Romano, Giuseppe A. Palumbo, Giacomo Bonanno and Francesco Di Raimondo
University of Catania
Italy

1. Introduction

The stomach is the most common extranodal site of non-Hodgkin lymphoma (NHL) accounting for 7.1 to 10% of adult NHL (Danzon et al., 2009). The most frequent histotypes of gastric lymphomas are MALT lymphomas that arise from the stomach-associated lymphatic tissue and the Diffuse Large B-Cell Lymphoma (DLBCL) (Koch et al., 2001).
Several studies have observed that in recent years both gastric-NHL incidence and survival are increasing (Danzon et al., 2009). Furthermore, the management of gastric lymphomas has changed during the last two decades with a strong reduction of surgery in flavor to conservative treatments (Yoon S.S. et al., 2004). Indeed, the progress in biologic understanding of the pathogenesis, the introduction of Helicobacter pylori (HP) eradication therapy and the introduction of conservative treatment have definitely changed the approach to the disease and gastrectomy is no longer the first choice (Fischbach, 2010). The role of HP is a consolidated finding and several studies have confirmed that a simple antibiotic therapy (AT) for HP eradication is an effective treatment for MALT lymphomas with limited extension (Fischback et al., 2004), whereas, for advanced gastric lymphomas, the golden standard of treatment is the antineoplastic chemotherapy with alkylating agents in monochemotherapy such as Clorambucil for MALT lymphomas and polichemotherapy together with immunotherapy such as R-CHOP for DLBCL (Zucca & Dreyling, 2010).
The loco-regional staging of gastric lymphomas with limited disease is important in order to better understand how to treat patients and endoscopic ultrasound (EUS) technique plays in this context a pivotal role by giving information for the prevision of response to HP eradication therapy since this therapy has shown to induce a high percentage of histological remission (up to 88%) when the disease is confined to mucosa and submucosa (Caletti et al., 2002).
However, the importance of EUS in assessing the response to treatment and the follow-up is controversial. During the last decade, some reports indicated the importance of EUS in evaluating the response to treatment and also in long-term follow-up of gastric lymphomas with limited disease (Yeh et al., 2003), whereas other recent reports indicated the importance of EUS also in the follow-up of local-advanced MALT lymphoma (Pavlović et al., 2005). That notwithstanding, the latest ESMO clinical guidelines for diagnosis, treatment and follow-up

of gastric lymphomas does not recommend the usage of EUS in assessing the response to treatment and the follow-up in these patients (Zucca & Dreyling, 2010).

Based on the fact that the importance of EUS in initial assessment in gastric lymphoma is incontrovertible and that its role in follow-up is not clearly established (Zucca & Dreyling, 2010), the present work is focused in better define its role in diagnosis and follow-up.

A review of the literature will evaluate the publications on reliability of EUS in the management of patients affected by gastric lymphoma. Finally, we will present our centre experience in the management of gastric lymphomas.

2. Primary gastrointestinal non Hodgkin's lymphomas: general concepts on epidemiology, histology and clinical presentation

Primary gastric NHL (PGL) accounts for 30-45% of extra nodal lymphomas in western countries (Feng et al., 2009) and 80% of extra-nodal lymphomas in eastern countries, with an incidence of 0.51 and 0.29 for male and female respectively, showing an upward trend in both incidence and survival (Danzon et al., 2009).

The age of patients at diagnosis is on average 51-66 years (Danzon et al., 2009; Feng et al., 2009) with a male-female ratio of 1:1.3, even if it depends on the histotype. The most frequent histotype is MALT lymphoma, a type of indolent disease, that arise from the marginal zone of "acquired" stomach-associated lymphatic tissue and the Diffuse Large B-Cell Lymphoma (DLBCL), a form of aggressive malignancy (Koch et al., 2001).

The differential diagnosis between these two lymphomas is based on morphological and immune-histo-chemical evaluation.

Macroscopically, PGL lies in the sub-mucosa layer and is morfologically characterized by small cells with dense/ moderately dispersed nuclear chromatin, not noticeable nucleoli, abundant pale cytoplasm and low proliferation rate, being similar to centrocytes. In one third of PGL of MALT type plasmacytic differentiation could be noticed. This cells infiltrate around reactive follicles in an external zone called "marginal zone" converging in a larger mass. Often, lympho- epitheliod degeneration occurs with lymphoma cells disrupting the epithelium organization with eosinophilic degeneration of epithelial cells (Swerdlow et al., 2008).

Occasionally, transformed centroblast may be present in the context of PGL of MALT type, but the presence of transformed cells with round and vescicular nuclei, scanty and amphophilic cytoplasm, organized in solid or sheet-like aggregates should testify the presence of DLBCL. Additionally, in some cases, a low grade component may be present in the context of high grade lymphoma, approximately in one fifth of cases (Koch et al., 2005).

Immunophenotypic assays can help in differential diagnosis between MALT lymphoma, DLBCL and reactive inflammatory processes, being CD20, CD21, CD35 positive CD5, CD10, CD23 negative Additionally, polimerase chain reaction (PCR), detecting the product of the translocation t(14;18)(q21;q21) may be useful in confirming the diagnosis of PGL (Swerdlow et al., 2008).

The behaviour of these histotype is quite different, being the MALT lymphoma usually localized with multiple localizations up to 25% of cases, meanwhile DLBCL often evolve infiltrating other layers of stomach with a rapidly growing mass with one or more nodal sites, with crucial implication in clinical manifestation and care.

The clinical presentation of PGL may vary according to the histological type of lymphoma. The majority of patients with PGL of MALT type present at diagnosis unspecific symptoms, related to the presence of lymphoma and the location of the malignancy.

In a report, the German group, in the context of the GIT NHL 01/92 study (Koch et al, 2001), showed that patients present especially epigastric pain (80.5%), loss of appetite (46.5%), loss of weight (23.2%), related either to ''B'' lymphoma symptoms either to the loss of appetite, fever and night sweats (11.9%). The median duration from beginning of symptoms to diagnosis was 93 days. General symptoms include fatigue, due to blood loss and consequent anemia. In some cases, the formation of ulcers in the stomach may determine hemorrhages and haematemesis or melena, especially in DLBCL.
Mainly, symptoms are divided into two different clusters: non-alarm symptoms and alarm symptoms (Andriani et al., 2006). Non-alarm symptoms include Epigastric/abdominal pain, dyspepsia, and heartburn; meanwhile alarm symptoms comprise weight loss, vomiting, haematemesis/melena, anemia, perforation (table 1).

	MALT	DLBCL
ALARM SYMPTOMS	(28%)	(54%)
NON ALARM SYMPTOMS	(72%)	(46%)

Table 1. Symptoms at presentation in PGL of MALT type and DLBCL (Andriani et al., 2010)

3. Role of endoscopic ultrasound in diagnosis of disease

The unspecific clinical presentation leads to an endoscopic evaluation revealing different patterns. These lesions are more frequent at antrum and gastric body (77%) respect to the fundus (8%), and only in 15% of cases they occur diffusely.
On the whole, three main patterns could be detected using gastroscopy (Kelessis et al, 2003):
1. Ulcerative (28-85%);
2. Polipoid (5-44%);
3. Diffuse infiltrative (5-44%).

Usually, DLBCLs have a macroscopic presentation that may lead clinicians to suspect malignancies prior to histological confirmation, appearing as exophytic masses (fig. 1) or ulcerative lesion (fig. 2-9) or petechial hemorrhages, meanwhile low grade lymphomas appear as flat lesions, and/or enlarged gastric folds, and/or ulcers and/or erosions (Zullo et al., 2010). It is also to be considered that these lesions are not specific of lymphomas, for example petechial haemorrhages can be found in FANS-related gastritis; therefore histological evaluation is mandatory (Fig. 3).
It is also noteworthy that endoscopic ultrasound (EUS) assay is of great help in determine the differential diagnosis of large gastric folds and can spare the performance of unnecessary invasive procedures. Indeed, large gastric folds are found in several benign situations, such as Zollinger-Ellison syndrome, Menetrier's disease or lymphoid hyperplasia and malignancies, such as adenocarcinoma. Recently, the application of diathermic snare has been proposed, but is not routinely performed because the risk of major complications, including hemorrhages and perforations. EUS findings are able to predict malignancies, especially the evaluation of gastric wall thickness (especially if ≥ 4 mm), the no preserved wall architecture and the enlargement of deep layers (Ginès t al., 2006). This is particularly useful in the diagnosis of plastic linitis, even if more additional studies are needed (Andriulli et al., 1990). Additionally, EUS keeps also a pivotal role in defining the diagnosis of PGL. In a recent report, Fusaroli & Caletti (Fusaroli and Caletti, 2006) observed that, in some series of gastric malignancies, traditional biopsies are positive in 50% of cases and the

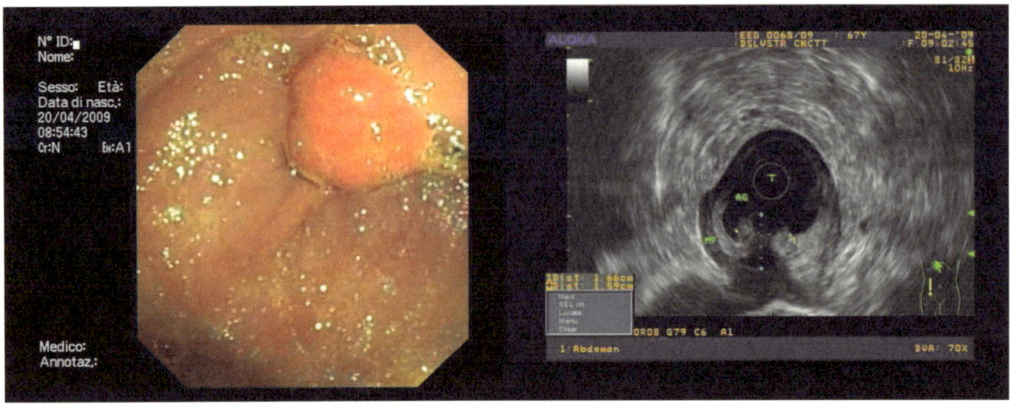

Fig. 1. Endoscopy: Polipoid lesion in the gastric antrum (left panel); histology: MALT Lymphoma; EUS (radial scanning) showing an irregularity of the gastric wall limited to the second layer (stage: T2 N0).

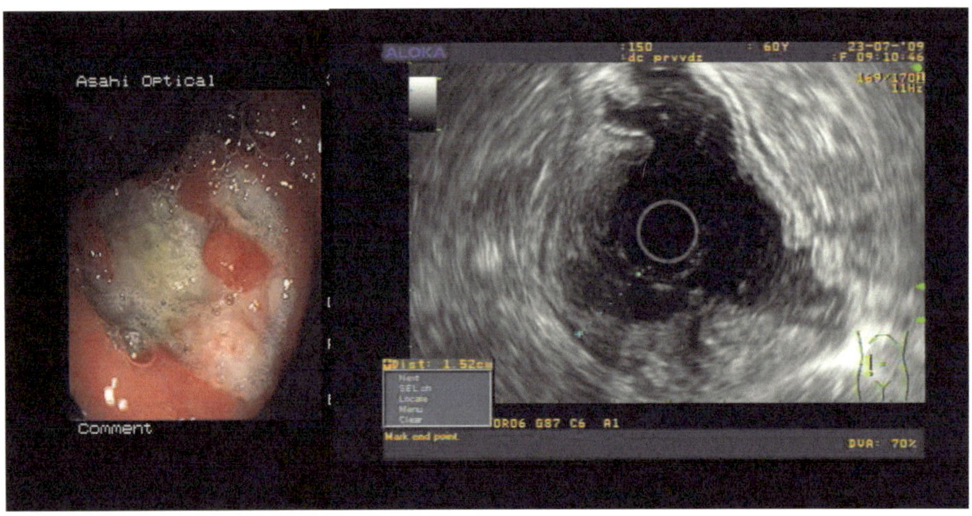

Fig. 2. Endoscopy: gastric ulcer (panel on the left); EUS (radial scanning): irregular circumferential thickening of the gastric body with disruption of the layers and penetration of the serosa (T3 N0). Horizontal extension of the lesion bigger than endoscopic appearance

usage of large forceps has slightly increased the diagnostic sensitivity. In this prospect, EUS features have improved the diagnostic accuracy up to 89% (Nagler, 2011), due to the peculiar echographic presentation of different malignancies, independently from the accuracy of the staging. Usually, gastric adenocarcinoma have a vertical extension with the involvement of all the layers of the gastric wall, differently from the PGL that have an horizontal growth pattern involving the gastric wall sparing the first layer. Due to this assertion, EUS is able to predict the presence of PGL more than endoscopy and biopsy alone. Furthermore, the detection of pathological nodes is a sign that induce a strong suspect of gastric malignancies. An additional advantage from using EUS in establishing diagnosis of PGL is related to the reduced risk of minor and major complication following biopsy, principally in presence of vascular alterations (Chen et al., 1999).

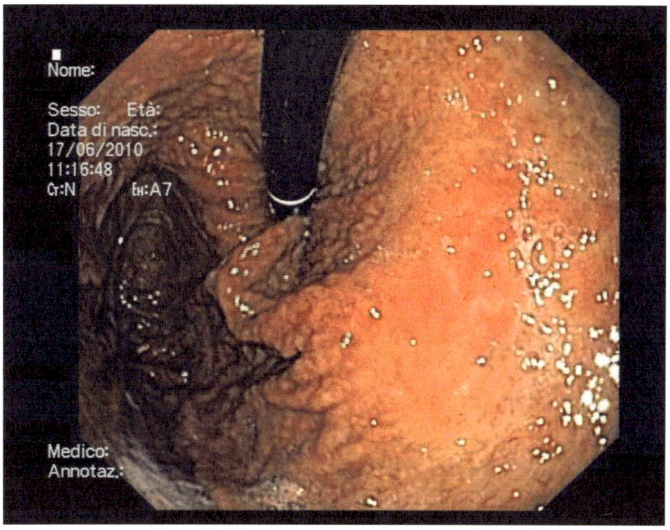

Fig. 3. Endoscopy: Micronodular gastritis. Histology revealed a low-grade MALT lynphoma

That notwithstanding, the bioptic evaluation represents the golden standard to define diagnosis of malignancies, especially in presence of sub-epithelial lesions (Karaca et al., 2010). Over the 70 publications about EUS in the management of PGL, researched using MeSH database, from 1996 to 2011, only 6 of them (8.5%) discussed the role of EUS in determining the diagnosis of PGL. In spite of a great initial emphasis, especially when the tumor is localized to the gastric wall (Chen et al., 1999; Yücel et al., 1999; Caletti et al., 2000), subsequent studies have not confirmed these findings, giving a major importance to the ability to augment, together with bioptic evaluation, the accuracy of diagnosis (Ginès et al., 2006; Karaca et al., 2010; Nagler et al., 2011).

Biopsy is usually taken in the context of the endoscopic lesions and also randomly, in at least 8-12 regions, in order to clarify the amount of gastric wall involved by the disease and if some aggregates have transformed into more aggressive types of lymphomas. Considering that the new-formed MALT tissue in the stomach lays in the sub-mucosa, biopsies must be taken in depth; otherwise the risk is to underestimate the diagnosis. However, the introduction of large-valve biopsy forceps has improved the rate in obtaining the bioptic tissue on which establish the diagnosis (Boot & Jong, 2002) and the application of fine needle ago-biopsy (FNAB) EUS-guided as well (Fusaroli & Caletti, 2007) (fig. 4).

Definitive diagnosis is based on morphological and immunophenotypic evaluation. In regard to PGL of MALT type, it has been developed a score, namely Wotherspoon score, useful to differentiate it from reactive inflamation, taking into account the presence of limpho-epithelioid lesions (LEL) and the formation of follicles (table 2).

Additionally, PCR for the detection of t(14;18)(q21;q21) can be also performed cause it confirms the occurrence of malignancy and, on the other hand, can assess the likelihood of response to the treatment. Furthermore, documentation of HP infection is mandatory and could be performed histologically, using Hematoxylin-Eosin and modified Giemsa staining, or with culture, urea breath test, antigen stool test or serological analysis.

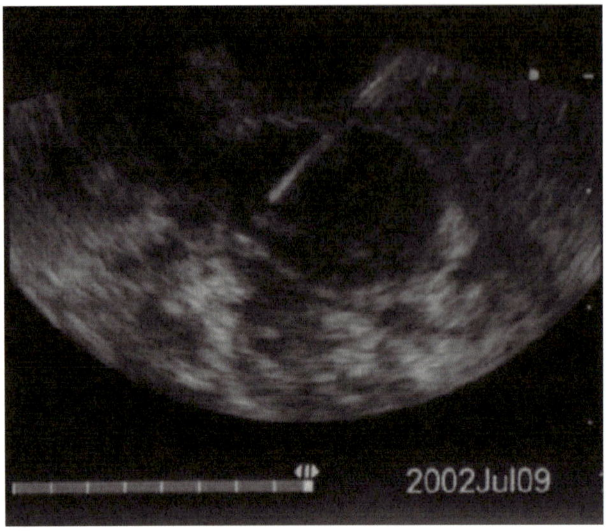

Fig. 4. EUS-guided FNAB: needle in perigastric node for cytological examination.

SCORE	DESCRIPTION	HISTOLOGY
0	Normal	Scattered plasma cells in lamina propria. No lymphoid follicles
I	Chronic active gastritis	Small clusters of lymphocytes in lamina propria. No lymphoid follicles. No LEL
II	Chronic active gastritis with florid lymphoid follicle formation	Prominent lymphoid follicles with surrounding mantle zone and plasma cells. No LEL
III	Suspicious lymphoid infiltrate, probably reactive	Lymphoid follicles surrounded by small lymphocytes that infiltrate diffusely in lamina propria and occasionally into epithelium
IV	Suspicious lymphoid infiltrate, probably lymphoma	Lymphoid follicles surrounded by marginal zone cells that infiltrate diffusely in lamina propria and into epithelium in small groups
V	MALT lymphoma	Presence of dense infiltrate of marginal zone cells in lamina propria with prominent LEL

Table 2. Wotherspoon's score for MALT lymphoma diagnosis (Hummel et al., 2006).

4. Endoscopic ultrasound in staging of disease

After diagnosis, the subsequent step is the staging of disease. This, together with the HP infection, is the most important factor in establishing the treatment needed and the prognostic status.

Usually, staging is based on three main classifications (table 3):

1. Ann Arbor classification modified by Mussshoff and Radaszkiewics (Radaszkiewicz et al., 1992);
2. Paris classification, that reproduce the TNM (Tumor-Node-Metastasis) classification for gastric cancer (Ruskoné-Fourmestraux et al., 2003);
3. Lugano classification (Rohatiner et al., 1994).

Lugano	TNM	Ann Arbor	Extension
I	T1-3 N0 M0	IE	Mucosa, sub-mucosa, muscolaris propria (fig.5-6-9)
II1 II2	T1-3 N1 M0 T1-3 N2 M0	IIE IIE	Peri-gastric nodes Distant nodes
III	T4 N0 MO	IIIE	Invasion of serosa and surrounding organs (Fig. 12)
IV	T1-4 N3 M0 T1-4 N0-3 M1	IIIE IVE	Extranodal dissemination or lymph node on both sides of diaphragm. Metastasis (e.g. bone marrow)

Table 3. Staging of PGL: comparison between different systems.

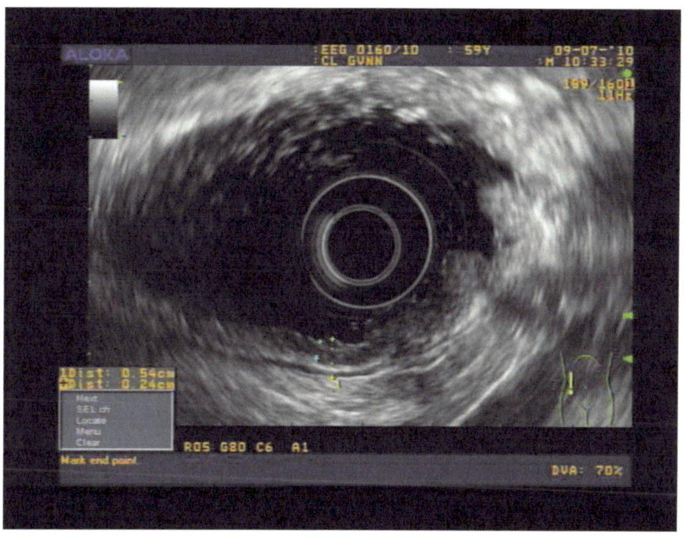

Fig. 5. EUS (radial scanning): thickening of the second layer of the gastric wall, corresponding to mucosa (stage: T1m N0)

Physical examination is useful in order to detect palpable nodes, masses in the abdomen and Waldeyer's ring involvement. Particular importance must be given to the general condition of patients, stratified with the ECOG performance status (PS), since it is a direct manifestation of the aggressiveness and stage of disease. The latest ESMO guidelines recommend additional work-up studies including complete blood counts, LDH and β2-microglobulin evaluation and a bone marrow aspirate and biopsy, even if a bone marrow involvement is rare.

Spiral-CT scan of neck, thorax, abdomen and pelvis with intravenous contrast is useful in order to detect masses in various body districts with a sensibility and specificity of 80% and

90% respectively, especially when performed with multiplanar reformations (Gligorievsky, 2009). Furthermore, 2-[fluorine-18] fluoro-2-deoxy-D-glucose (FDG)-positron emission tomography (PET) has an important role in staging and prognostic evaluation of DLBCL, but not in MALT lymphomas and is not recommended in the initial staging of PGL (Yi et al. 2010). Endoscopic Ultrasound (EUS) represents with no doubt the golden standard in determine the loco-regional staging of PGL, in particular in the era of HP eradication therapy in early stage disease.

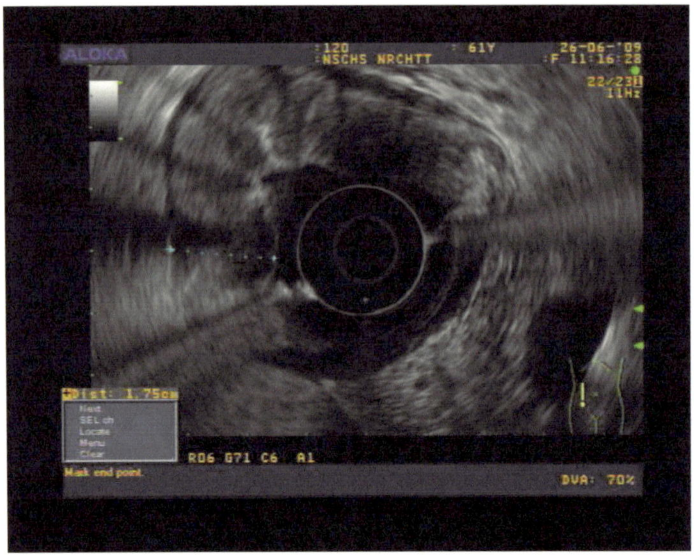

Fig. 6. EUS (radial scanning) demonstrated an irregular circumferential thickening of the gastric body with disruption of layers except for serosa (stage: T2 N0).

Due to the importance of EUS in establishing the most appropriate treatment in PGL, many papers has been published during the last decades, together with the number of publication about EUS in general (Fusaroli et al., 2010) (fig. 7).

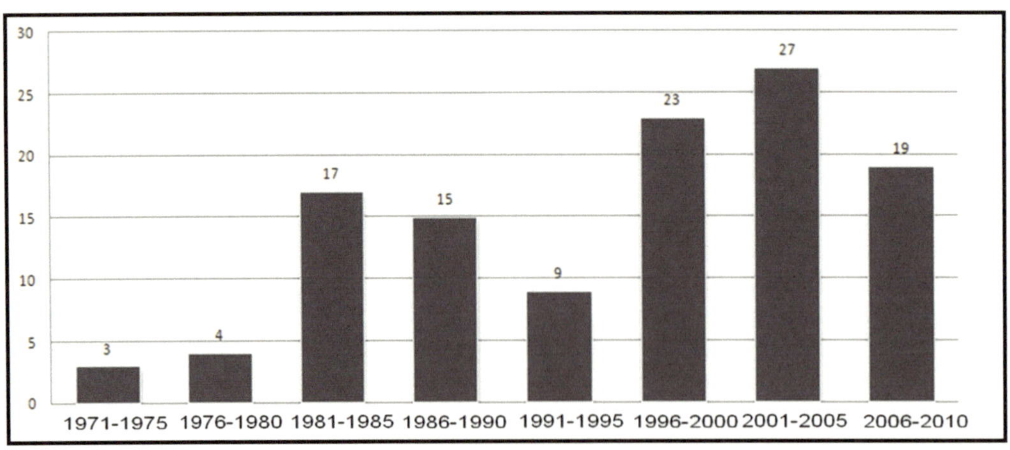

Fig. 7. Trend of published papers concerning the usage of EUS in the management of PGL.

A bibliographic research in MeSH database, using the key words [Stomach], [Lymphoma, Non-Hodgkin] and [Ultrasonography] has revealed a total amount of 117 papers published. The majority of them have been published from the second half of '90s when has been introduced for the first time by Sackmann, in 1997, the concept that early stage PGL responds to eradication treatment (Sackmann et al., 1997).

Particularly, the last decade has viewed an escalating number of published materials, compared to previous decades with a great quantity of prospective and retrospective studies (fig. 8).

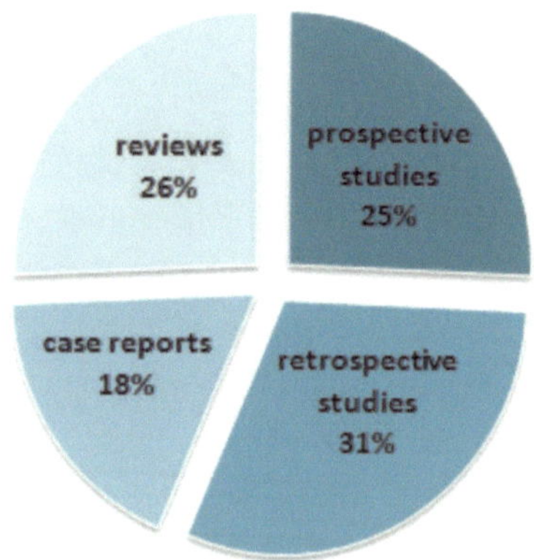

Fig. 8. Pie chart describing the typology of published papers concerning EUS in the management of PGL in the last decade.

First publications on the reliability of EUS in staging of PGL raised during the early '90's (Caletti et al., 1993) reported an accuracy of 80-92% and 77-90% for T and N stage respectively. These data were not confirmed by a successive study (Fischbach et al., 2002), involving 34 centers that reported an accuracy of 59% in detecting early stages and 71% in detecting the nodes involvement. These differences are probably due to the fact that EUS is an operator-dependent technique (Janssen, 2009). In general, EUS can define pathologic lymph node, defined as size greater than 10mm, sharply demarcated border, echopoor structure, rounded contour (Catalano et al., 1994), better than local extension.

Due to this conflicting data, an inter-observer agreement in diagnosis and staging with EUS of gastric lesions has been investigated. Firstly, Gress et al., described how the agreement factor, called k factor, in diagnosing sub-epithelial masses is lower (k=0.34) compared to the examination of superficial lesions (k=0.53-0.8). Additionally, the rate of disagreement were higher between low experienced endosonographers; therefore the lowest the number of EUS performed, the higher the discordance (Gress et al., 2001). At the same time, the Italian group, in the context of the staging of PGL of MALT type, found a fair agreement for T description (k=0.38) and substantial agreement in N definition (k=0.63). The lowest agreement was in the definition of intermediate stage (k=0.33-0.35) (Fusaroli et al., 2002).

Some studies have also indicated that the usage of miniprobe (fig. 9) would have improved the accuracy in detecting lesions (Lügering et al., 2001), but additional studies are needed. Interestingly, Varas et al. defined, in a subset of 24 patients, an accuracy of EUS in defining T factor of 91%, whereas the usage of miniprobes has given an accuracy of 88% and this mismatch was higher in evaluating the N factor confirming the high clinical impact of EUS (Varas et al., 2006).

As a general rule, EUS has entered in the clinical practice of staging evaluation (Di Raimondo et al., 2007;Pavlović et al. 2005) and has been indicated as an *"obligatory part of the staging procedure"* (Fischbach, 2010). Thus, in the 2010 ESMO guidelines (Zucca & Dreayler, 2010), EUS has been indicated as the most appropriate technique in defining the loco-regional staging.

Conversely, EUS staging is not mandatory for DLBCL (Fischbach & Al-Taie, 2010), being it treated as a systemic disease; even though a growing number of reports is showing its clinical utility.

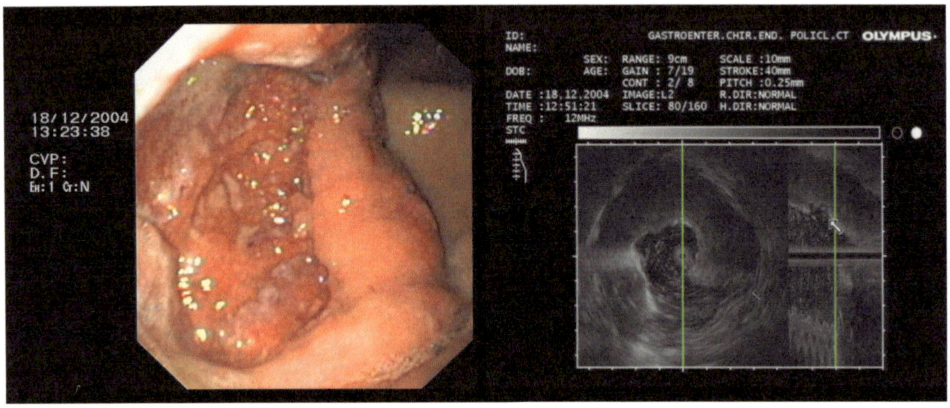

Fig. 9. Endoscopic view of ulcerated lesion of the gastric body. Histology revealed a high-grade gastric lymphoma (left panel); EUS (miniprobe): showing a circumferential irregularity of gastric wall limited at the second layer (stage: T2 N0) (right panel).

5. Prognostic assessment and treatment: how endoscopic ultrasound staging can help in tailoring patient management

Surely, the stage of disease assumes a great prognostic significance, being it related with survival either in pre- either post- HP eradication era; above all the bone marrow involvement represents a factor of poor outcome, together with the advanced loco-regional stage and depth of infiltration (Radaszkiewicz et al., 1992). Before the introduction of HP-eradication therapy, the presence of an early stage disease represented the major indicator of response to surgery, while in HP-eradication era it designates the response to the HP-therapy itself.

Nevertheless, the most important factor in risk assessment remains the loco regional staging and EUS preserves a great importance due to the fact that it is able to indicate, with accuracy superior to other techniques, the precise loco-regional stage of disease and consequently the required treatment (Pavlović et al. 2005).

Indeed, PGL of MALT type, when confined to mucosa and sub-mucosa layers responds to HP eradication therapy without any need of chemotherapy, meanwhile DLBCL are usually treated as general disease with chemo-immuno-therapy, even if recent case reports indicated the regression of locally staged DLBCL after HP eradication (Montalban et al., 2001, Tari et al., 2009).

Independently from the stage and dissemination, transformation to DLBCL occurs in about 10% of the cases (Zucca et al., 2008). Usually, DLBCL shows a prognosis worsen than MALT lymphoma. However, loco-regional stage remains a central prognostic factor also in DLBCL, having patients with advanced stage (II2-III according to Lugano classification) an overall survival (OS) of 71% at 5 years, whereas patients in early stage (I-II1according to Lugano classification) have a greater OS.

Reference	n	Staging procedure	% CR	Time to CR (months)	No. of relapses
Wotherspoon et al., 1993;	6	US	83	---	---
Savio et al., 1996;	12	CT	84	2-4	0
Pinotti et al., 1997;	45	CT	67	3-18	2
Neubauer et al., 1997;	50	CT+EUS	80	1-9	5
Nobre-Leitão et al., 1998;	17	CT+EUS	100	1-12	1
Steinbach et al., 1999;	23	CT+EUS	56	3-45	0
Montalban et al., 2001;	19	CT+EUS	95	2-19	0
Ruskoné-Fourmestraux et al., 2001;	46	CT+EUS	79	2-18	2
Stathis et al., 2009	105	CT	76	5-32	16

Table 4. Response to antibiotics in early-stage gastric MALT lymphoma. US: ultrasonography; CT: computed tomography; EUS: endoscopic ultrasonography; n: number of patients enrolled in the study; CR: Complete remission; No. of relapses: number of relapses

The GIT NHL 02/96 study, confirming the results of the previous study GIT NHL 01/92, revealed that surgery is no longer the better strategy in early-stage low- and high-grade gastric lymphomas (Koch et al., 2005), except when perforation, bleeding or obstruction take place, proving these findings in a cohort of 363 patients. Firstly, the great impact of the stomach-preserving treatment has been suggested by Fischbach in a prospective non-randomized trial, reporting a survival rate from 89% to 96% at 2 years for low-grade lymphomas and from 83% to 88% for high-grade lymphomas (Fischbach et al., 2000). Subsequently, randomized trials confirmed the superiority of a stomach-conservative approach compared to surgery in early stage DLBCL (Martinelli et al., 2009) and PGL of MALT type.

Interestingly, the Taiwan Cooperative Oncology Group (TCOG) performed two prospective studies, the T1296 study in low grade PGL and DLBCL(MALT) study in high grade PGL, involving 41 and 24 patients respectively. They obtained 80% of complete remission among patients involved in the T1296 study and 64% in patients enrolled in the study DLBCL(MALT), both groups being treated with HP eradicating therapy.

The same could be said about advanced-stage PGL, where the surgical approach is no longer the first choice. On the whole, for advanced gastric lymphomas, the golden standard of treatment is the antineoplastic chemotherapy with alkylating agents in monochemotherapy such as Clorambucil for MALT lymphomas and polichemotherapy together with immunotherapy such as R-CHOP for DLBCL (Zucca & Dreyling, 2010).

With regard to relapsed low-grade early stages PGL MALT lymphomas, independently from the HP eradication, radiotherapy represents a very good treatment option, increasing the survival rate to 85-100% at 5 years. Additionally, radiotherapy could be an option in HP negative MALT lymphomas. In high-grade lymphomas radiotherapy is usually performed in presence of partial remission of disease after chemotherapy or in presence of relapse (Aleman et al., 2010).

Of particular interest is the fact that early stage MALT PGL respond to the HP eradication in about 90% of cases, sparing chemotherapy to these patients (Andriani et al., 2009). Several regimens have been proposed, but the best strategy should be based on the expected antibiotic resistance. The first-choice regimen is triple therapy, but other regimens are effective as well.

Certainly, after the first 6 cases published in 1993 by Wotherspoon et al in *the Lancet*, HP eradication has become the best studied therapeutic approach with a large number of reported studies confirming that histological regression of the lymphoma can be achieved in the majority of cases (Wotherspoon et al., 1993) (table 4).

That notwithstanding, about 10% of patients do not respond to HP eradication and for these patients radiotherapy has been proposed as a good option.

6. Response evaluation: histology vs endoscopic ultrasound

Response assessment to treatment lacks of standard reproducible criteria. However, histological evaluation on mapping biopsies, considering histologic Wotherspoon score (table 2), has gained a great role in determining the response evaluation being it strictly related with the clinical outcome. Patients with score ≤ 2 achieve a complete remission, while patients with score = 3 a partial response and patients with a score ≥ 4 have a persistent lymphoma. Recently, the European Gastro-Intestinal Lymphoma Study (EGILS) has proposed the new recommendation on the management of PGL, including EUS in establishing the response assessment. Basically, complete remission (CR) is characterized by the absence of EUS abnormalities with negative E-Bx (Fig. 10) in two subsequent evaluations, Partial remission (PR) is defined as restoration of EUS with histological persistence of lymphoma but no clinical signs of progression, Stable disease (SD) is defined by constant presence of disease at EUS and/or histology, Progressive disease (PD) is defined by expansion of endoscopic findings, or transformation into high grade lymphoma in case of MALT lymphomas, Relapse (Rel) is defined as recurrence of lymphoma documented with histology after a reached complete remission (Ruskoné-Fourmestraux et al. 2011).

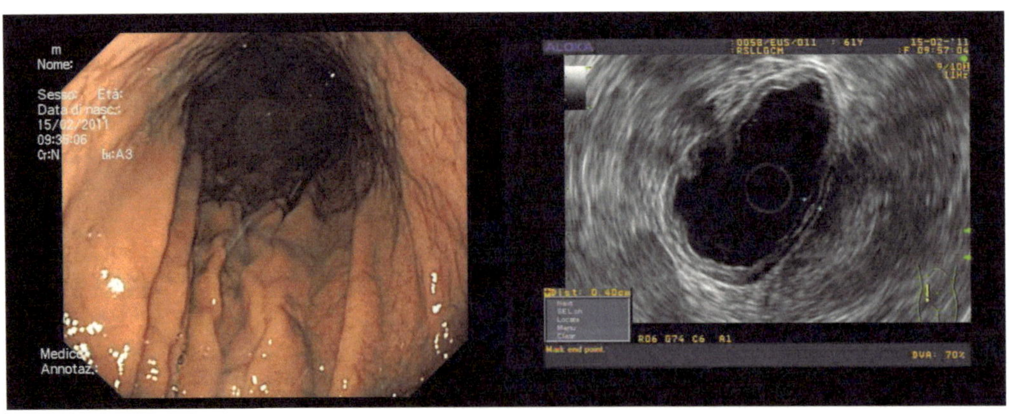

Fig. 10. Endoscopy: gastric body after eradication therapy. No histologic signs of MALT Lymphoma (left panel); EUS (radial scanning) showing a complete restoration of the gastric wall after eradication therapy (right panel).

7. Follow-up: is endoscopic ultrasound clinically helpful?

Several follow-up studies have confirmed that the achievement of complete response corresponds with an augmentation of OS and PFS. The TCOG group confirmed this finding in two prospective clinical trial, the T1296 study for low-grade lymphomas and the DLBCL(MALT) study for high grade, showing an OS of 94% and 87% at 5- and 7- years of follow-up respectively for patients with MALT lymphoma, while DLBCL patients showed a OS of 92% and 92% at 5- and 7-years correspondingly. In these trials, patients with DLBCL that achieved complete remission have shown no relapse of disease or lymphoma-related death, meanwhile patients with MALT lymphoma, without high-grade component, showed a relapse rate of 13% in a 70 months follow-up period.

Similarly, the German group, in a multicentric prospective study involving 417 patients (Fischbach et al., 2002), demonstrated that recurrence of disease occurs in 3.9% of MALT lymphoma and 4.7% of DLBCL. Additionally, in another multicentric trial on early stage MALT lymphoma, patients with histologically proven residual disease, have shown no recurrence of disease, except one of them that presented a transformation to DLBCL. Thus a postremission "watch and wait" strategy without further treatment can be safely adopted. Interestingly, it has been prospected that early-stage HP-negative PGL that respond to Hp-eradication treatment can be securely managed with the same "watch and wait" plan (Fischbach, 2010).

However, a general consensus in the management of follow-up does not exist (Zucca & Dreyler, 2010). The ESMO group suggest to perform a strict endoscopic follow-up with multiple biopsies 2-3 months after treatment and then twice a year for two years. In certain cases, histological relapse can occur, but still a "watch and wait" approach seems to be not dangerous, even if the level of evidence is IV and the grade of recommendation is D.

Basically, there is a lack of concordance between the histological evaluation and EUS in follow-up due to the fact that even if the EUS can detect the disappearance of gastric-wall lesion, histology can identify foci of residual disease, defined as a Wotherspoon score >2. On the contrary, in some cases endoscopy with mapping biopsies can give negative results for residual disease, whereas EUS is positive. That can be due to the real persistence of disease that biopsies cannot detect because the depth of the infiltration or the occurrence of fibrotic tissue subsequent to the treatment (Fig. 11-12) or the presence of lesions other than lymphoma, posing the same problems when diagnosis have to be established. Residual thickness of the gastric wall could represent a scar following the chemotherapy, especially in patients affected by DLBCL (fig. 12) where it is well documented that fibrosis remains after therapy in patients with nodal presentation of disease (Canellos et al., 1988).

In the last years few studies have taken into consideration the reliability of EUS in the follow-up management of PGL (table 5).

An early report indicated that post-treatment EUS documented an abnormal thickness of the wall in three out of 11 patients affected by MALT and two of the three patients had residual lymphoma (Pavlick et al., 1997). In one case of MALT lymphoma, persistence of EUS changes was able to predict relapse of disease in absence of a "positive" biopsy. Therefore, authors concluded that the persistence of wall thickness at EUS is an indication for repeating biopsies in order to detect persistence of disease or early relapse (Levy et al, 1997). These and other small studies would indicate that EUS is a useful tool for follow-up evaluation and indicate that for patients in remission, with a restoration of normal gastric wall, a recurrent wall thickening at EUS might be indicative for relapse. However, more recent studies, conducted in larger series, have reduced the importance of EUS in the setting of follow-up. A study indicated that the accuracy of EUS in evaluating remission of disease was inferior to histology, with a concordance between histology and EUS present in 64% of patients. In addition, the EUS findings returned to normal in a much more prolonged time in respect to gastroscopy with biopsy. After a prolonged follow-up, however, an EUS complete remission occurred in almost every patient (Püspök et al., 2002). On the contrary, another study confirmed that EUS is reliable in determining tumor regression or relapse with a concordance between EUS and endoscopic biopsies of about 80% (Lügering et al., 2001). During 2003, two other reports stated that EUS is a reliable tool in determining the response evaluation and the early detection of disease reappearance, thus avoiding the performance of invasive procedures (Hoepffner et al., 2003; Yeh et al., 2003). In addition, the Serbian group found a stringent correlation between EUS and histology in patients treated both with HP-eradicating therapy and/or chemotherapy ± radiotherapy (Pavlović et al. 2005).

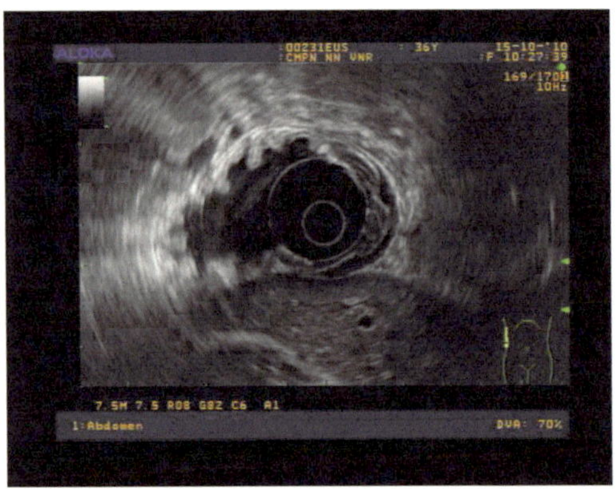

Fig. 11. Post-eradication therapy: The fourth layer persists thickened.

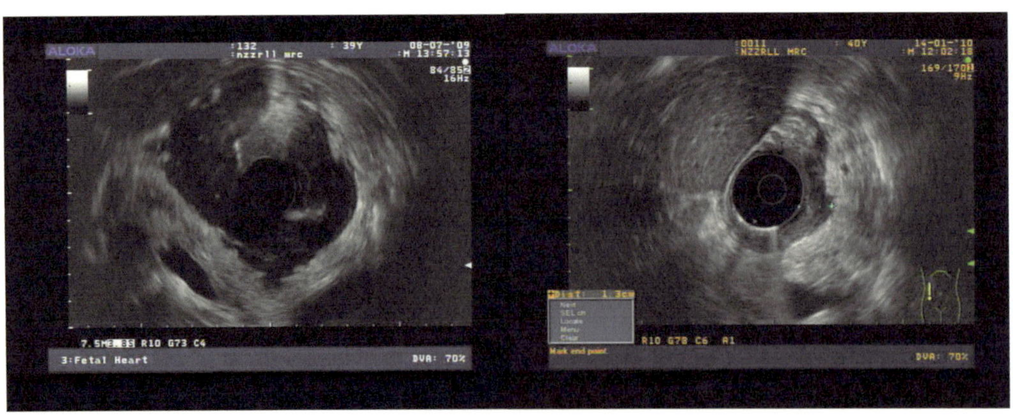

Fig. 12. EUS (radial scanning): left panel showing an high-grade gastric lymphoma infiltrating all layers of the gastric wall and the left lobe of the liver (stage: T4 N0); right panel indicates the persistence of residual abnormalities after 6 months post- chemotherapy (stage: T3 N0), even if the histology confirmed the complete response to the chemotherapy.

Author	Year	N	Follow-up (months)	Concordance EUS and histology	Time to reach histological response	Time to reach EUS response
Pavlick	1997	11	2	90.9%	///	///
Lévy	1997	15	17 (4-48)	50%	///	///
Lügering	2001	24	22 (17-28)	79.16%	///	///
Püspök	2002	33	15 (3-48)	64%	21.9	41.7
Yeh	2003	20	24 (3-51)	82.4%	///	///
Hoepffner	2003	22	21 (4-51)	///	///	///
Pavlović	2005	26	///	100% ; 78% *	///	///
Di Raimondo	2007	23	44 (25-71)	33%	8	20
***patients treated with HP-eradication therapy and chemotherapy ± radiotherapy respectively**						

Table 5. studies concerning the reliability of EUS in the follow-up of PGL.

8. Follow-up evaluation: experience of our group

Our experience is not confirmatory of the aforementioned studies. In fact, in order to evaluate the role of EUS in follow-up management, our group carried out a retrospective study in gastric lymphoma patients with the aim to compare EUS with conventional endoscopy and biopsy. In our series, after a complete remission, two patients experienced a relapse and this event was not predicted by EUS nor by E-Bx. More important, we found that EUS was concordant with biopsies in only one third of patients. In addition, the EUS findings returned to normal with a considerable delayed time in respect to gastroscopy with biopsy, even after a prolonged follow-up (fig.13).

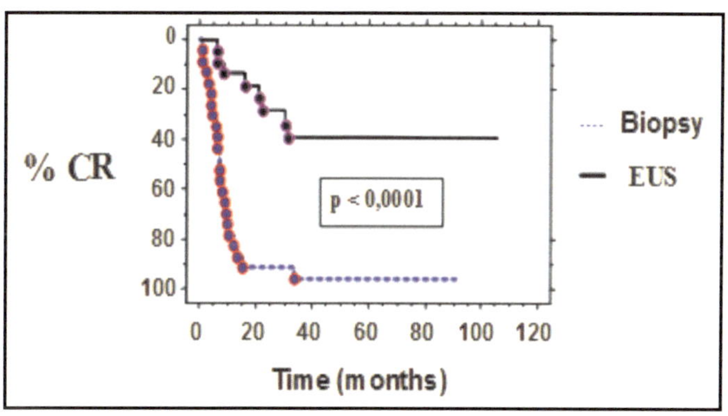

Fig. 13. Time required for achieving a complete remission by endoscopy with biopsy (E-Bx) and endoscopic ultrasound (EUS) (Di Raimondo et al. 2007)

Our series was composed by 23 patients, 11 female and 12 male, afferent at Division of Hematology, University of Catania, Italy, from January 1994 to December 2003, treated with a stomach conserving approach and with at least two EUS evaluation in the follow-up. The median age at diagnosis was 60 years ranged between 26 and 79. Sixteen patients had a low grade gastric lymphoma; while seven had a high-grade lymphoma, of whom one with a MALT lymphoma component.

Diagnosis was based on morphological and immunophenotypic analysis, according to WHO classification, from gastric biopsies performed with endoscopy with biopsy (E-Bx). HP infection has been assessed by using histochemistry or urea breath test and/or the antigen stool test and has resulted as positive in the total amount of patients with low grade lymphoma (12/12) and in only 1 patient with high grade lymphoma.
At diagnosis a total of 6 patients presented alarm symptoms, 4 with low grade lymphoma and 2 with high grade lymphoma. The ulcerative pattern was the mainly represented at gastroscopy, being present in 12 patients out of 23.
Patients have been staged at baseline with computed tomography (CT) scan of neck, thorax and abdomen, EUS and bone marrow biopsy. EUS staging was carried out according to TNM (tumour-node-metastasis) classification and the Lugano staging system (Table 6).
Response evaluation was based on the Wotherspoon score on bioptic samples. Endosonographic remission was defined as wall thickness ≤ 4 mm with a restoration of a normal layer pattern.

		TNM					
		T1 N0	T2 N0	T3 N0	T1-3 N1	T1-3 N2	T1-4 N0-3
LUGANO CLASSIFICATION	I	3	6	1			
	II1				6		
	II2					3	
	IIIE						4
	IVE						

Table 6. Extension of disease according to TNM and Lugano classification.

HP eradication with triple therapy regimen was employed in 6 patients with localized MALT lymphoma. Oral alkylating agents (either clorambucil or cyclophosphamide) or purine analogues (fludarabina, cladribine) were given, as second line treatment, in 3 out of 6 patients that failed to achieve the complete remission after AT and, as first line therapy, in 7 patients with extended MALT lymphoma. Patients with DLBCL were treated with R-CHOP (Rituximab, cyclophosphamide, doxorubicin, vincristine, and prednisone) or CHOP-like regimens with or without radiotherapy.
One patient died for hepatic failure and four more patients had a secondary neoplasia, on average 4 years after the achieved complete remission (1 colon carcinoma, 1 gastric carcinoma, 1 anaplastic NHL and 1 MALT lymphoma of small intestine).
Follow-up was conducted with endoscopic biopsies (E-Bx) in any abnormal area, or randomly if none, with EUS at variable intervals according to clinical judgment.
The echoendoscopists were unaware of the results of histology and the pathologists were unaware of the results of EUS.
At the end of initial treatment a CR was documented by biopsy in 15 (65%) patients. At the same time only two patients showed a normalization of EUS (P = 0.0002). Patients were then evaluated with EBs and EUS every 3/6 months and with a more prolonged follow-up (four patients) or the addition of further chemotherapy (two patients) a total of six patients in PR turned to CR so that the final number of patients in CR by E-Bx has increased to 21 (91%). At the same time, although EUS showed a reduction of median value of thickness of gastric

wall from 1 to 0.6 cm (P = 0.0031), only seven patients (30%) had a normal EUS (P < 0.0001). Complete remission, documented with E-Bx, was achieved in 18 patients with EUS restoration significantly delayed respect to E-Bx findings (26 vs 6 moths) (table 7).

TIME TO REACH CR		E-Bx		EUS	
TOTAL	MEDIAN	6		26	
	RANGE	2	19	6	56
MALT	MEDIAN	5		21	
	RANGE	2	19	6	56
HIGH GRADE	MEDIAN	6		N.A.	
	RANGE	2	10		

Table 7. Time required for achieving a complete remission by endoscopy with biopsy (E-Bx) and endoscopic ultrasound (EUS). CR: Complete Remission, N.A.: Not Available.

All the patients with MALT lymphoma, which responded to the treatment and maintained the response, eventually reached the EUS complete remission at the end of a prolonged follow-up, except for one of them that presented EUS abnormalities also after a follow-up of 114 months. On the contrary, only one patient with high grade lymphoma reached the EUS complete remission, after 30 months of follow-up.

Thus, it is possible that disappearance of lymphoma cells is a very slow process that takes several years to extinguish once the initiating factors have been eliminated. In any case, persistence of EUS abnormalities, irrespective of the fact that it indicates fibrosis or minimal residual disease, did not seem to have a clinical relevance being not predictive of relapse and should not be used as a guidance for further treatment.

A total of 120 EUS were performed, the majority of them (97/120) within the first five years of follow-up, with a discordance rate of 61.6%. Particularly, the discordance rate was 68% during the first five years of follow-up but it was reduced to 34.7%, in the subsequent period; on the contrary, the concordance rate shows an upward trend at 10-years follow-up, from 32% to 65%. However, taking into account the histotype, this trend seems to be confirmed for MALT lymphomas but not for DLBCL where the discordance rate, after 10 years of follow-up, remains higher than the concordance rate (Fig. 14).

On the whole, the prolonged follow-up confirmed our previous findings. In fact, EUS can detect the complete remission with a significant delay compared to E-Bx in both types of lymphoma. Additionally, EUS restoration of normal stomach layers occurs after many years from the achieved complete remission in patients with MALT lymphoma; while in patients with DLBCL EUS continues to show an abnormal pattern, despite the obtained complete remission.

9. Conclusion

The introduction of EUS in the management of PGL has radically changed the approach to these patients. Nowadays, EUS keeps a pivotal role in defining the sub-mucosal lesions and large gastric folds, also determining the differential diagnosis prior to the histological evaluation. The precise staging delineated by EUS assumes a critical importance in defining the prognosis and in turn tailors the therapy; nevertheless, EUS seems to be not very useful to define the response assessment, since it can show the restoration of gastric layers with a great delay compared to the histological evaluation.

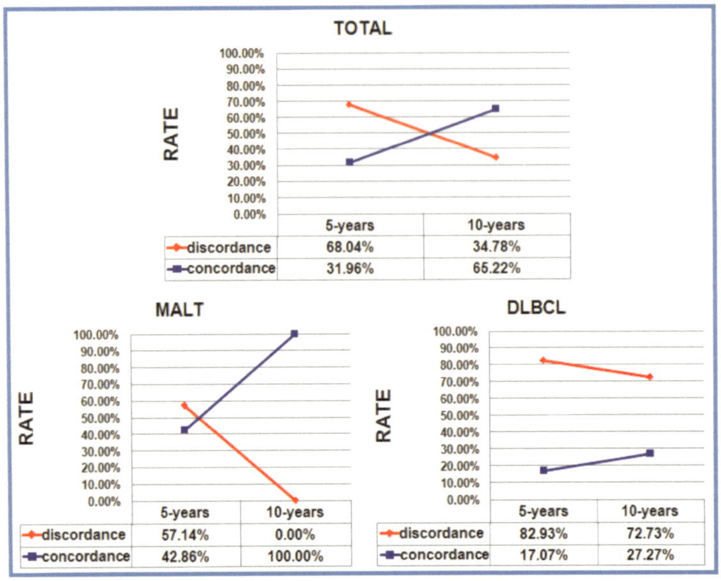

Fig. 14. Trend, at 5- and 10- years follow-up, of Discordance (red line) and Concordance (blue line) rate between E-Bx and EUS fining in the total set of patients (top panel), in patients with MALT lymphoma (left panel on the bottom) and in patients with DLBCL (right panel on the bottom).

Finally, the trustworthiness of EUS in follow-up is questionable. The latest ESMO guidelines do not recommend the performance of EUS in the follow-up. We have shown that it is not reliable in DLBCL, where most patients maintained a complete remission even with persistent EUS abnormality. In MALT patients, the role of EUS during the follow up period could be more important since we have noticed several changes in the EUS findings with a more prolonged follow up. Our study is, however, retrospective and also lies in a small number of cases. A prospective study should be carried out with an adequate number of patients so as to distinguish between DLBCL and MALT since the two diseases have different therapeutic approaches. We think that until now patients with gastric lymphoma should be treated with a conservative approach and they should be followed with both EUS and E-Bx in order to have a longer follow-up and more information on the role of EUS in detecting early relapse..

10. References

Aleman, B.M.; Haas, R.L. & van der Maazen, R.W. (2010) Role of radiotherapy in the treatment of lymphomas of the gastrointestinal tract. *Best Practice & Research Clinical Gastroenterology*, Vol. 24, No. 1 (February 2010), pp.24–34, ISSN 1521-6918.

Andriani, A.; Zullo, A.; Di Raimondo, F.; Patti, C.; Tedeschi, L.; Recine, U.; Caruso, L.; Bonanno, G.; Chiarenza, A.; Lizzani, G.; Miedico, A.; Romanelli, A.; Costa, A.; Linea, C.; Marrone, C.; Mirto, S.; Mistretta, A.; Montalbano, L.; Restivo, G.; Vinci, M.; Bibas, M.; Hassan, C.; Stella, F.; Cottone, M. & Morini S. (2006) Clinical and endoscopic presentation of primary gastric lymphoma: a multicentre study.

Alimentary pharmacology and therapeutics.Vol. 23, No. 6, (15 March 2006), pp. 721-726, ISSN 1365-2036.

Andriani, A.; Miedico, A.; Tedeschi, L.; Patti, C.; Di Raimondo, F.; Leone, M.; Schinocca, L.; Romanelli, A.; Bonanno, G.; Linea, C.; Giustini, M.; Hassan, C.; Cottone, M. & Zullo, A. (2009)Management and long-term follow-up of early stage H. pylori-associated gastric MALT-lymphoma in clinical practice: an Italian, multicentre study (2009) *Digestive and liver disease : official journal of the Italian Society of Gastroenterology and the Italian Association for the Study of the Liver.* Vol. 41, No. 7, (July 2009), pp. 467-473, ISSN 1878-3562.

Andriulli ,A.; Recchia, S.; De Angelis, C.; Mazzucco, D.; Berti, E.; Arrigoni, A. & Verme, G. (1990). Endoscopic ultrasonographic evaluation of patients with biopsy negative gastric linitis plastica. *Gastrointestinal endoscopy,* Vol. 36, No. 6, (November-December 1990), pp. 611-615, ISSN 1097-6779.

Boot, H. & de Jong, D. (2002) Diagnosis, treatment decisions, and follow up in primary gastric lymphoma. *Gut,* Vol. 51, No. 5, (November 2002), pp. 621-622, ISSN 1468-3288

Caletti, G.; Ferrari, A.; Brocchi, E. & Barbara, L. (1993). Accuracy of endoscopic ultrasonography in the diagnosis and staging of gastric cancer and lymphoma. *Surgery,* Vol. 113, No. 1, (January 1993), pp. 14-27, ISSN 1532-7361.

Caletti, G.; Fusaroli, P.; Togliani, T.; Bocus, P. & Roda, E. (2000) Endosonography in gastric lymphoma and large gastric folds. *European journal of ultrasound : official journal of the European Federation of Societies for Ultrasound in Medicine and Biology,* Vol. 11, No. 1, (March 2000), pp. 31-40, ISSN 0929-8266.

Caletti, G.; Zinzani P.L.; Fusaroli P.; Buscarini E.; Parente F.; Federici T.; Peyre S.; De Angelis C.; Bonanno G.; Togliani T. ; Pileri S.; Tura S. & The Italian Gastric Lymphoma Study Group (2002). The importance of endoscopic ultrasonography in the management of low-grade gastric mucosa-associated lymphoid tissue lymphoma. *Alimentary Pharmacology and therapeutics,* Vol. 16, No. 10, (October 2002), pp. 1715-1722, ISSN 0269-2813.

Canellos, G.P. (1988). Residual mass in lymphoma may not be residual disease. *Journal of clinical oncology : official journal of the American Society of Clinical Oncology,* Vol 6, No. 6, (June 1988), pp. 931–933, ISSN 1527-775.

Catalano, M.F.; Sivak, M.V.; Rice, T.; Gragg, L.A. & Van Dam J. (1994) Endosonographic features predictive of lymph node metastasis. *Gastrointestinal Endoscopy,* Vol. 40, No. 4, (July-August 1994), pp. 442-446, ISSN 1097-6779.

Chen, T.K.; Wu, C.H.; Lee, C.L.; Lai, Y.C.; Yang, S.S. (1999) Endoscopic ultrasonography in the differential diagnosis of giant gastric folds. *Journal of the Formosan Medical Association,* Vol. 98, No. 4, (April 1999), pp. 261-264, ISSN 0929-6646.

Danzon, A.; Belot, A.; Maynadie, M.; Remontet, L.; Dupont, A.C.G.; Carbonnel, F. & The Association FRANCIM (2009). Incidence and survival of gastric non-Hodgkin's lymphoma: A population-based study from the Association of the French Cancer Registries (FRANCIM). *Acta Oncoogica,* Vol. 48, No. 7, (January 2009), pp. 977-983, ISSN 0284-186X.

Di Raimondo, F.; Caruso, L.; Bonanno, g.; Naso, P.; Chiarenza, A.; Fiumara, P.; Bari A.; Palumbo, G.A.; Russo A. & Giustolisi R. (2007). Is endoscopic ultrasound clinically useful for follow-up of gastric lymphoma. *Annals of oncology : official journal of the*

European Society for Medical Oncology / ESMO, Vol. 18, No. 2, (February 2007), pp. 351-356, ISSN 0923-7534.

Feng, L.; Zhang, G.; Hu, Z.; Zou, Y.; Chen, F.; Zhang, G. & Tang, L. (2009). Diagnosis and treatment of 81 patients with primary gastrointestinal lymphoma. *Journal of Central South University. Medical sciences,* Vol. 34, No. 7, (Julie 2009), pp. 582-588.

Fischbach, W.; Goebeler-Kolve, M.E. & Greiner, A. (2002) Diagnostic accuracy of EUS in the local staging of primary gastric lymphoma: results of a prospective, multicenter study comparing EUS with histopathologic stage. *Gastrointestinal Endoscopy,* Vol. 56, No. 5, (November 2002), ISSN 1097-6779.

Fischbach, W.; Goebeler-Kolve, ME; Dragosics, B; Greiner, A. & Stolte, M. (2004). Long term outcome of patients with gastric marginal zone B cell lymphoma of mucosa associated lymphoid tissue (MALT) following exclusive Helicobacter pylori eradication therapy: experience from a large prospective series. *Gut,* Vol. 53, No. 1, (January 2004), pp. 34-37, ISSN 1468-3288.

Fischbach, W. (2010). Long-term follow-up of gastric lymphoma after stomach conserving treatment. *Best Practice & Research Clinical Gastroenterology,* Vol. 24, No. 1 (February 2010), pp. 71–77, ISSN 1521-6918.

Fischbach, W. & Al-Taie, O. (2010). Staging role of EUS. *Best Practice & Research Clinical Gastroenterology,* Vol. 24, No. 1, (February 2010), pp. :13-17, ISSN 1532-1916.

Fusaroli, P.; Buscarini, E.; Peyre, S.; Federici, T.; Parente, F.; De Angelis, C.; Bonanno, G.; Meroni, E.; Napolitano, V.; Pisani, A.; Sottili, S.; Togliani, T. & Caletti, G. (2002). Interobserver agreement in staging gastric malt lymphoma by EUS. Gastrointestinal Endoscopy, Vol. 55, No. 6, (May 2002), pp. 662-668, ISSN 1097-6779.

Fusaroli, P. & Caletti, G. (2006). EUS in the Evaluation of Gastric Wall Layer Abnormalities - Non-Hodgkin Lymphoma and Other Causes, In: *Endosonography,* Robert H. Hawes MD, Paul Fockens MD PhD, pp. 127 - 146, Sounders Elsevier, ISBN: 1437708056 , Philadelphia.

Fusaroli, P. & Caletti, G. (2007). Endoscopic ultrasonography, *Endoscopy,* Vol. 39, No. 1, (January 2007), pp.17-20, ISSN 1438-8812.

Fusaroli, P.; Kypreos, D.; Alma Petrini, C.A. & Caletti, G. (2010). Scientific Publications in Endoscopic Ultrasonography: Changing Trends in the Third Millennium, *Journal of clinical gastroenterology,* Vol. 00, No. 00, (November 2010), ISSN 1539-2031.

Gligorievsky, A. (2009). CT evaluation of gastric lymphoma. *Contributions / Macedonian Academy of Sciences and Arts, Section of Biological and Medical Sciences,* Vol.30, No. 2, (December 2009), pp. 125-138, ISSN 0351-3254.

Gress, F.; Schmitt, C.; Savides, T.; Faigel, D.O.; Catalano, M.; Wassef, W.; Roubein, L.; Nickl, N.; Ciaccia, D.; Bhutani, M.; Hoffman, B. & Affronti, J. (2001) Interobserver agreement for EUS in the evaluation and diagnosis of submucosal masses. *Gastrointestinal Endoscopy,* Vol. 53, No. 1, (January 2001), pp. 71-76, ISSN 1097-6779.

Ginès, A.; Pellise, M.; Fernández-Esparrach, G.; Soria, M.T.; Mata, A.; Membrillo, A.; Martínez-Pallí, G.; Solé, M.M.; Llach, J.; Bordas, J.M. & Piqué, J.M. (2006). Endoscopic ultrasonography in patients with large gastric folds at endoscopy and biopsies negative for malignancy: predictors of malignant disease and clinical impact, *The American journal of gastroenterology,* Vol. 101, No. 1, (January 2006), pp. 64-69, ISSN 1572-0241.

Hoepffner, N.; Lahme, T.; Gilly, J.; Koch, P.; Foerster, E.C. & Menzel, J. (2003). Endoscopic ultrasound in the long-term follow-up of primary lymphomas of the stomach under conservative therapy. *Zeitschrift für Gastroenterologie*, Vol.41, No. 12, (December 2003), pp. 1151-1156, ISSN 1439-7803.

Hummel, M.; Oeschger, S.; Barth, T.F.; Loddenkemper, C.; Cogliatti, S.B.; Marx, A.; Wacker, H.H.; Feller, A.C.; Bernd, H.W.; Hansmann, M.L.; Stein, H. & Möller, P. (2006). Wotherspoon criteria combined with B cell clonality analysis by advanced polymerase chain reaction technology discriminates covert gastric marginal zone lymphoma from chronic gastritis. *Gut*, Vol. 55, No. 6, (June 2006), pp. 782-787, ISSN 1468-3288.

Janssen, J. (2009). The impact of EUS in primary gastric lymphoma. *Best practice & research. Clinical gastroenterology*, Vol. 23, No. 5, (October 2009),pp. 671-678, ISSN 1532-1916.

Karaca, C,; Turner, B.G.; Cizginer, S.; Forcione, D. & Brugge, W. (2010). Accuracy of EUS in the evaluation of small gastric subepithelial lesions. *Gastrointestinal endoscopy*, Vol. 71, No. 4, (April 2010), pp. 722-727, ISSN: 1097-6779.

Kelessis, N.G.; Vassilopoulos, P.P.; Tsamakidis, K.G.; Bai, M.G.; Avital, S. & Rosenthal, R.J. (2003) Is gastroscopy still a valid diagnostic tool in detecting gastric MALT lymphomas? A dilemma beyond the eye. Mucosa-associated lymphoid tissue. *Surgical* endoscopy, Vol. 17, No. 3, (March 2003), pp. 469-74, ISSN 1432-2218

Koch, P.; del Valle, F.; Berdel, W.E.; Willich, N.A.; Reers, B.; Hiddemann, W.; Grothaus-Pinke, B.; Reinartz, G.; Brockmann, J.; Temmesfeld, A.; Schmitz, R.; Rübe, C.; Probst, A.; Jaenke, G.; Bodenstein, H.; Junker, A.; Pott, C.; Schultze, J.; Heinecke, A.; Parwaresch, R.& Tiemann M. (2001) Primary Gastrointestinal Non-Hodgkin's Lymphoma: I. Anatomic and Histologic Distribution, Clinical Features, and Survival Data of 371 Patients Registered in the German Multicenter Study GIT NHL 01/92. *Journal of clinical oncology : official journal of the American Society of Clinical Oncology*, Vol. 19, No. 18, (September 2001), pp. 3861-3873, ISSN 1527-7755.

Koch, P.; Probst, A.; Berdel, W.E.; Willich, N.A.; Reinartz, G.; Brockmann, J.; Liersch, R.; del Valle, F.; Clasen, H.; Hirt, C.; Breitsprecher, R.; Schmits, R.; Freund, M.; Fietkau, R.; Ketterer, P.; Freitag, E.M.; Hinkelbein, M.; Heinecke, A.; Parwaresch, R. & Tiemann, M. (2005) Treatment results in localized primary gastric lymphoma: data of patients registered within the German multicenter study (GIT NHL 02/96). *Journal of clinical oncology : official journal of the American Society of Clinical Oncology*, Vol. 1, No. 23, (October 2005) pp. 7050-7059, ISSN 1527-7755.

Lévy, M.; Hammel, P.; Lamarque, D.; Marty, O.; Chaumette, M.T.; Haioun, C.; Blazquez, M. & Delchier, J.C. (1997) Endoscopic ultrasonography for the initial staging and follow-up in patients with low-grade gastric lymphoma of mucosa-associated lymphoid tissuetreated medically. *Gastrointestinal Endoscopy*, Vol. 46, No. 4, (October 1997), pp. 328-333, ISSN 1097-6779.

Lügering, N.; Menzel, J.; Kucharzik, T.; Koch, P.; Herbst, H.; Tiemann, M. & Domschke, W (2001). Impact of miniprobes compared to conventional endosonography in the staging of low-grade gastric malt lymphoma. *Endoscopy*, Vol. 33, No. 10, (October 2001), pp. 832-827, ISSN 1438-8812.

Martinelli, G.; Gigli, F.; Calabrese, L.; Ferrucci, P.F.; Zucca, E.; Crosta, C.; Pruneri, G.; Preda, L.; Piperno, G.; Gospodarowicz, M.; Cavalli, F. & Moreno Gomez, H. (2009) Early stage gastric diffuse large B-cell lymphomas: results of a randomized trial comparing chemotherapy alone versus chemotherapy + involved field radiotherapy. (IELSG 4). *Leukemia & Lymphoma*, vol. 50, No. 6, (June 2009), pp. 925-931, ISSN 1029-2403.

Montalban, C.; Santon, A.; Boixeda, D. & Bellas, C. (2001) Regression of gastric high grade mucosa associated lymphoid tissue (MALT) lymphoma after Helicobacter pylori eradication. *Gut*, Vol. 49, No. 4, (October 2001), pp. 584-587, ISSN 1468-3288.

Nagler, A.K.; Aslanian, H.R. & Siddiqui, U.D. (2011) Endoscopic ultrasound and gastric lesions. *Journal of clinical gastroenterology*, Vol. 45, No. 3, (March 2011) pp. 215-21, ISSN 1539-2031.

Neubauer, A.; Thiede, C.; Morgner, A.; Alpen, B.; Ritter, M.; Neubauer, B.; Wündisch, T.; Ehninger, G.; Stolte, M. & Bayerdörffer, E. (1997) Cure of Helicobacter pylori infection and duration of remission of low-grade gastric mucosa-associated lymphoid tissue lymphoma. *Journal of National Cancer Institute*, Vol. 89, No., 18, (September 1997), pp. 1350-5, ISSN 1460-2105.

Nobre-Leitão, C.; Lage, P.; Cravo, M.; Cabeçadas, J.; Chaves, P.; Alberto-Santos, A.; Correia, J.; Soares, J. & Costa-Mira, F. (1998) Treatment of gastric MALT lymphoma by Helicobacter pylori eradication: a study controlled by endoscopic ultrasonography. *The American journal of gastroenterology*, Vol. 93, No. 5, (May 1998), pp. 732-736, ISSN 1572-0241.

Pavlick, A.C.; Gerdes, H. & Portlock, C.S. (1997) Endoscopic ultrasound in the evaluation of gastric small lymphocytic mucosa-associated lymphoid tumors. Journal of Clinincal Oncology : official journal of the American Society of Clinical Oncology, Vol. 15, No. 5, (May 1997), pp. 1761-1766, ISSN 1527-7755.

Pavlović, A.R.; Krstic, M.; Tomic, D.; Bjelovic, M.; Jesic, R. & Suvajdzic N. (2005). Endoscopic ultrasound (EUS) in initial assessment and follow-up of patients with MALT lymphoma treated drug therapy. *Acta chirurgica Iugoslavica*, Vol. 52, No. 1, pp. 83-89, ISSN 0354-950X.

Pinotti, G.; Zucca, E.; Roggero, E.; Pascarella, A.; Bertoni, F.; Savio, A.; Savio, E.; Capella, C.; Pedrinis, E.; Saletti, P.; Morandi, E.; Santandrea, G. & Cavalli F. (1997) Clinical features, treatment and outcome in a series of 93 patients with low-grade gastric MALT lymphoma. *Leukemia & Lymphoma*, Vol.26, No. 5-6, (August 1997), ISSN 1029-2403.

Püspök, A.; Raderer, M,; Chott, A.;.Dragonics, B.; Gangl, A. & Schofl, R. (2002) Endoscopic ultrasound in the follow up and response assessment of patients with primary gastric lymphoma. *Gut*, Vol. 51, No. 5, (November 2002), pp. 691–694, ISSN 0017-5749 .

Radaszkiewicz, T.; Dragosics, B. & Bauer, P.(1992) Gastrointestinal malignant lymphomas of the mucosa-associated lymphoid tissue. Factors relevant to prognosis. *Gastroenterology*, Vol 102, No. 5, (May 1992), pp. 1628-1638, ISSN 1528-0012.

Rohatiner, A.; d'Amore, F.; Coiffier, B.; Crowther, D. ; Gospodarowicz, M.; Isaacson, P.; Lister, T. A.; Norton, A. ; Salem, P.; Shipp M. & R. Somers (1994). Report on a workshop convened to discuss the pathological and staging classifications of gastrointestinal tract lymphoma. *Annals of oncology : official journal of the European Society for Medical Oncology / ESMO*, Vol. 5, No. 5, (May 1994), pp. 397-400, ISSN 1569-8041.

Ruskoné-Fourmestraux, A.; Lavergne, A.; Aegerter, P.H.; Megraud, F.; Palazzo, L.; de Mascarel, A.; Molina, T. & Rambaud, J.L. (2001). Predictive factors for regression of gastric MALT lymphoma after anti-Helicobacter pylori treatment. Gut, Vol. 48, No. 3, (March 2001) pp. 297-303, ISSN 1468-3288.

Ruskoné-Fourmestraux, A.; Dragosics, B.; Morgner, A.; Wotherspoon, A. & De Jong, D. (2003) Paris staging system for primary gastrointestinal lymphomas, Vol. 52, No. 6, (June 2003), pp. 912-913, ISSN 1468-3288.

Ruskoné-Fourmestraux, A.; Fischbach, W.; Aleman, B.M.; Boot, H.; Du, M.Q.; Megraud, F.; Montalban, C.; Raderer, M.; Savio, A. & Wotherspoon, A.; on behalf of the EGILS group (2011). EGILS consensus report. Gastric extranodal marginal zone B-cell lymphoma of MALT. *Gut*, (February 2011), ISSN 1468-3288, [Epub ahead of print].

Sackmann, M,; Morgner, A.; Rudolph, B.; Neubauer, A.; Thiede, C.; Schulz, H.; Kraemer, W.; Boersch, G.; Rohde, P.; Seifert, E.; Stolte, M. & Bayerdoerffer E. (1997). Regression of gastric MALT lymphoma after eradication of Helicobacter pylori is predicted by endosonographic staging. MALT Lymphoma Study Group, *Gastroenterology*, Vol. 113, No. 4, (October 1997), pp. 1087-1090 ISSN 1528-0012.

Savio, A.; Franzin, G.; Wotherspoon, A.C.; Zamboni, G.; Negrini, R.; Buffoli, F.; Diss, T.C.; Pan, L. & Isaacson, P.G. (1996) Diagnosis and posttreatment follow-up of Helicobacter pylori-positive gastric lymphoma of mucosa-associated lymphoid tissue: histology, polymerase chain reaction, or both? *Blood*. Vol. 87, No. 4, (Februry 1996), pp. 1255-1260, ISSN 1528-0020.

Stathis, A.; Chini, C.; Bertoni, F.; Proserpio, I.; Capella, C.; Mazzucchelli, L.; Pedrinis, E.; Cavalli, F.; Pinotti, G. & Zucca, E. (2009) Long-term outcome following Helicobacter pylori eradication in a retrospective study of 105 patients with localized gastric marginal zone B-cell lymphoma of MALT type. *Annals of oncology : official journal of the European Society for Medical Oncology / ESMO*, Vol. 20, No. 6, (June 2009), pp. 1086-1093, ISSN 1569-8041.

Steinbach, G.; Ford, R.; Glober, G.; Sample, D.; Hagemeister, F.B.; Lynch, P.M.; McLaughlin, P.W.; Rodriguez, M.A.; Romaguera, J.E.; Sarris, A.H.; Younes, A.; Luthra, R.; Manning, J.T.; Johnson, C.M.; Lahoti, S.; Shen, Y.; Lee, J.E.; Winn, R.J.; Genta, R.M.; Graham, D.Y. & Cabanillas, F.F. (1999). Antibiotic treatment of gastric lymphoma of mucosa-associated lymphoid tissue. An uncontrolled trial. *Annals of Internal Medicine*, Vol. 131, No. 2 (20 July 1999), pp. 88-95, ISSN 1539-3704.

Swerdlow S.H.; S.H.; Campo, E.; Harris, N.L.; Ja_E.S.; Pileri,S.A.; Stein, H.; Thiele, J. & Vardiman, J.W. (October 2008) *WHO Classification of Tumours of Haematopoietic and Lymphoid Tissue* (4th edition), World Health Organization, ISBN 9789283224310.

Tari, A.; Asaoku, H.; Kashiwado, K.; Yoshino, T.; Kitadai, Y.; Tanaka S & Fujihara, M. (2009). Predictive value of endoscopy and endoscopic ultrasonography for regression of gastric diffuse large B-cell lymphomas after Helicobacter pylori eradication. *Digestive endoscopy : official journal of the Japan Gastroenterological Endoscopy Society*. Vol. 21, No. 4, (October 2009), pp. 219-227, ISSN 1443-1661.

Varas, M.J.; Fabra, R.; Abad, R.; Turró, J.; Espinós, J.C.; Bargalló, D. & Miquel, J.M. (2006). Endoscopic staging of low-grade gastric MALT lymphoma. *Revista española de enfermedades digestivas : organo oficial de la Sociedad Española de Patología Digestiva*, Vol. 98, No. 3, (March 2006), pp. 189-195, ISSN 1130-0108.

Yeh, H.Z.; Chen, G.H.; Chang, W.D.; Poon, S.K.; Yang, S.S.; Lien, H.C.; Chang, C.S. & Chou, G. (2003). Long-term follow up of gastric low-grade mucosa-associated lymphoid tissue lymphoma by endosonography emphasizing the application of a miniature ultrasound probe. *Journal of gastroenterology and hepatology*, Vol. 18, No. 2, (February 2003), pp. 162-167, ISSN 0815-9319.

Yi, J.H.; Kim, S.J.; Choi, J.Y.; Ko, Y.H.; Kim, B.T. & Kim W.S. (2010). 18F-FDG uptake and its clinical relevance in primary gastric lymphoma. *Hematological oncology*, Vol. 28, No. 2, (June 2010), pp. 57-61, ISSN 1099-1069.

Yoon, S.S.; Coit D.G.; Portlock C.S. & Karpeh M.S. (2004). The diminishing role of surgery in the treatment of gastric lymphoma. *Annals of Surgery*, Vol. 240, No. 1, (July 2004), pp 28–37, ISSN 0003-4932.

Yücel, C.; Ozdemir, H. & Işik, S. (1999). Role of endosonography in the evaluation of gastric malignancies. *Journal of ultrasound in medicine : official journal of the American Institute of Ultrasound in Medicine*, Vol. 18, No. 4, (April 1999), pp. 283-238, ISSN 1550-9613.

Wotherspoon, A.C.; Doglioni, C.; Diss T.C.; Pan L.; Moschini A.; de Boni M. & Isaacson P.G. (1993). Regression of primary low-grade B-cell gastric lymphoma of mucosa-associated lymphoid tissue type after eradication of Helicobacter pylori. *The Lancet*, Vol. 342, No. 8871, (September 1993), pp. 575-577, ISSN 0140-6736.

Zucca, E.; Bertoni, F.; Stathis, A. & Cavalli, F. (2008). Marginal Zone Lymphomas. *Hematology/Oncology Clinics of North America*, Vol. 22, No. 5,(October 2008), pp. 883-901, ISSN 1558-1977

Zucca, E. & Dreyling, M. (2010). Gastric marginal zone lymphoma of MALT type: ESMO Clinical Practice Guidelines for diagnosis, treatment and follow-up. *Annals of Oncology*, Vol. 21, No. 5, (May 2010), pp. v175-v176, ISSN 0923-7534.

Zullo, A.; Hassan, C.; Andriani, A.; Cristofari, F.; Cardinale, V.; Spinelli, G.P.; Tomao, S. & Morini, S. (2010) Primary low-grade and high-grade gastric MALT-lymphoma presentation. *Journal of clinical gastroenterology*. Vol. 44, No. 5, (May-June 2010), pp. 340-344.

13

Endoscopic Ultrasound Elastography in Inflammatory Bowel Disease

Nadan Rustemovic, Irena Hrstic and Silvija Cukovic-Cavka
School of Medicine Zagreb, University of Zagreb
Division of Gastroenterology and Hepatology, Zagreb
Croatia

1. Introduction

The diagnosis of inflammatory bowel disease (IBD) is based on clinical, endoscopic, radiologic and histologic criteria[1]. There are two main IBD phenotypes - Crohn's disease (CD) and ulcerative colitis (UC). In some circumstances, especially when disease extension is restricted to the colon or in cases of acute severe pancolitis, recognition of specific IBD phenotype is very difficult. Recognition of the exact IBD phenotype is essential for guiding therapeutic decisions and detection of complications that warrant treatment.

Endoscopic examination is the mainstay in the diagnosis of IBD. Endoscopic appearance (distribution and shape of lesions) helps to differentiate CD from UC in most cases. Pathohistologic analysis confirms the elements of chronic inflammation but it is frequently not diagnostic. Patients with UC may have atypical histological features such as microscopic inflammation of the ileum, patchiness of inflammation and rectal sparing at the time of diagnosis prompting physicians to make the diagnosis of CD in UC cases. Other endoscopic findings such as cobble stoning, segmental colitis, ileal stenosis and ulceration, perianal disease and pathologically confirmed multiple granulomas in the small bowel or colon strongly suggest a diagnosis of CD.

The progress in genetics, serological markers and imaging studies will lead to more reliable determination of exact IBD phenotype in the future[2]. In the meantime, it is reasonable to explore other diagnostic options for better differentiation between different IBD phenotypes. We think that endoscopic ultrasound (EUS) elastography is a promising method to achieve this goal, picture 1 and 2. It is a new endoscopic procedure which can differentiate the stiffness of normal and pathological tissue by ultrasound. This finding is based on B-mode scanning during compressions[3]. There are some data on elastography applied on the GI tract, biliary tract, kidney, muscle, breast and the heart[3-5].

Primary sclerosing cholangitis (PSC) is a chronic liver disease of unknown etiology, characterized by cholestasis, inflammation, fibrosis and stricture formation of the biliary ducts. The pathophysiology of PSC is a complex multistep process included unclear immunological mechanisms, genetic susceptibility and various defects of the biliary epithelial cells.

The disease is rare in the general population but is strongly associated with inflammatory bowel disease. The prevalence of IBD, predominantly ulcerative colitis, among PSC patients is approximately 70-90% while only 5% of patients with UC develop PSC. The percentage of

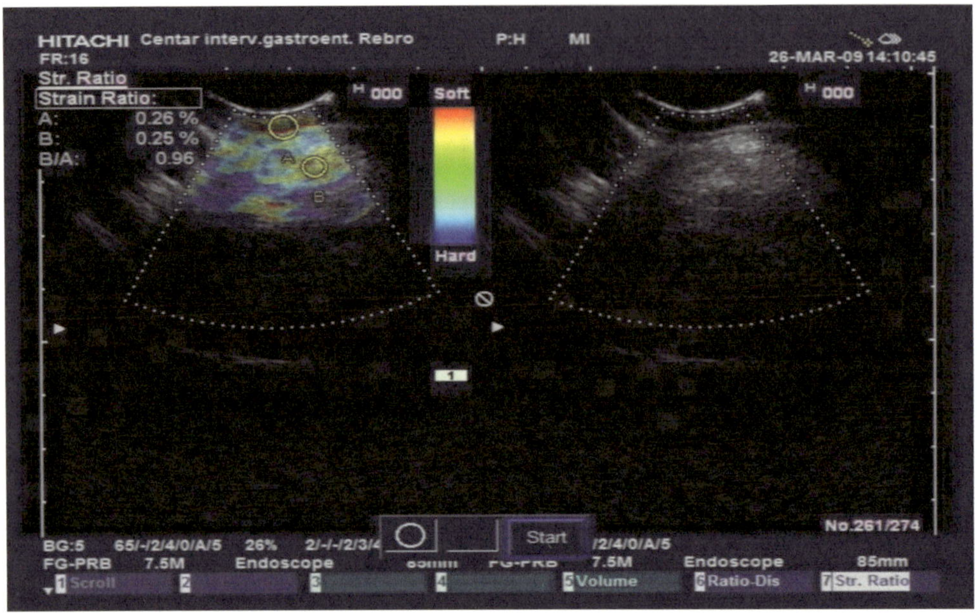

Picture 1. TRUS elastography in a UC patient

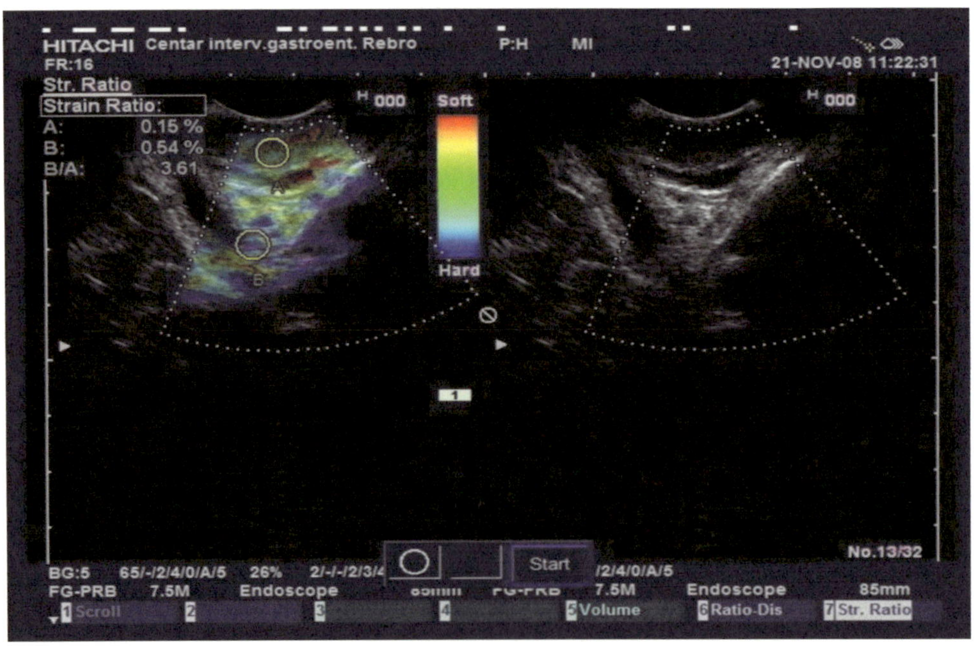

Picure 2. TRUS elastography in a CD patient

Crohn's disease patients affected by PSC is much smaller. Recently, it was recognized that PSC-IBD is a distinct IBD phenotype. Ulcerative colitis associated with PSC is usually mild, quiet, is associated with rectal sparing, more intensive right sided disease, and backwash ileitis and has a significant risk of developing pouchitis after colectomy.

In advanced cases symptoms include icterus, itch and lethargy but almost 45% of patients have no symptoms and increasing numbers of asymptomatic patients are being identified.
Primary sclerosing cholangitis is generally aggressive disorder and can progress in cirrhosis. In that setting, liver transplantation is the only therapeutic option with cure potential because median survival without liver transplantation after diagnosis is approximately 12 years.
PSC is associated with a 10%-15% lifetime risk of developing cholangiocellular carcinoma which often presents in advanced stage with a poor prognosis. Primary sclerosing cholangitis also has a risk of developing colorectal dysplasia and neoplasia in IBD. Treatment with high dose ursodeoxycholic acid has chemoprotective effects against potential neoplasia.
Magnetic resonance cholangiography (MRC) and endoscopic retrograde cholangiography (ERC) are diagnostic procedures which confirm multifocal strictures and dilatation of biliary ducts, characteristic for PSC. Both procedures, ERC and MRC are comparable for diagnosing PSC but there are conflicting data regarding the role of ERCP in patients with PSC. It seems that elective ERCP has a modest risk of ERCP-related complications in patients with PSC. However, ERCP in severe ill IBD patients increases the probability of post procedure complications. Because of its noninvasive nature, MRCP may have advantages over invasive cholangiography when diagnosis is the main goal of the procedure.
According to evident well-documented risk of malignant disease during the life course, early identification of PSC patients is very important for establishing adequate surveillance strategy.
Elastography is a method which can differentiate the stiffness of normal and pathological tissue by ultrasound which is based on B-mode scanning during compressions, picture 3 and 4.

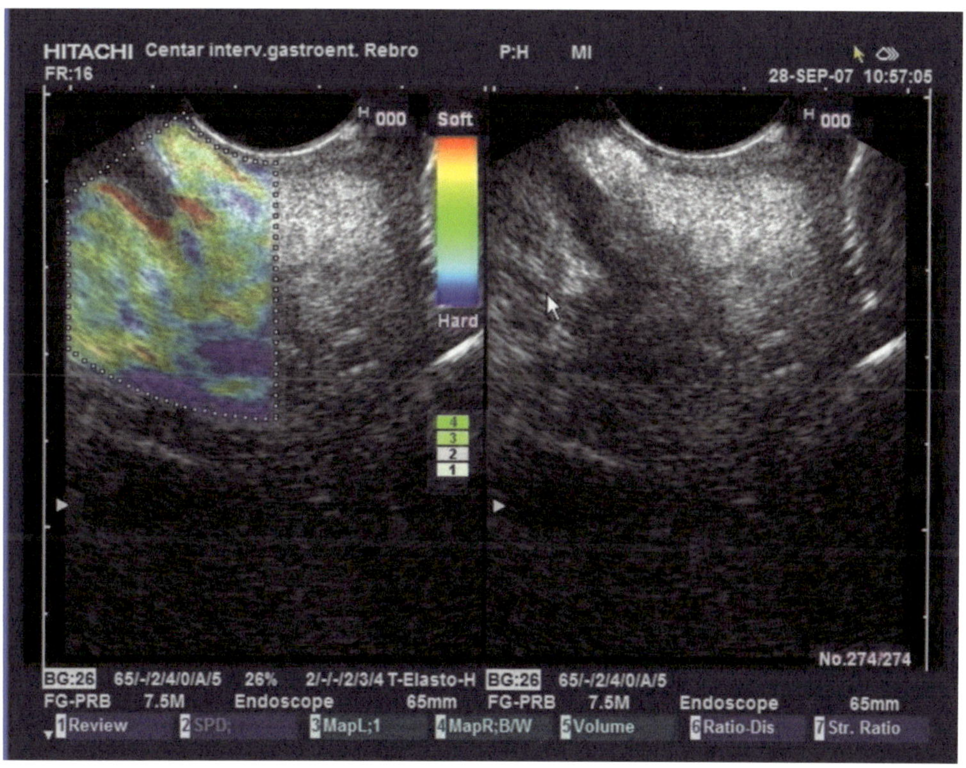

Picture 3. Normal bile duct.

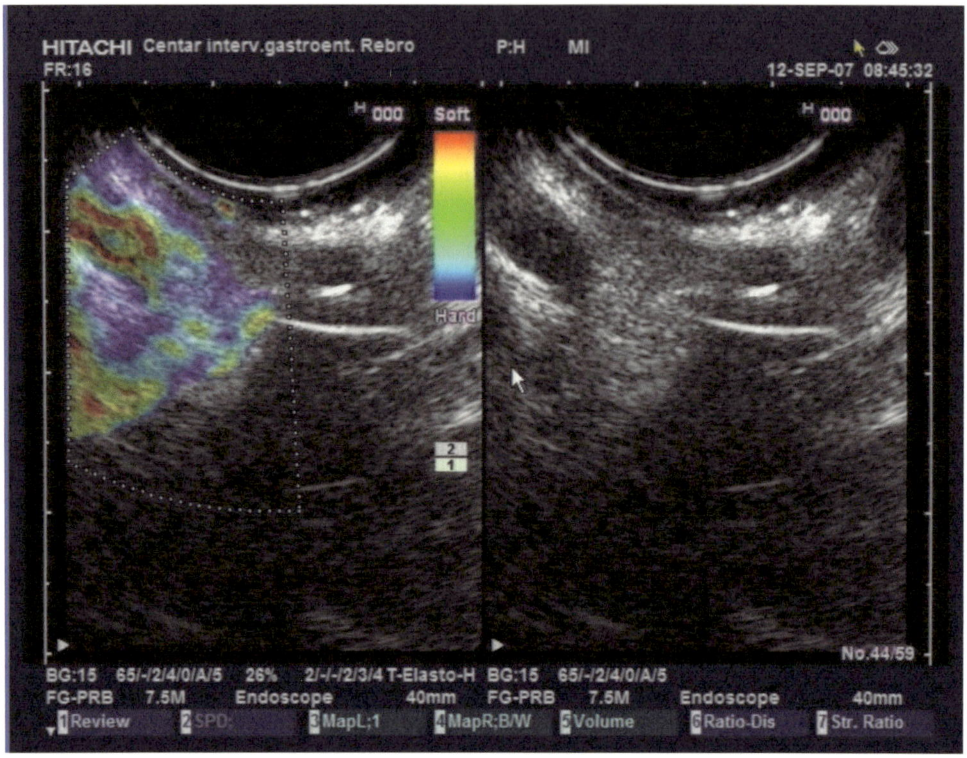

Picture 4. PSC patient.

Regarding to the fact that imaging of ultrasound tissue elasticity is a way to distinct normal from abnormal tissue we analyzed the role of EUS elastography in assessing ductus choledochus properties in patients with and without PSC. EUS elastography has a potential to define tissue characteristics but specificity has to be improved[4].

Based on the idea that imaging of ultrasound tissue elasticity is a way to differentiate tissue characteristics, we hypothesized that EUS elastography has the role in assessing the thickness of bowel wall in patients with IBD and in differentiation between types of colonic inflammation in Crohn's colitis and ulcerative colitis[6,7] based on the fact that CD is a transmural disease and UC is limited to the mucosa and submucosa of the bowel wall.

2. Discussion

There are numerous papers in the current literature on the issue of EUS elastography. The method was initially inaugurated to distinguish benign from malignant pancreatic lesions[6,9,10]. Although it cannot replace biopsy and histological confirmation of cancer, „virtual biopsy" done by EUS elastography could provide good information of the consistency of the tissue of interest[11].

We hypothesized that „virtual biopsy" technique might be implemented in differentiating colonic tissue between CD and UC[4,12]. IBD phenotyping is clinically very important because of three specific reasons. Firstly, Crohn's colitis and UC have different risk of complications (fistulas, strictures, extraintestinal manifestations) that require specific therapeutic approach.

Secondly, regarding the drugs, there is a clear difference in the efficacy of mesalazine in active Crohn's colitis and ulcerative colitis[15,16]. Delay of introduction of immunosuppressive agents in misdiagnosed patients with Crohn's colitis can be deleterious. Thirdly, accurate determination of disease phenotype is important in cases were surgical intervention becomes necessary, since continent proctocolectomy is inappropriate method in Crohn's colitis where pelvic reservoir in case of unrecognized CD gets complicated by fistulas, stenosis and pelvic sepsis[17]. To conclude, present serologic and genetic markers cannot always confirm the phenotypic diagnosis and predict the clinical course in IBD patients [18, 19, 20]. EUS elastography could be, therefore, a new diagnostic option with the potential to recognize differences in the UC tissue and Crohn's colitis tissue.

In order to clearly define the differences between the colonic wall in CD and UC, our investigation was focused on the characteristics of the rectal wall and perirectal tissue, observed by the EUS elastography with SR calculation. Perirectal tissue in UC patients is supposed to be soft, without inflammation. In CD patients, „hard tissue" reflects the transmural nature of inflammation. These qualitative and quantitative elastography data could lead to accurate differentiation of IBD phenotypes.

Our pilot study revealed a significant difference in rectal wall thickness between IBD group as a whole and controls which is in agreement with other reports from the literature[21,22]. Interestingly, we also found a significant difference in rectal wall thickness between CD patients without rectal involvement and controls. The significance of this finding in our pilot study is unclear but it could suggest a possible predictive role of TRUS elastography in CD. Bearing in mind the fact that CD can involve any part of the GI tract, it would be interesting to identify such patients early in the course of the disease and follow them prospectively to see whether rectal involvement or perianal disease will develop. In UC patients, a significant difference in rectal wall thickness but not strain ratio was found between active UC patients and controls. This finding reflects the fact that inflammatory process in UC is confined to the mucosa and submucosa leading to the thickening of the rectal wall in acute inflammation but without changes in perirectal tissue as measured by strain ratio. A significant difference was detected in rectal wall thickness and strain ratio between CD and UC patient group reflecting the difference in pathogenetic mechanisms driving these diseases with CD being characterized by transmural inflammation as opposed to UC. Finally, we detected a significant difference in both rectal wall thickness and strain ratio between CD patients with rectal involvement and UC patients with active disease.

There was unfortunately significant difference in age between control group and IBD group. The results of TRUS elastography show that control group and UC group had comparable strain ratios, while CD group had statistically higher strain ratio. Based on the available literature, there are no significant changes in the rectal wall thickness with aging[23,24].

We believe that the results of our study confirm the potential usefulness of TRUS elastography in determining the exact phenotype of IBD. Currently, about 10% of patients with inflammation restricted to the colon can not be accurately classified using standard diagnostic techniques[25,26]. More importantly, 4-6 % of patients with presumably UC undergoing proctocolectomy with ileoanal anastomosi and pelvic pouch formation turned out to have CD resulting in significant morbidity and high rate of pouch failure[27,28]. Although we found a significant difference in rectal wall thickness and significant difference in strain ratio between CD patients with rectal involvement and active UC patients, our study has a limitation due to a small number of patients included. There is a need for a prospective study with inclusion of a greater number of patients and for the construction of receiver operating characteristics (ROC) curve to definitely assess the value of TRUS elastography in IBD.

3. Conclusion

TRUS elastography with strain ratio calculation provides valuable information regarding the stiffness of the rectal and perirectal tissue and can help to differentiate CD from UC. Our study indicates that TRUS elastography could be one of the perspective and promising diagnostic tools in IBD. A prospective study on a large cohort of patient is necessary to consolidate and confirm the results and establish the role of TRUS in distinguishing Crohn's colitis and UC. In addition, one of the important benefits of EUS elastography in the long run could be the possibility of identifying individuals at risk of developing a transmural disease, thereby facilitating appropriate action for prevention of disease complications.

4. References

[1] Nikolaus S, Schreiber S. Diagnostics of inflammatory bowel disease. Gastroenterology 2007;133;1670-1689.

[2] North American Society for Pediatric Gastroenterology Hepatology, and Nutrition; Colitis Foundation of America, Bousvaros A, Antonioli DA Colletti RG, Dubinsky MC, Glickman JN, Gold BD, Griffiths AM, Jevon GP, Higuchi LM, Hyams JS, Kirschner BS, Kugathasan S, Baldassano RN, Russo PA. Differentiating ulcerative colitis from Crohn disease in children and young adults: report of a working group of the North American Society for Pediatric Gastroenterology, Hepatology, and Nutrition and the Crohn's and Colitis Foundation of America. J Pediatr Gastroenterol Nutr 2007;44:653-74.

[3] Odegaard S, Nesje LB, Hoff DA, Gilja OH, Gregersen H. Morphology and motor function of the gastrointestinal tract examined with endosonography. World J Gastroenterol 2006;12:2858-2863.

[4] Rustemovic N, Cukovic-Cavka S, Opacic M, Petrovecki M, Hrstic I, Radic D, Ostojic R, Pulanic R, Vucelic B. Endoscopic ultrasound elastography as a method for screening the patients with suspected primary sclerosing cholnagitis. Eur J Gastroenterol Hepatol 2010;22:748-753.

[5] Corpechot C, El Naggar A, Poujol-Robert A, Ziol M, Wendum D, Chazouilleres O, de Ledinghen V, Dhumeaux D, Marcellin P, Beaugrand M, Poupon R. Assessment of biliary fibrosis by transient elastography in patients with PBC and PSC. Hepatology 2006;43:1118-1124.

[6] Giovannini M, Hookey LC, Bories E, Pesenti C, Monges G, Delpero JR. Endoscopic ultrasound elastography: the first step towards virtual biopsy? Preliminary results in 49 patients. Endoscopy 2006;38:344-348.

[7] Saftoiu A, Vilman P. Endoscopic ultrasound elastography-- a new imaging technique for the visualization of tissue elasticity distribution. J Gastrointestin Liver Dis 2006;15:161-165.

[8] Baron JH, Connell AM, Lennard-Jones JE. Variation between observers in describing mucosal appearances in proctocolitis. Br Med J 1964;1:89-92.

[9] Giovannini M, Thomas B, Erwan B, Christian P, Fabrice C, Benjamin E, Genevieve M, Paolo A, Pierre D, Robert Y, Walter S, Hanz S, Carl S, Christoph D, Pierre E, Jean-Luc VL, Jacques D, Peter V, Andrian S. Endoscopic ultrasound elastography for evaluation of lymph nodes and pancreatic masses: a multicenter study. World J Gastroenterol. 2009;15:1587-1593.

[10] Saftoiu A, Vilmann P, Gorunescu F, Gheonea DI, Gorunescu M, Ciurea T, Popescu GL, Iordache A, Hassan H, Iordache S. Neural network analysis od dynamic sequences of EUS elastography used for the differential diagnosis of chronic pancreatitis and pancreatic cancer. Gastrointest Endosc 2008;68:1086-1094.

[11] Gill KR, Wallace MB. EUS elastography for pancreatic mass lesions: between image and FNA? Gastrointest Endosc 2008;68:1095-1097.

[12] Rustemovic N, Hrstic I, Opacic M, Ostojic R, Jakic-Razumovic J, Kvarantan M, Pulanic R, Vucelic B. EUS elastography in the diagnosis of focal liver lesions. Gastrointest Endosc 2007;66:823-824.

[13] M'koma AE, Seeley EH, Washington MK, Schwartz DA, Muldoon RL, Herline AJ, Wise PE, Caprioli RM. Proteomic profiling of mucosal and submucosal colonic tissues yields protein signatures that differentiate the inflammatory colitides. Inflamm Bowel Dis 2010 Aug 30 [Epub ahead of print]

[14] Vucelic B. Inflammatory bowel diseases: controversies in the use of diagnostic procedures. Dig Dis 2009;27(3):269-77.

[15] Travis SP, Stange EF, Lémann M, Oresland T, Bemelman WA, Chowers Y, Colombel JF, D'Haens G, Ghosh S, Marteau P, Kruis W, Mortensen NJ, Penninckx F, Gassull M; for the European Crohn's and Colitis Organisation (ECCO). European evidence-based Consensus on the management of ulcerative colitis: Current management. Journal of Crohn's and Colitis 2008;2:24-62.

[16] Dignass A, Van Assche G, Lindsay JO, Lémann M, Soderholm J, Colombel JF, Danese S, D'Hoore A, Gassull M, Gomollon F, Hommes DW, Michetti P, O'Morain C, Oresland T, Windsor A, Stange EF, Travis SP; European Crohn's and Colitis Organisation (ECCO). The second European evidence-based consensus on the diagnosis and management of Crohn's disease: Current management. Journal of Crohn's and Colitis 2010;428-62.

[17] Shen B, Fazio VW, Remzi FH, Lashner BA. Clinical approach to diseases of ileal pouch-anal anastomosis. Am J Gastroenterol 2005;100(12):2796-807.

[18] Arai R. Serologic markers: impact on early diagnosis and disease stratification in inflammatory bowel disease. Postgrad Med 2010;122(4):177-85.

[19] Dotan I. New serologic markers for inflammatory bowel disease diagnosis. Dig Dis 2010;28(3):418-23.

[20] Vermeire S, Van Assche G, Rutgeerts P. Role of genetics in prediction of disease course and response to therapy. World J Gastroenterol 2010;16(21):2609-15.

[21] Rasmussen SN, Riis P. Rectal wall thickness measured by ultrasound in chronic inflammatory diseases of the colon. Scand J Gastroenterol 1985;20:109-114.

[22] Lew RJ, Ginsberg GG. The role of endoscopic ultrasound in inflammatory bowel disease. Gastrointest Endosc Clin N Am 2002;12:561-571.

[23] Huh CH, Bhutani MS, Farfan EB, Bolch WE. Individual variations in mucosa and total wall thickness in the stomach and rectum assesed via endoscopic ultrasound. Physiol Meas 2003;24:N15-22.

[24] Karahan OI, Dodd GD 3rd, Chintapalli KN, Rhim H, Chopra S. Gastrointestinal wall thickening in patients with cirrhosis: frequency and patterns at contrast-enhanced CT. Radiology 2000;215:103-107.
[25] Vind I, Riis L, Jess T, Knudsen E, Pedersen N, Elkjaer M, Bak Andersen I, Wewer V, Norregaard P, Moesgaard F, Bendtsen F, Munkholm P, DCCD study group. Increasing incidences of inflammatory bowel disease and decreasing surgery rates in Copenhagen City and County, 2003-2005: a population-based study from Danish Crohn colitis database. Am J Gastrenterol 2006;101:1274-1282 .
[26] Stewenius J, Adnerhill I, Ekelund G, Floren CH, Fork FT, Janzon L, Lindström C, Mars I, Nyman M, Rosengren JE. Ulcerative colitis and indeterminate colitis in the city of Malmo, Sweden. A 25-year incidence study. Scand J Gastroenterol 1995;30:38-43.
[27] Melton GB, Fazio VW, Kiran RP, He J, Lavery IC, Shen B, Achkar JP, Church JM, Remzi FH. Long-term outcomes with ileal pouch-anal anastomosis and Crohn's disease: pouch retention and implications of delayed diagnosis. Ann Surg 2008;4:608-616.
[28] Braveman JM, Schoetz DJ Jr., Marcello PW, Roberts PL, Coller JA, Murray JJ, Rusin LC. The fate of the ileal pouch in patients developing Crohn's disease. Dis Colon Rectum 2004;47:1613-1619.

14

Foundamentals and Applications of Abdominal Doppler

Pablo Gomez Ochoa[2], Delia Lacasta[2], Ivan Sosa[1], Manuel Gascon[2], Juan Jose Ramos[2] and Luis Miguel Ferrer[2]
[1]*Great Western Referrals*
[2]*Animal Pathology Department, Veterinary Faculty of Zaragoza, University of Zaragoza,*
[1]*United Kingdom*
[2]*Spain*

1. Introduction

Since the Doppler effect was firstly described by Christian Doppler in 1842, it has been applied in many different fields. In human medicine has been extremely helpful in monitoring the fetal viability or assessing the carotid flow, and it is currently being used in most of the disciplines.

In veterinary medicine, the Doppler effect is a helpful tool in abdominal ultrasound, and essential in the echocardiography exam. Its principle can be defined as the apparent shift in transmitted frequency, reflected back to the source off a target, which occurs as a result of the movement of this target. When this effect is applied in ultrasonography, the red blood cells (RBC's) are the moving targets, and the apparent shift in the frequency of the sound reflected back to the transducer is proportional to their velocity and direction of the movement. The software of the ultrasound machine displays this values in a color code (Color Doppler) or in a graphic, (spectral trace of the Pulsed wave Doppler (PW) or Continuous wave Doppler (CW)).

In Color Doppler, a given color is usually assigned to the direction of flow; red is flow toward, and blue is flow away from the transducer (Figure 1).

The center of the color bar, displayed in the screen, is black and represents zero flow. In addition to simple direction, velocity information is also displayed. Progressively increasing velocities are encoded in varying ranges of either red or blue. The more dull the hue, the slower the velocity. The brighter the hue, the faster the relative velocity. Color Doppler is also used to display turbulent flow (showing a mosaic of many colors) and allows an operator to discriminate between normal and abnormal flow states. Color Doppler is useful for assessing relatively big areas, whilst PW (Pulsed Wave) and CW (Continous Wave) Doppler are used for assessing smaller areas of interest. Since Color Doppler is a type of pulsed wave Doppler, it suffers from the same limitations.

Before explaining the difference between CW and PW, explaining the concept of spectral trace is required. This is the graphic representation of velocity flow profile against time. Depending of the number of cells crossing the amount of signal increases (Figure 2).

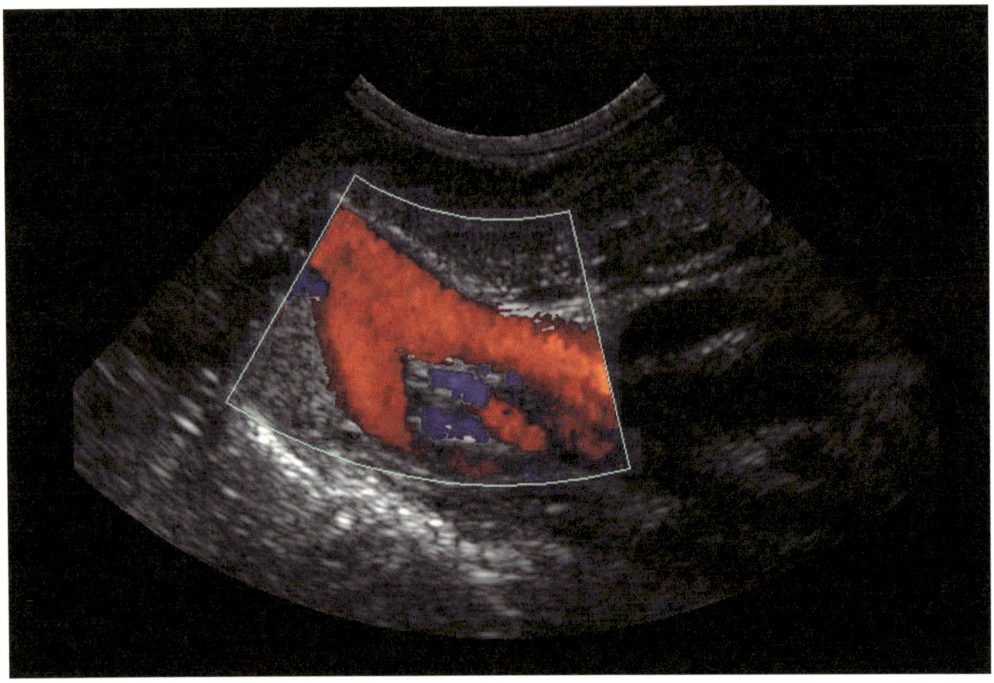

Fig. 1. Color Doppler window depicting the mesenteric veins.

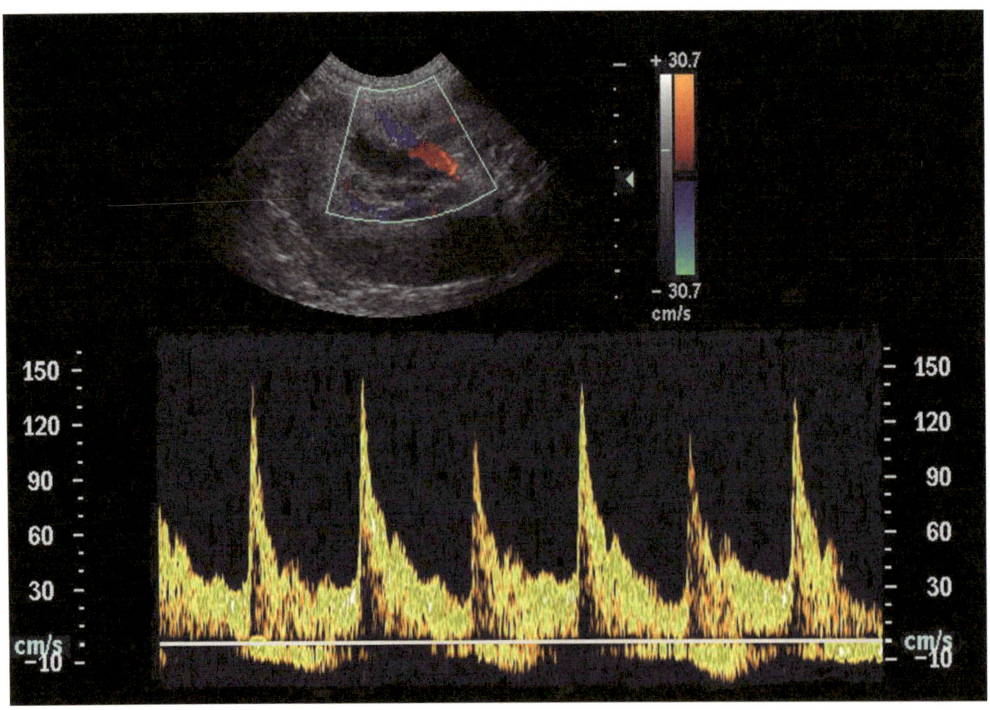

Fig. 2. Spectral trace of an interlobar artery in a kidney

The CW Doppler, is an older technology in which the ultrasound waves are continuously emitted from, and received back by the same transducer so very high velocities can be measured (Figure 3). PW Doppler systems uses only one transducer that alternates packed transmission and reception of ultrasound. The main advantage of PW Doppler compared with CW Doppler, is its ability to provide Doppler shift data selectively from a small segment along the ultrasound beam, referred to as the "sample volume", which it can be controlled by the operator (Figure 4). An ultrasound pulse is sent into the tissues travels for a given time and reflected back by a moving red cell. This ultrasound pulse returns to the transducer over the same time interval but at a shifted frequency. The location of the sample volume it is very important because the speed of ultrasound in the tissues does not change and the roundtrip travel time will differ. In this dependence on the location of the window lies the main disadvantage of PW Doppler, since it will not be possible to accurately measure high blood flow velocities, such as may be encountered in certain types of valvular and congenital heart diseases. This limitation is technically known as "aliasing" and results in an inability to record velocities above 1.5 to 2 m/sec, depending on the depth (Figures 5, 6). Although this artefact is very important in echocardiography, it will be rarely found in abdominal ultrasound, since the velocity of the blood flow in the abdominal vessels is usually lower than 1m/s.
Another main advantage of PW Doppler is the fact that some imaging may be carried on alternately with the Doppler and thus the sample volume may be shown on the actual two-dimensional display for guidance.

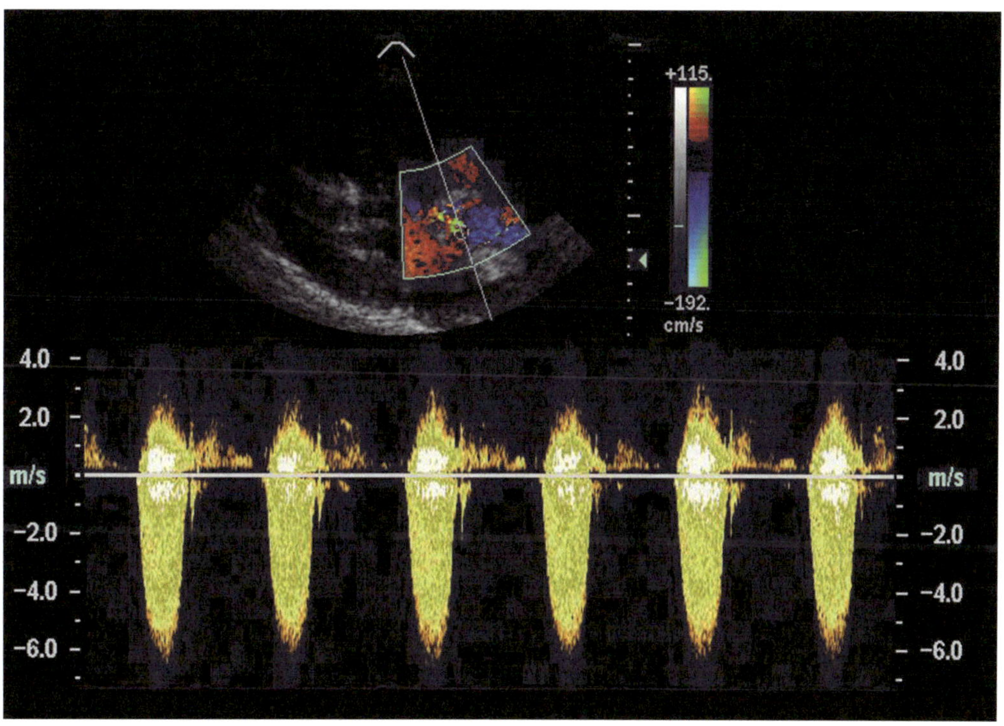

Fig. 3. Continous wave Doppler in a severe aortic stenosis. A high velocity profile (6m/s) is depicted.

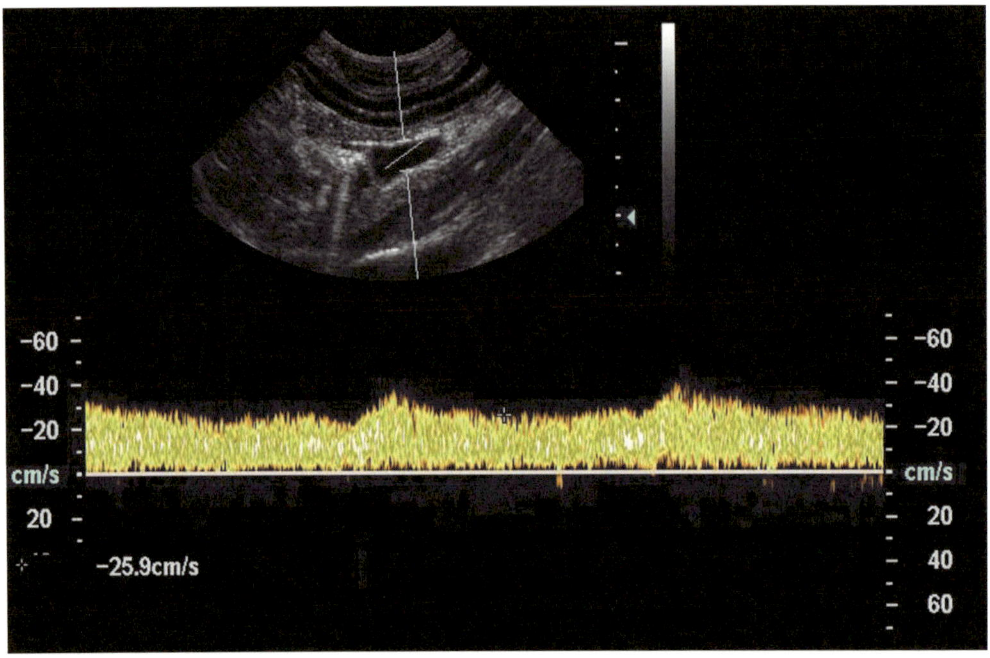

Fig. 4. Pulsed wave Doppler in a normal portal vein. Using the sample volume the sonographer is able to define the studied volume, in this case it has a width of 4 mm.

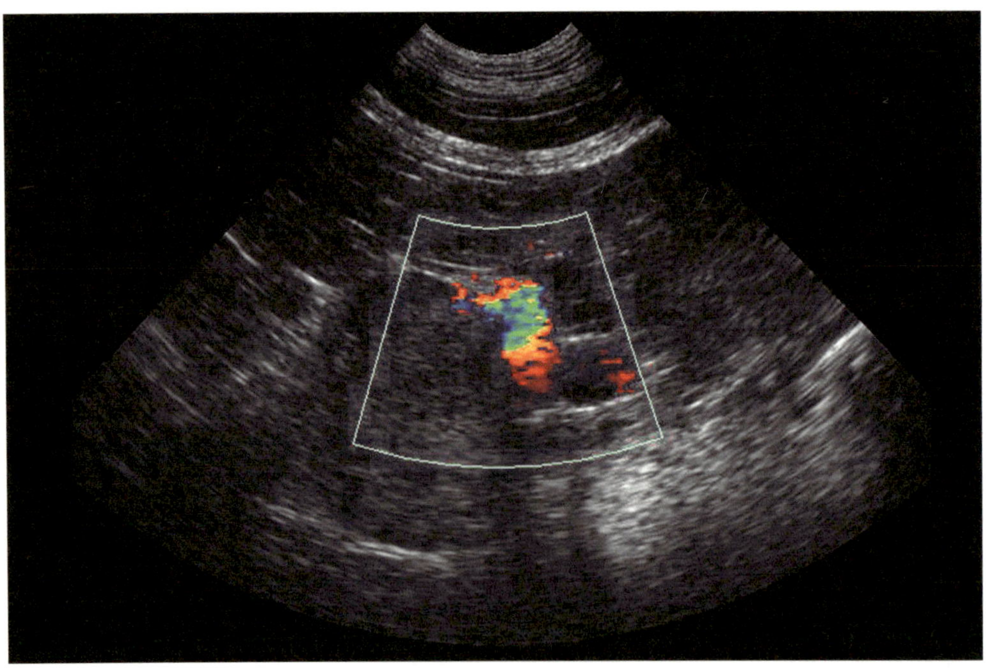

Fig. 5. Aliasing. The velocity overwhelms the máximum limit in the velocity profile (red-yellow), depicting the botom of the negative velocities (green-blue). However the blood dierction does not change.

The spectral trace from PW and CW are also different. When there is no turbulence in the blood flow analized, PW will generally display a laminar (narrow band) spectral trace. However CW rarely displays such a narrow band of flow velocities, because all the various velocities encountered by the ultrasound beams are detected by CW.
PW is usually used when a specific area of abnormal flow is located. Then, If it is important to know the accurate measurement of elevated flow velocity, CW Doppler should be used.

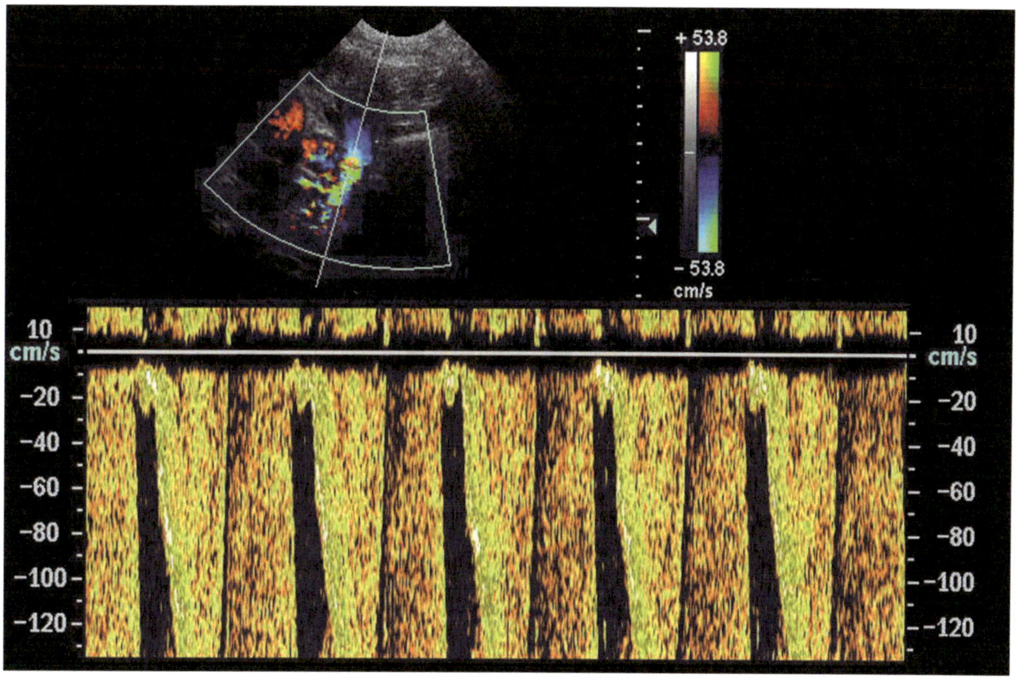

Fig. 6. Non-optimised spectral trace obtained by means of pulsed Doppler. The PRF (pulsed repetition frequency) is to low.

A relatively easy and systematic way to achieve a good spectral trace of a vessel can be summarised as follows:

1. Location of the vessel or area to scan by B mode.
2. Obtain a good view from the area. If the grey scale is not adequate, the Doppler signal will not be optimal.
3. Activate Color Doppler. Unlike in echocardiography, in abdominal ultrasound is preffered to use a higher permanence to be able to identify small structures. The PRF scale should be the adequate to fill up the vessels, being used a combination of high gain and low PRF.
4. Activate PW Doppler. Volume sample should be adjusted to the size of the vessel (usually between 2 and 4 mm).
5. Adjust the angle of insonation. It is convenient to remember that the angle of the probe related to the direction of the vessel will change the values of velocity registered. Refering the reader to the literature provided at the end of this chapter, physics of the Doppler effect will not be explained in depth, but angles between 0 and 60 degrees are recommended to register a reliable velocity.

6. Optimization of the spectral trace. In most of the ultrasound machines, the size of the screen adapts automatically. Changes in the baseline and scale of the velocity will be necessary to obtain the best image.

2. Aplications of Doppler in abdominal ultrasound

The most straightforward application using Doppler in abdominal ultrasound is assessing, by color Doppler the presence or lack of blood flow in a vascularised structures. It is an essential imperative to have a profound knowledge of the machine as well as to set up the settings properly. With this, it can be relatively easy differenciate for example between an haematoma from another lesion, or identify a thrombosis in a vessel wherein can be difficult with the bidimensional mode (Figure 7).

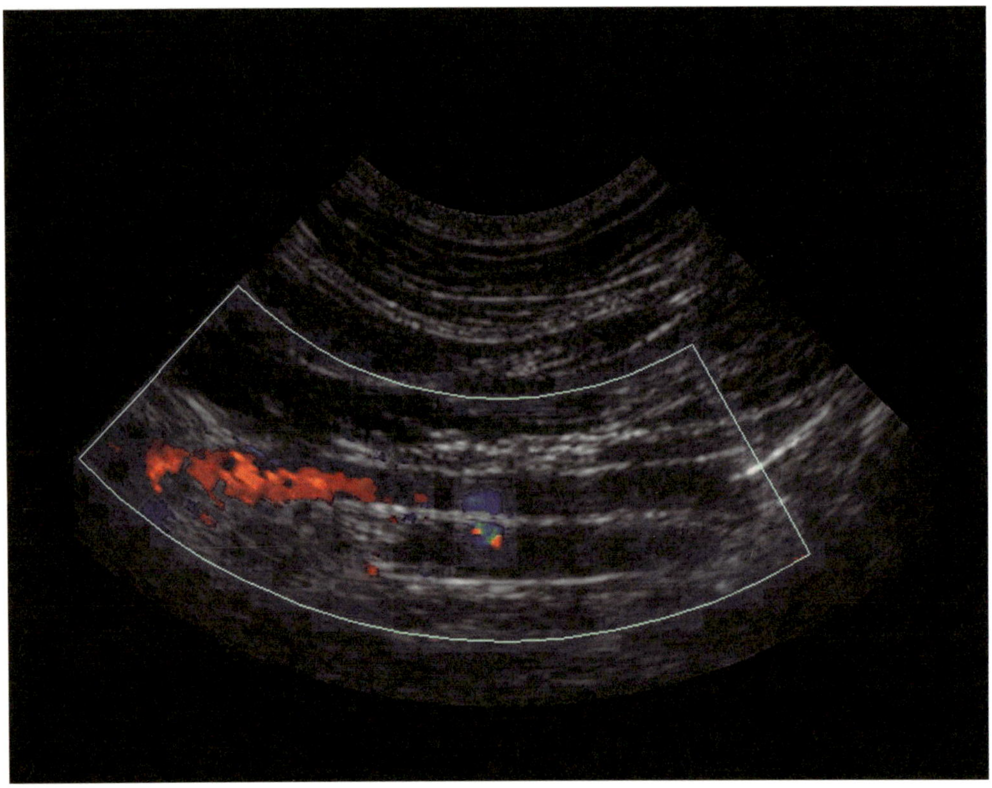

Fig. 7. Trombus in the medial iliac artery. The blood flow is interrupted.

It may also be useful when is necessary localise areas less vascularised to perform aspirations or biopsies. However, when the PRF scale is set up too low in order to improving the identification of small vessels flowing at less than 10cm/s, movements or the breathing can produce artefacts in the window making difficult the interpretation. Other tools, like the Power Doppler (Figure 8), vascular Doppler or B-Flow (currently included in most of the machines), can be very helpful due to its high sensitivity, although they are still affected by the same artefacts. The study of the spectral display of the great abdominal vessels is widely reported in the veterinary literature. Each artery and vein have distinctive trace depending on the vascular beed they supply or areas they connect. As a example, it is totally different the trace of the caudal vena cava, influenced by the respiration and the pressure in the right atrium, than the portal vein, much more stable, due to the similar pressures between the areas connected by this vessel (Figure 9).

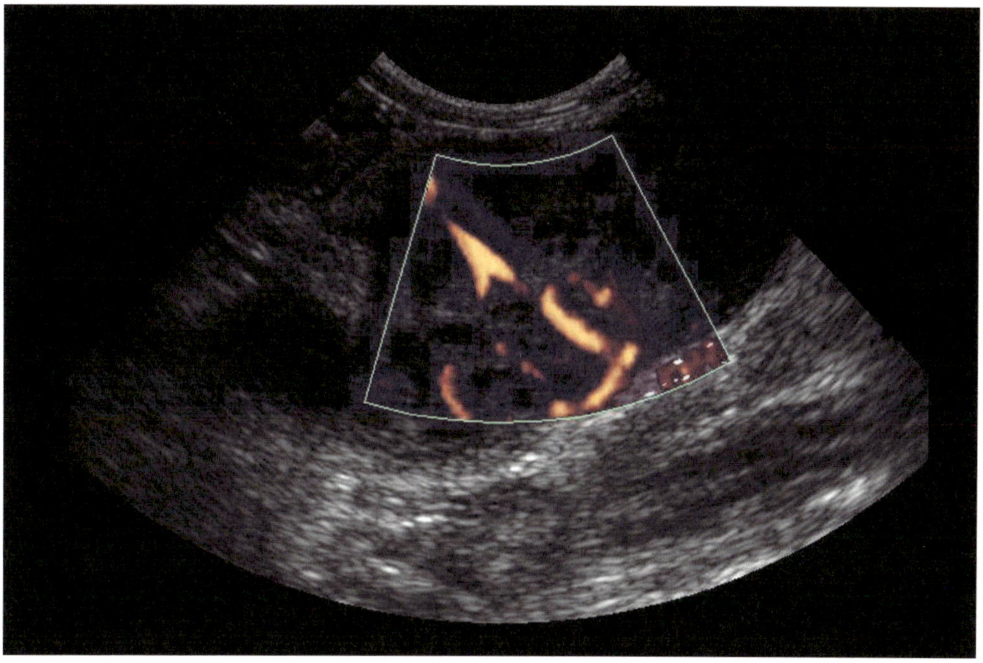

Fig. 8. Metastasic Abdominal lymph node. The vessels could not be displayed using color Doppler, however the Power Doppler used in the image had sensitivity enough

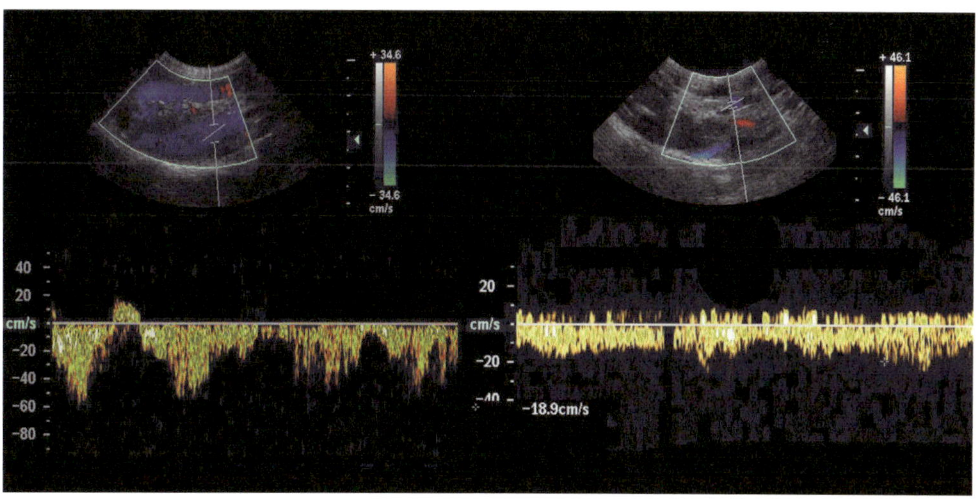

Fig. 9. Left side of the image caudal vena cava spectral trace showing the typical bi- or tri phasic pattern. In the right side portal vein spectral trace.

3. Doppler study in portal hypertension

By means of portal vein Doppler spectral trace it can be easy to diagnose and to monitore portal hypertension (PH). PH is a constant increasing of the venous pressure in the portal system, and it is the main cause of ascites in small animals. For the diagnose of this disease is necessary a broad clinical approach including biochemistry and electrolyte profiles, radiography and the analysis of the free abdominal fluid, although all these diagnostic methods will roughly help as a criteria for the monitoring of the disease. It is in this field where the ultrasound, specially the Doppler study will provide a new tool for its study in small animals. Development of PH is due to the obstruction of the blood flow, initially distending the vascular beed previous to the site of the obstruction. This place will be used as a criteria for the classification of the PH, including: Prehepatic PH (when the vascular area affected is located previous to the hepatic hilus) (Figure 10), Intrahepatic PH (hepatic structures affected) and Posthepatic PH (when the problem is located in the hepatic veins, caudal vena cava or right side of the heart). Prehepatic PH is rare in small animals, and although in the acute forms -portal thrombosis- is associated to fatal prognosis at short term, chronic evolution (pe external compression, neoplasia, etc) is less aggressive and allows for the development of compensatory mechanisms. Intrahepatic PH is the most common type of PH in dogs and cats, being less common in the latest. Almost always is due to abnormal sinusoidal circulation produced either in fibrosis or nodular regeneration in hepatic cirrhosis. Although this is the most frequent mechanism, any diffuse hepatic disease (hepatitis, lipidosis, neoplasia, etc…) may induce portal hypertension. Posthepatic PH is less frequent, and is usually due to the increasing of the resistence in hepatic veins or caudal vena cava, although it can be also produced secondary to alterations in the right side of the heart (constrictive pericarditis, heart worm disease, etc…) .

The study of the portal system by B mode ultrasound provides information about the integrity and shape of the portal vein, and when Doppler is used, we can also obtain quantitative and qualitative information of the flow and velocity. However, the result of the ultrasonographic study can by frustrating if previous factors are not considered, for example the inadequate preparation of the animal, being this the main factor for the proper viewing of the prehepatic tract of the portal vein. When performing the ultrasonographic study, two positions are usually used depending on the window chosen: Left lateral recumbency is the most adequate position for dogs and cats, placing the probe in the 11th or 12th intercostal space, or caudal to the last rib. When the animal is placed in dorsal recumbency, it is easy to access the ventral window caudal to the xiphoid process. The *porta hepatis* is the best place for aquirying the spectral trace, but the sonographer has to consider as a main concern a proper angle correction. Remaining below 60° is acceptable for a reliable velocity profile (Figure 11). The normal trace is quite stable with little or no waves, and we can consider a normal mean velocity for dogs betweeen 12 to 17cm/s and between 10 to 12cm/s in cats. The Doppler evaluation should investigates as well the direction of this flow.

Although the findings in the PH obviously depends on the type (Figure 12), there is a common and reliable one, the decrease in the mean velocity. The flow should be decreased in aproximately a 50% (below 17 ml/min/kg) and the velocity under 10 cm/s. Another consecuence that can be found in a prolonged PH is the development of collateral vessels, known as adquired portosystemic shunts (Figure 13).

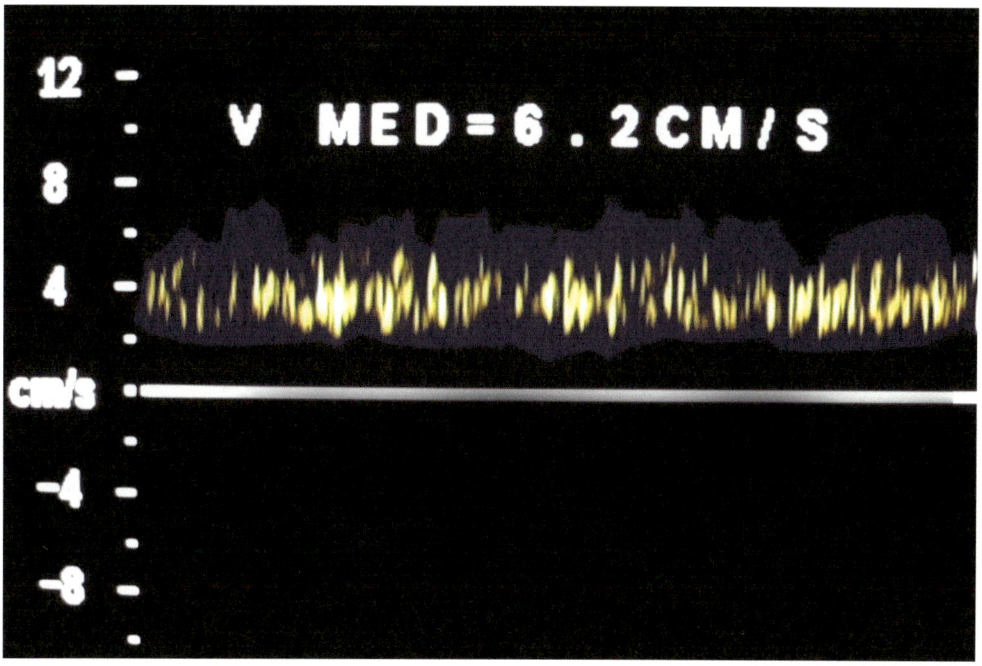

Fig. 10. Spectral trace from a German Shepherd dog with portal hypertension due to a pancreatic carcinoma

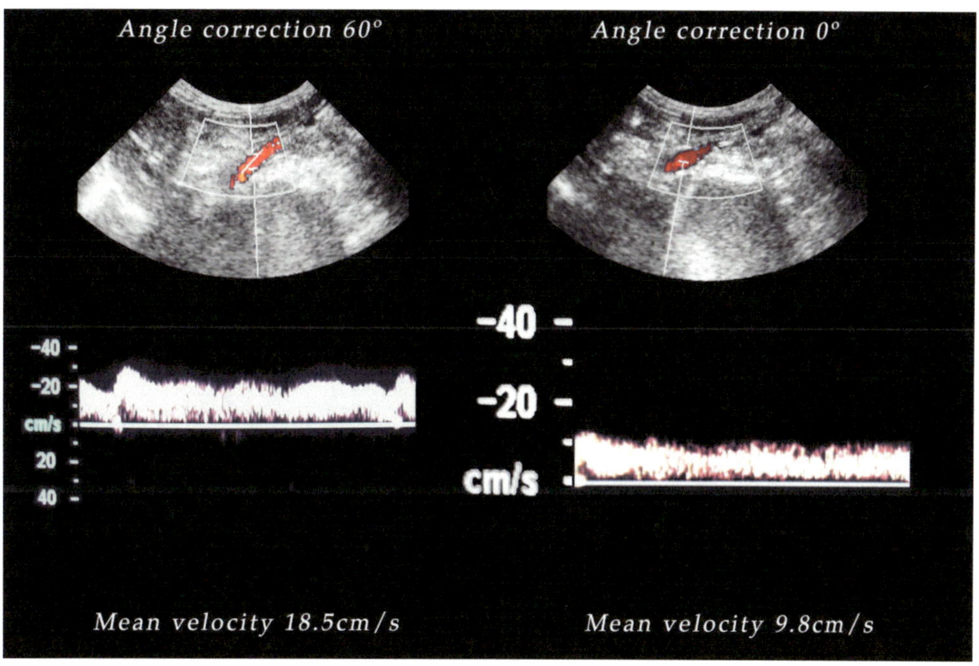

Fig. 11. Different velocity profile retrieved from the same patient using the right angle correction (left) and the wrong one (right)

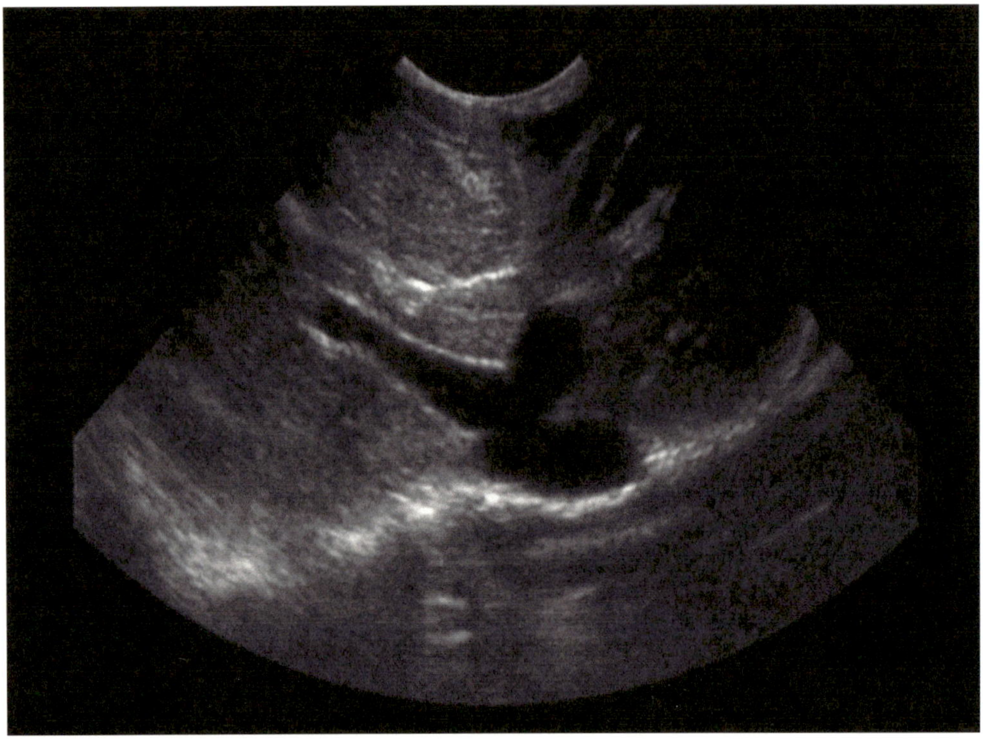

Fig. 12. Portal hypertension in a caval syndrome. The image shows the congestive liver, huge hepatic veins related to portal vessels.

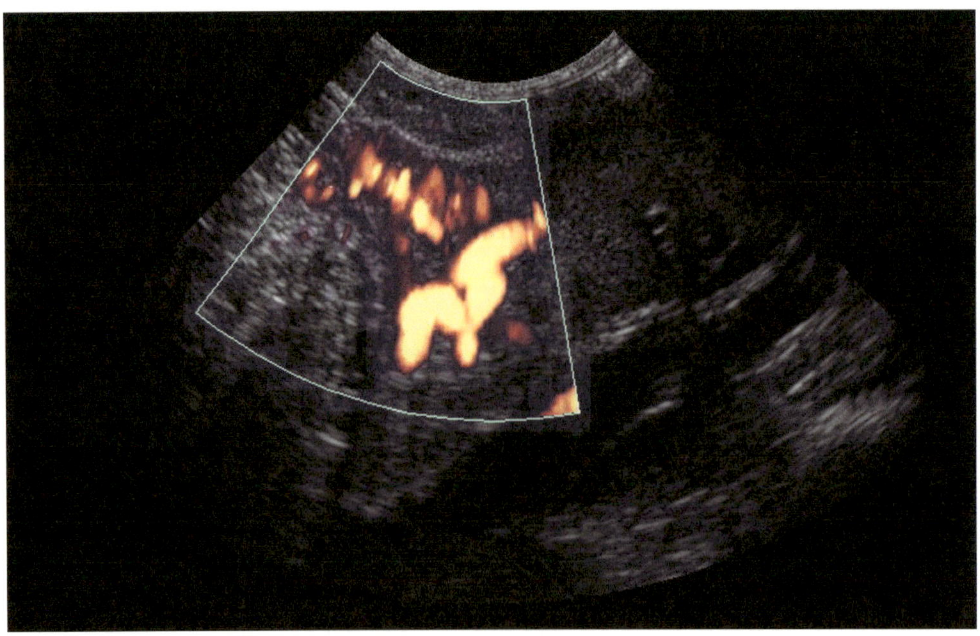

Fig. 13. Tortuous vessels corresponding to nephro-splenic shunts in a dog with chirrosis

4. Doppler assessment of affected lymph nodes

Lymphadenopathy is a common finding in a wide range of diseases. Benign conditions are those related to inflammation induced by infection, trauma, etc. In malignant conditions it is possible to distinguish between primary tumour (lymphoma) and tumour dissemination (metastases). Therefore, lymphadenopathy is a non-specific lesion that merely indicates the presence of a pathologic process. For this reason and taking into account that both conditions can be found in the same patient (e.g. mammary carcinoma in a bitch with cystitis) the real pathologic status of the lymph node must be ascertained. Diagnosis mainly consists of physical examination, which is very subjective and non-specific, needle aspirations and biopsies. These are feasible techniques when dealing with superficial lymph nodes; however they have some inconveniences for abdominal lymph nodes. Sonography plays an important role in this field, being able to explore size, shape and internal appearance. Nevertheless, ultrasonographic changes such as echotexture or size are often inconclusive, the same as guided cytological aspiration (Figure 14).

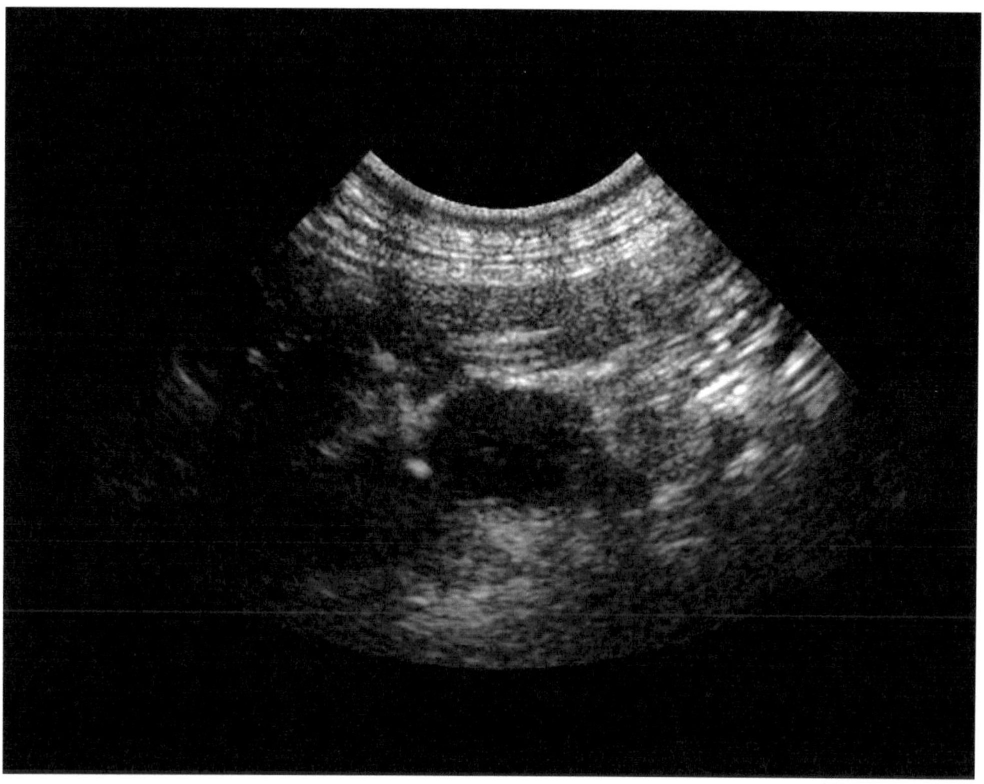

Fig. 14. Fine needle aspiration in a mesenteric lymph node. The 22G needle is clearly visualizad from the right side entering the jejunal lymph node

From a clinical point of view, taking a biopsy of every single lymph node that looks bigger or shows an altered echo pattern would be unpractical. To circumvent these difficulties another diagnostic tool could be used, the Doppler pulse wave analysis of lymph node vessels. This has proved its efficacy in canine superficial lymph nodes, in abdominal ones and in many human medical studies. The first step in the protocol is to look for an internal

lymph node vessel using color Doppler, turning to Power Doppler when necessary. The vessel is later insonated using pulsed wave Doppler to obtain the spectral trace, measuring two semiquantitative indices: Resistive (RI) and Pulsatility (PI). These indices show the relation between arterial flow and the vascular bed. The RI or Pourcelot Index is calculated as follows: (Systolic Peak Velocity - Minimum Diastolic Velocity)/ Systolic Peak Velocity, and the PI or Gosling-King Index is calculated applying this formula: (Systolic Peak Velocity - Minimum Diastolic Velocity)/ Mean Velocity. The final number is obtained using the mean of three arterial insonations in the same lymph node. Two groups of lymph nodes are proposed, benign (healthy plus reactive) and malignant (tumoral or metastasic) a proposed cut-off using the ROC curves had been demonstrated.
The values under which an iliac lymph node is considered benign are 0.6750 for RI and 1.025 for PI. The mean PIs obtained for mesenteric lymph nodes (jejunal) were 0.81, 0.87 and 1.32 for healthy, reactive and tumoral or metastasic ones respectively. The mean RI for the same ones were 0.58, 0.60 and 0.79 respectively. Tumoral or metastasic ones were singnificantly different for PI and RI. The proposed cut-off obtained from the ROC curves with a sensitivity of 100% was 1.23 for the PI and 0.76 for the RI, upper values in a mesenteric lymph node pinpoint to a malignant cause (Figures 15,16).

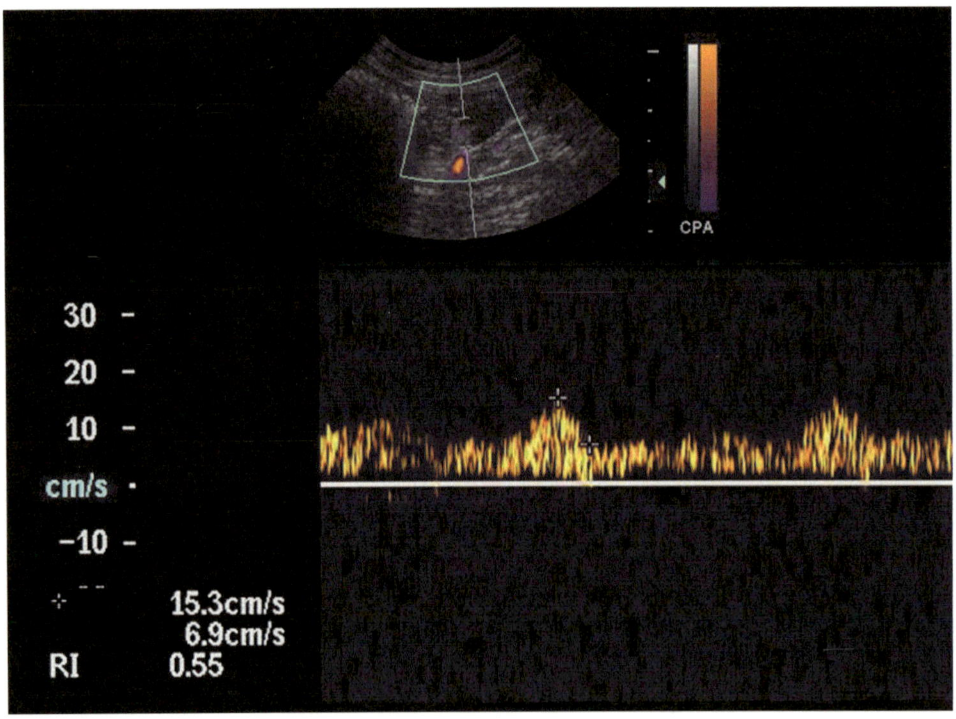

Fig. 15. Spectral trace from a reactive mesenteric lymph node, showing a RI of 0.55

5. Doppler study in renal arteries

The study of the arcuates arteries is the last importat aplication discussed in this chapter. Like the arteries of the lymph nodes, its study reflects the vascular bed. It is essential to obtain a clear spectral trace where three waves are displayed and reliable results can be

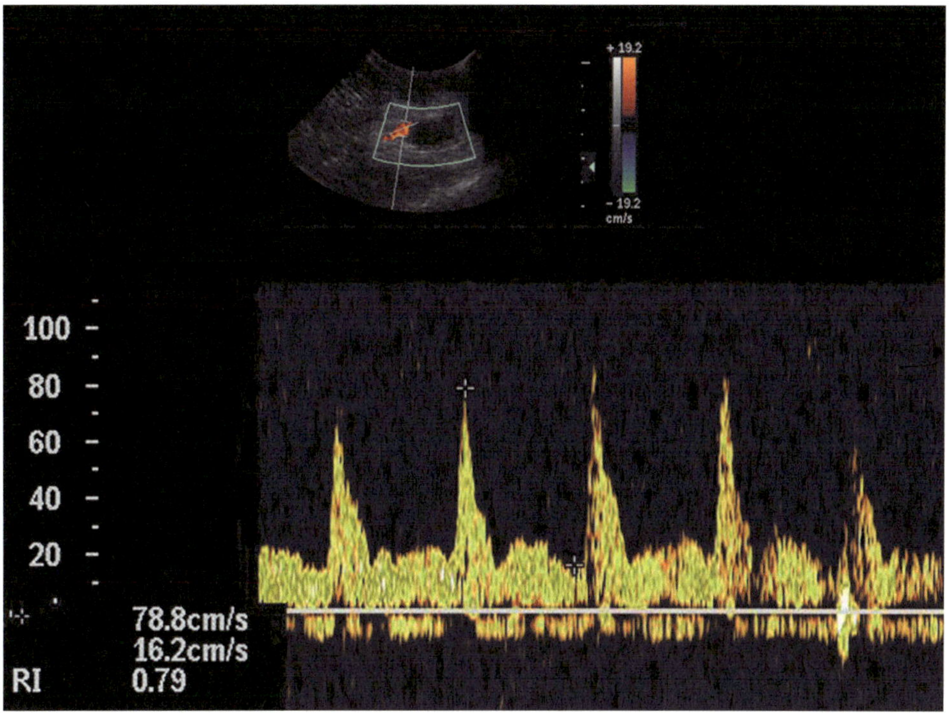

Fig. 16. Spectral trace from a metastasic mesenteric lymph node from a ovaric carcinoma, showing a RI of 0.79

achieved. The resistive index is obtained as the same way as for the lymph nodes and usually indicating the maximal systolic and the minimal diastolic velocities is enough in most of the ultrasound machines to calculate it automatically (Figure 17). Results over 0.75-0.8 are considered abnormal in both dogs and cats. There are processes other than renal diseases that can affect the resistivity index like anaemia, hypovolemic status or hypertension. Thus, further investigation in small animals is necessary to achieve more reliable conclusions, due to most of the published literature proceed from human beings. Since the resistive index is harmless, quick, simple and repeatable, and there are no many available tools for monitoring renal disease, this index should be used as a routine tool in chronic renal failure, diabetes and hyperadrenocorticism. In cats, a raise in this index seems to be linked to tubular damage (Figure 17), although further investigation is necessary in both dogs and cats to relate the type of pathologic lesions with the alteration of this index and clinical signs. As a clinical example, data of a recent study in dogs with Leishmaniosis and different stages of renal damage, showed that the resistive index could be used as an indicator of the progression, with high sensibility but low specificity. In this study all the animals with raised indexes showed advanced renal damage and proteinuria. However, many other dogs with renal damage appeared with a normal resisitve index.

The introduction of the Doppler within the routinary abdominal protocol is necessary, and provides a higher diagnostic accuracy. In coming years new applications of its use will appear as a powerful tool for the diagnosis and monitoring of the diseases in small animals.

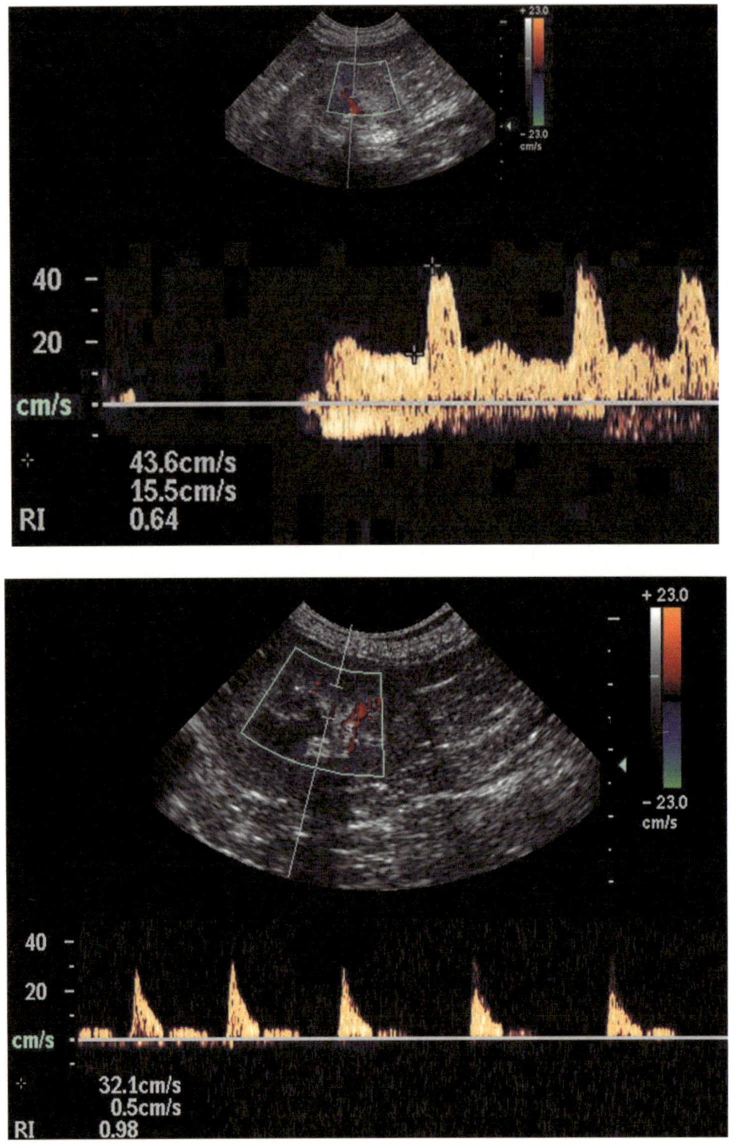

Fig. 17. Normal arquate artery, the spectral trace depicted a low resistence artery, meanwhile in the right there is arquate artery from a cat with advance chronic renal faliure.

6. References

Arndt JW, Oyama MA, Agitated saline contrast echocardiography to diagnose a congenital heart defect in a dog. J Vet Cardiol 2008;10:129-32.

Burns PN, The physical principles of Doppler and spectral analysis. J Clin Ultrasound 1987;15:567-90.

Chang DB, Yuan A, Yu CJ, Luh KT, Kuo SH, Yang PC, Differentiation of benign and malignant cervical lymph nodes with color Doppler sonography. AJR Am J Roentgenol 1994;162:965-8.

Choi MY, Lee JW, Jang KJ, Distinction between benign and malignant causes of cervical, axillary, and inguinal lymphadenopathy: value of Doppler spectral waveform analysis. AJR Am J Roentgenol 1995;165:981-4.

d'Anjou MA, Penninck D, Cornejo L, Pibarot P, Ultrasonographic diagnosis of portosystemic shunting in dogs and cats. Vet Radiol Ultrasound 2004;45:424-37.

Dragoni F, Cartoni C, Pescarmona E, Chiarotti F, Puopolo M, Orsi E, Pignoloni P, De Gregoris C, Mandelli F, The role of high resolution pulsed and color Doppler ultrasound in the differential diagnosis of benign and malignant lymphadenopathy: results of multivariate analysis. Cancer 1999;85:2485-90.

Kinns J, Mai W, Association between malignancy and sonographic heterogeneity in canine and feline abdominal lymph nodes. Vet Radiol Ultrasound 2007;48:565-9.

Koma LM, Spotswood TC, Kirberger RM, Becker PJ, Influence of normovolemic anemia on Doppler characteristics of the abdominal aorta and splanchnic vessels in Beagles. Am J Vet Res 2005;66:187-95.

Koma LM, Kirberger RM, Scholtz L, Doppler ultrasonographic changes in the canine kidney during normovolaemic anaemia. Res Vet Sci 2006;80:96-102.

Lamb CR, Burton CA, Carlisle CH, Doppler measurement of hepatic arterial flow in dogs: technique and preliminary findings. Vet Radiol Ultrasound 1999;40:77-81.

Langenbach A, McManus PM, Hendrick MJ, Shofer FS, Sorenmo KU, Sensitivity and specificity of methods of assessing the regional lymph nodes for evidence of metastasis in dogs and cats with solid tumors. J Am Vet Med Assoc 2001;218:1424-8.

Lee YW, Pulsed Doppler ultrasonographic evaluation of portal blood flow in dogs with experimental portal vein branch ligation. J Vet Med Sci 1999;61:59-61.

Llabres-Diaz FJ, Ultrasonography of the medial iliac lymph nodes in the dog. Vet Radiol Ultrasound 2004;45:156-65.

Mastorakou I, Robbins ME, Bywaters T, Resistance and pulsatility Doppler indices: how accurately do they reflect changes in renal vascular resistance. Br J Radiol 1993;66:577-80.

Nelson TR, Pretorius DH, The Doppler signal: where does it come from and what does it mean? AJR Am J Roentgenol 1988;151:439-47.

Novellas R, Ruiz de Gopegui R, Espada Y, Effects of sedation with midazolam and butorphanol on resistive and pulsatility indices in healthy dogs. Vet Radiol Ultrasound 2007;48:276-80.

Novellas R, Espada Y, Ruiz de Gopegui R, Doppler ultrasonographic estimation of renal and ocular resistive and pulsatility indices in normal dogs and cats. Vet Radiol Ultrasound 2007;48:69-73.

Novellas R, de Gopegui RR, Espada Y, Increased renal vascular resistance in dogs with hepatic disease. Vet J 2008;178:257-62.

Nyman HT, Kristensen AT, Flagstad A, McEvoy FJ, A review of the sonographic assessment of tumor metastases in liver and superficial lymph nodes. Vet Radiol Ultrasound 2004;45:438-48.

Nyman HT, Kristensen AT, Skovgaard IM, McEvoy FJ, Characterization of normal and abnormal canine superficial lymph nodes using gray-scale B-mode, color flow mapping, power, and spectral Doppler ultrasonography: a multivariate study. Vet Radiol Ultrasound 2005;46:404-10.

Nyman HT, Nielsen OL, McEvoy FJ, Lee MH, Martinussen T, Hellmen E, Kristensen AT, Comparison of B-mode and Doppler ultrasonographic findings with histologic features of benign and malignant mammary tumors in dogs. Am J Vet Res 2006;67:985-91.

Nyman HT, Kristensen AT, Lee MH, Martinussen T, McEvoy FJ, Characterization of canine superficial tumors using gray-scale B mode, color flow mapping, and spectral Doppler ultrasonography--a multivariate study. Vet Radiol Ultrasound 2006;47:192-8.

Nyman HT, O'Brien RT, The sonographic evaluation of lymph nodes. Clin Tech Small Anim Pract 2007;22:128-37.

Prieto S, Gomez-Ochoa P, de Blas I, Gascon M, Aceña M, Corda A, Sosa I, Gregori T, Couto CG, Pathologic correlation of resistive and pulsatility indices in canine abdominal lymph nodes. The Veterinary Radiology &Ultrasound 2009;In Press:

Rivers BJ, Walter PA, Letourneau JG, Finlay DE, Ritenour ER, King VL, O'Brien TD, Polzin DJ, Estimation of arcuate artery resistive index as a diagnostic tool for aminoglycoside-induced acute renal failure in dogs. Am J Vet Res 1996;57:1536-44.

Rivers BJ, Walter PA, Letourneau JG, Finlay DE, Ritenour ER, King VL, O'Brien TD, Polzin DJ, Duplex Doppler estimation of resistive index in arcuate arteries of sedated, normal female dogs: implications for use in the diagnosis of renal failure. J Am Anim Hosp Assoc 1997;33:69-76.

Rivers BJ, Walter PA, Polzin DJ, King VL, Duplex Doppler estimation of intrarenal pourcelot resistive index in dogs and cats with renal disease. J Vet Intern Med 1997;11:250-60.

Rubaltelli L, Proto E, Salmaso R, Bortoletto P, Candiani F, Cagol P, Sonography of abnormal lymph nodes in vitro: correlation of sonographic and histologic findings. AJR Am J Roentgenol 1990;155:1241-4.

Skidmore R, Woodcock JP, Physiological interpretation of Doppler-shift waveforms--I. Theoretical considerations. Ultrasound Med Biol 1980;6:7-10.

Smeets AJ, Zonderland HM, van der Voorde F, Lameris JS, Evaluation of abdominal lymph nodes by ultrasound. J Ultrasound Med 1990;9:325-31.

Spaulding KA, A review of sonographic identification of abdominal blood vessels and juxtavascular organs. Vet Radiol Ultrasound 1997;38:4-23.

Steinkamp HJ, Mueffelmann M, Bock JC, Thiel T, Kenzel P, Felix R, Differential diagnosis of lymph node lesions: a semiquantitative approach with color Doppler ultrasound. Br J Radiol 1998;71:828-33.

Steinkamp HJ, Teichgraber UK, Mueffelmann M, Hosten N, Kenzel P, Felix R, Differential diagnosis of lymph node lesions. A semiquantitative approach with power Doppler sonography. Invest Radiol 1999;34:509-15.

Szatmari V, Nemeth T, Kotai I, Voros K, Sotonyi P, Doppler ultrasonographic diagnosis and anatomy of congenital intrahepatic arterioportal fistula in a puppy. Vet Radiol Ultrasound 2000;41:284-6.

Szatmari V, Sotonyi P, Voros K, Normal duplex Doppler waveforms of major abdominal blood vessels in dogs: a review. Vet Radiol Ultrasound 2001;42:93-107.

Taylor KJ, Ramos I, Carter D, Morse SS, Snower D, Fortune K, Correlation of Doppler US tumor signals with neovascular morphologic features. Radiology 1988;166:57-62.

15

Use of Ultrasound to Assess Drug Efficacy in Orthotopic Rat Models of HCC

Cedo M. Bagi, Terri Swanson and Theresa Tuthill
Pfizer, Research and Development, Groton
U.S.A.

1. Introduction

1.1 Imaging in drug development

The development of novel therapeutics follows a typical path from chemical and biological activities in the laboratory through extensive clinical testing and if successful, to the commercialization of a drug for a given labeled indication. The attrition, the failure of a new product to successfully complete all stages of drug testing, is a key metric for defining productivity in the pharmaceutical industry. The lack of therapeutic efficacy and poor safety profiles are the leading causes of attrition. Several solutions to better address attrition have been proposed in order to enhance our knowledge regarding efficacy, safety and mechanism of action in pre-clinical and early clinical setups, all in order to minimize late-stage attrition and make informed decisions regarding the likelihood of the novel compounds to successfully complete all stages of drug development and become a product. Clinical imaging has the potential to provide key biomarkers and to enable decision-making in drug development. Although, imaging is a complementary technology to biofluid-derived biomarkers, its non-invasive nature provides unique information regarding quantitative measurement of function at particular anatomical localization and is highly desirable in order to strengthen our confidence in positive clinical outcome. Imaging, therefore, has considerable potential to build upon well-established serum and urine biomarkers in order to better validate predictive values of biofluid-derived biomarkers in both the pre-clinical and clinical environments. In oncology, imaging techniques are complementary to methods that use biomarker techniques to detect presence of tumor tissue, tumor progression and response to therapy because imaging modalities provide precise anatomical localization of the tumor tissue(s) that generates biomarkers measured in fluids. Ultrasonography (US) is one of the emerging technologies that possess several key advantages over other molecular imaging modalities. These include frequency-dependent high spatial resolution, real-time imaging, both anatomical and molecular information in the single imaging session, freedom from ionizing radiation, inexpensive implementation, affordability worldwide, and finally, well-published preclinical and clinical use of US technology. Therefore, research teams can easily access information regarding adequate use and predictive value of ultrasound technology to address the specific project needs [1,2].

1.2 HCC and tumor models

Hepatocelluar carcinoma (HCC) is the fifth most common cancer and the third cause of cancer-related death globally that resists conventional chemotherapy and radiotherapy [3-5]. Also, the liver is, in addition to lungs and bones, one of the most common sites of metastases of other tumors, in particular colorectal, pancreatic and ovarian cancers. Conventional cytotoxic chemotherapy does not significantly prolong survival of patients with primary liver tumors or liver metastases, therefore new therapeutic approaches are needed in order to curb the local growth of solid tumors as well as micrometastases of HCC. Given the complexity of the interactions between tumor cells and surrounding stroma and uniqueness of microvascularization of the liver, there is a strong rationale to combine agents with different mechanisms of action when treating HCC, but also to simultaneously target tumor cells and surrounding stroma in order to make the tumor microenvironment less friendly (fertile) for growth of solid tumors or development of micro-metastases. In this chapter we describe the difference in vascularization between xenograft and orthotopic preclinical models of HCC and use of ultrasonogrophy to assess tumor and organ vasculature. Additionally, we emphasize the unique value of contrast enhanced ultrasonography to monitor tumor growth and change in tumor vasculature over time in order to assess effect of applied therapies.

1.3 Angiogenesis in tumors

Angiogenesis is a critical process in local tumor growth and in the invasion and development of distant metastases [6,7]. Research investigating molecular pathways of tumor angiogenesis has led to the identification of a number of key molecules involved in the stimulation of new vessel growth from existing host vasculature. Several of these molecules, such as vascular endothelial growth factor and its main receptor 2 (VEGFR2) have become targets for antiangiogenic drugs [8,9]. However, successful application of novel therapies that target tumor vasculature will require accurate selection of susceptible tumors and precise evaluation of early treatment response using adequate preclinical models. Previous work has shown that angiogenesis can be successfully characterized *in vivo* by using ultrasonography with microbubble contrast agents bearing anti-integrin antibodies adhered to fibroblast growth factor-stimulated vessels [10-12].

2. Preclinical models of hepatocellular carcinoma

Preclinical experimentation allows for simultaneous longitudinal implementation of various technologies and biomarkers to monitor the tumor take rate, growth and response to treatment as well as to confirm and correlate histological and histochemical results at various time points with serum or imaging biomarkers, which cannot always be determined in HCC patients.

2.1 Tumor vasculature in xenograft HCC model

The vast majority of *in vivo* oncology studies are performed in xenograft models, subcutaneously placed tumor cells in immunodeficient mice or rats. Xenograft models are relatively easy to perform since tumor cells are injected in subcutaneous tissue of mice or rats and simple caliper measurement of tumor size provides insight regarding tumor take rate, growth and the compound efficacy (Figure 1). Since human malignancies never start or metastasize to subcutaneous regions of the body, the xenograft models lack many critical characteristics of human cancers including lack of preexisting organ vasculature and interaction between the tumor cells and cells of the organ where tumor initiated or metastasized. Therefore, the main goal of studies using xenograft models is to confirm that the "targeted" therapy under investigation hits the intended target that should be present in the tumor cell line used in the particular study. In this model there are no pre-existing blood vessels and the newly formed tumor vasculature is fairly simple and consists of nutritional arteries designed to provide oxygen and nutrients to the tumor (Figure 1). Consequently, antiangiogenic therapy in the HCC xenograft models seems to be very effective against the tumor growth [13]. In general, the xenograft models are very informative and allow for several types of measurements to be performed simultaneously including caliper measurements, IVIS imaging, ultrasonography with and without the contrast agents, PET and MRI imaging, measurements of serum or urine biomarkers and finally deployment of many histological and histochemical methods. Recently, several groups have demonstrated that quantification of intra-tumoral flow of an ultrasound contrast agent with gray-scale imaging can be used for monitoring tumor vascular response to anti-angiogenic therapy in animal models, a technique that can also be used in the clinic [13-16]. In those studies data obtained with ultrasonography paralleled tumor volume data obtained by caliper measurement and showed good correlation with tumor histology, allowing assessment of necrotic and perfused tumor areas *in vivo*.

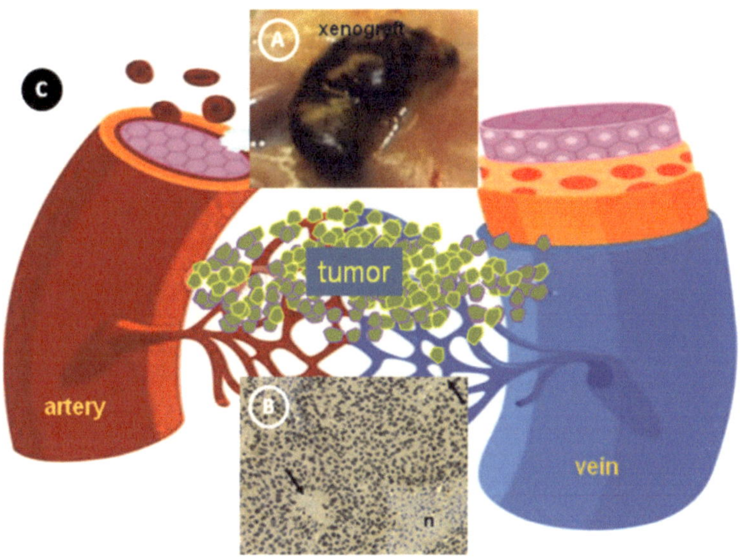

Fig. 1. Image of a xenograft of HCC tumor (A), histological appearance of the tumor (B) with arrows indicating a blood vessel, and schematic representation of the nutritional blood supply to the tumor (C).

2.2 Tumor vasculature and liver vasculature in orthotopic HCC model

Orthotopic HCC models of liver tumors are labor-intensive to perform as they require surgical inoculation of tumor cells into the liver (or spleen) and the use of sophisticated imaging technologies and/or biofluid based biomarkers to monitor the tumor take rate, tumor growth and effects of therapy on tumor progression [17]. Because in orthotopic HCC models the tumor is placed in the organ of origin, studies performed in those models provide more realistic and clinically relevant data regarding compound systemic and tumor exposure, efficacy and safety.

The local vasculature of the liver is extremely complex and is composed of nutritional and functional blood supplies that in addition to neo-vasculature created by the tumor itself, collectively support tumor growth within the liver (Figure 2). The hepatic artery accounts for only about 65% of the oxygen supply to the liver [18,19]. Slow circulation in the liver and an intense nutritional (hepatic artery) and functional (portal vein) vascular network allows the tumor to establish, survive and eventually metastasize [20,21]. The blood flow to the liver tumor is carried almost exclusively by systemic arterial vessels [22,23]. However, oxygen and nutrient supply through the portal vein is respectable, and it has been hypothesized that outside edges of the tumor use this alternate route to survive and spread to surrounding tissues [24] causing these tumors to be very resistant to antiangiogenic therapies. Finally, vascularization in the liver of cancer patients can be further complicated by liver cirrhosis [25-27]. Due to technical and other difficulties to reliably describe the exact anatomical location of the tumor within the liver, tumor size and growth propensity, presence or lack of secondary tumors, as well as tumor response to therapy, scientists that utilize orthotopic HCC models in their research as well as clinicians almost entirely depend on imaging modalities, including various ultrasound methods.

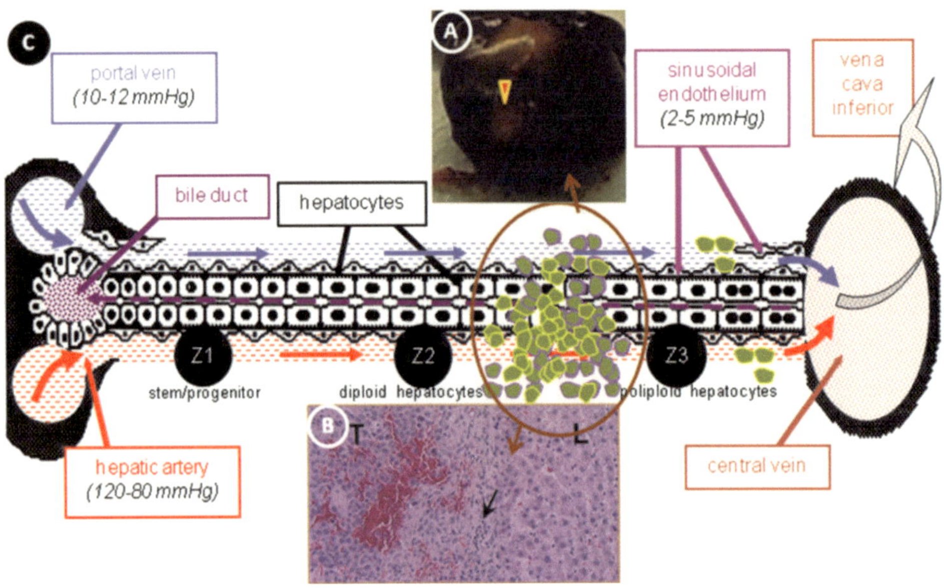

Fig. 2. Overview of a rat liver (A) with orthotopic HCC tumor (arrow head), histological appearance of intrahepatic tumor (B) depicting borderline area (arrow) between the tumor (T) and normal liver tissue (L) and schematic representation (C) of the nutritional (hepatic artery) and functional (portal vein) blood supply in the liver and the intrahepatic tumor, emphasizing differences in blood pressure between the two blood systems.

2.3 Delivery of contrast and/or drug in orthotopic HCC model

One of the most clinically effective ways to deliver drugs to the liver is through the hepatic artery because it allows continuous infusion directly into the arterial bed from which the tumor derives nearly all of its blood supply [27,28]. The use of orthotopic animal models allows for cannulation of the hepatic artery and portal vein to deliver drugs directly to the liver, thus mimicking the clinical arrangement. Due to technical difficulties associated with intra-arterial drug delivery, the most common way of dosing animals in preclinical studies is via tail-vein injections. Even though tail-vein injections have little similarity with the clinical setup, this method is acceptable as long as the frequency of repeated dosing does not cause local tissue damage and necrosis. However, a single bolus injection of a drug or contrast agent through the hepatic artery or portal vain is more desirable since it mimics human setup and delivers much better results. The differences in the microbubble concentrations in the liver following tail-vain, portal vein and hepatic artery delivery are shown in Figures 3.

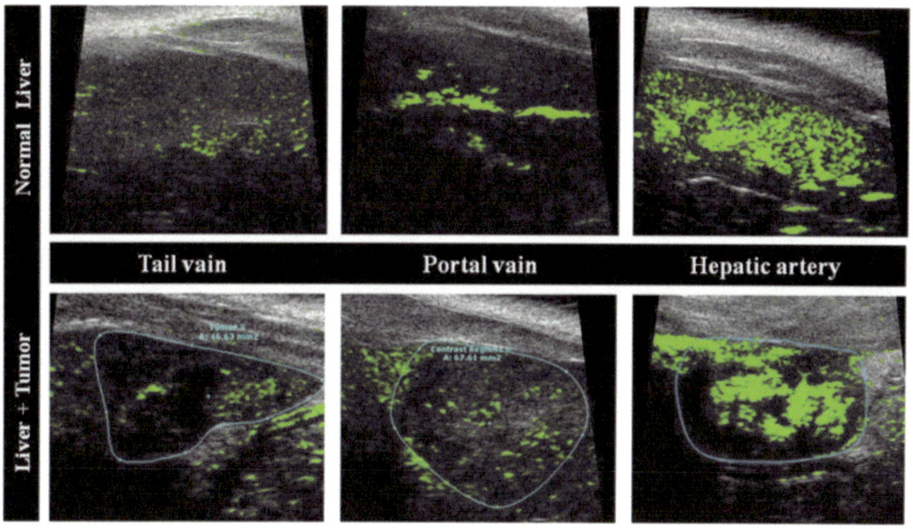

Fig. 3. Ultrasound images of normal rat livers and tumor bearing livers following bolus injection of microbubbles (50 μL) into the tail vein, portal vein, or hepatic artery. Take of the microbubble contrast (green) by the liver is very high if the injection is made through hepatic artery or portal vein, but poor if injection is made through the tail vein.

Microbubble contrast technology is known to be an extremely useful tool for non-invasive assessment of liver vascular structure [29]. Contrast Enhanced Ultrasound Imaging (CEUS) is used in both preclinical and clinical studies to diagnose liver tumors and/or liver metastases, to monitor disease progression, to deliver drugs and to assess the efficacy of antitumor therapies [16,30,31].

3. Tumor assessment using ultrasound imaging

Through both structural and functional imaging, ultrasound can provide an integrated suite of tools to characterize and monitor tumor changes. For pre-clinical use, the low-cost and real-time capabilities allow for high throughput of analyzed animals. In addition, developed imaging biomarkers are often translatable into humans for use in clinical trials.

3.1 Assessment of tumor volume

The resolution of an ultrasound B-scan image increases with frequency, though depth penetration is diminished due to attenuation. For small-animal imaging, frequencies in the range of 20 to 50 MHz can provide sharp images of anatomical structure for depths down to 1cm. At 40 MHz, the resolution is on the order of 50 μm [32]. In both xenograft and orthotopic rodent models, tumors can be viewed with well defined boundaries, allowing for quantitative measurement of volume size.

Though 3D matrix array probes are slowly becoming more available, accurate volume measurements can be obtained with a mechanical sweep of a 2D array. With the tumor bearing rodent fixed on a platform, a stepping motor translates the transducer across the region of interest. Post-processing of the 2D image sets includes manual outlining of the tumor on individual slices to estimate the volume. For small tumors (less than 2 mm^3), the coefficient of variation for tumor volume measurements has been shown to be on the order of 10% [33]. Delineation of tumor boundaries can be further improved with use of the contrast (Figure 4).

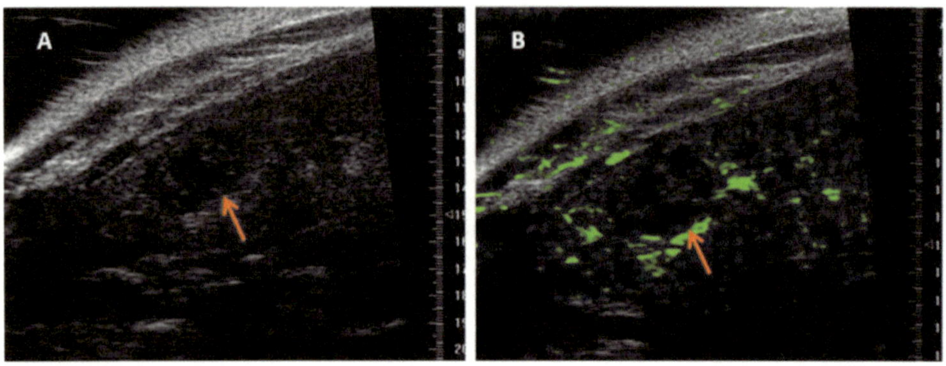

Fig. 4. Contrast enhanced ultrasound improves tumor identification and measurement. The left image (A) was taken without contrast, and although a shadow is visible (arrow), the tumor is difficult to identify. After contrast administration (B) a tumor mass (arrow) is clearly defined and can be readily quantified.

3.2 Assessment of tumor vascularity using Doppler

Since angiogenesis is a major enabling factor of tumor growth, the ability to image and monitor tumor vascularity is of primary interest in oncology applications of US technology. Doppler ultrasound is the standard modality for measuring blood flow. As a transducer emits an acoustic pulse, the echoes from moving scatters are shifted in frequency. In brief, the pulsed-wave Doppler sends short pulse bursts and gates the return signal corresponding to a specific depth. The display of tumor vasculature shows the velocity spectrum as a function of time. This technique is most useful for looking at velocity profiles of flow in macrovessels such as hepatic veins and arteries (Figure 5).

Power Doppler, which uses the integrated power of the Doppler signal, does not provide directional flow information, but is angle independent and more sensitive to slow flow than frequency-shift-based color Doppler. By using the clinical scanners, vessels as small as 100 μm diameter can be clearly visualized. Quantification is typically based on calculating the percentage of colorized-pixels in a region of interest. Power Doppler has been shown to have a strong correlation (r=0.98) with tumor blood vessels as determined by histological staining [34]. Regional variations, rim versus tumor core, can also be evaluated as well as heterogeneity of tumor vasculature.

3.3 Assessment of tumor perfusion using contrast imaging

Within the past decade, ultrasound contrast agents have been increasingly used to characterize vascular dynamics. The current generation of contrast agents is composed of 1-10 μm sizedmicrobubbles with a perfluorocarbon or hexafluoride gas core surrounded by a lipid shell. Injected into the blood stream, microbubbles are stable in the circulatory system for over 10

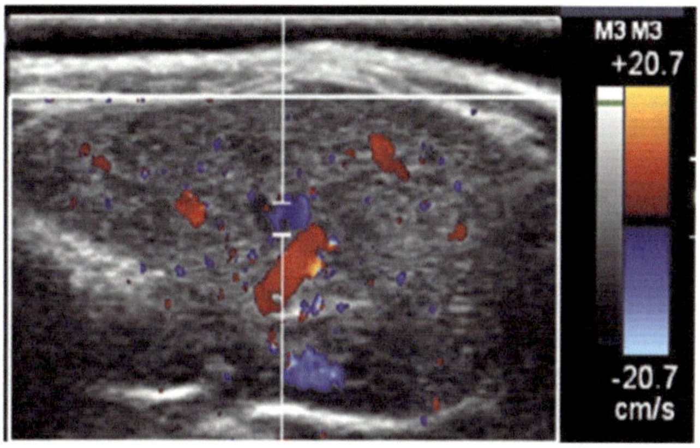

Fig. 5. Example of color Doppler imaging of the normal rat liver. Color Doppler shows directional flow allowing for visualization of the hepatic artery tree and portal vein. A pulse wave Doppler range gate is placed over the colorized vessel to measure flow velocity.

minutes, and unlike MRI contrast agents, the microbubbles remain in intravascular compartment until excreted from the system. Two methods are available when using the contrast agent to assess tumor perfusion; power Doppler and dynamic contrast imaging:

Use of power Doppler. When insonified by a high power ultrasound pulse, microbubbles disintegrate emitting a non-linear signal detectable with Doppler. Power Doppler imaging using contrast agents and a high mechanical index allows detection of vessels down to capillary size and is independent of flow velocities [35]. Total vessel fraction within a tumor can thus be computed from a 3D sweep and the ratio of colorized pixels to the total number of pixels within the tumor can be calculated.

Use of dynamic contrast imaging. The injection of a bolus of contrast can be monitored with low power (less than 0.1) mechanical index. Simultaneous recording of the intensity changes of the contrast agent as a function of time will provide information on blood flow in a region of interest during the entire time of imaging. In brief, the uptake curve can be fitted to an exponential function using the formula $y=A(1-e^{-\beta t})$ where A is proportional to the microvascular cross-sectional area, and β corresponds to velocity [36]. The product of these two parameters can then be used to quantify perfusion. Additional parameters that have been used in tumor assessment include peak enhancement, area under the curve, and wash-in-time [37]. The values obtained can be averaged across the tumor or evaluated on a pixel-by-pixel case to create parametric maps that demonstrate tumor heterogeneity.

The separation of fast flow (from larger functional vessels) and slow flow (from the microvasculature) can provide further insight to vasculature changes from treatment. In a study of an anti-angiogenic drug in a human/mouse chimera model, the quantification of CE-US imaging wash-in parameters revealed that the prevalence of fast blood flow, but not slow flow (associated with small, leaky vessels), was suppressed in treated tumors compared with control tumors [38].

4. Ultrasound imaging of tumor growth kinetics

4.1 Changes in tumor volume and tumor composition

In both the xenograft and orthotopic models B-mode imaging using high-frequency ultrasound can provide valuable data on the volume of the tumor. Traditional tumor volume measurement in xenograft models uses caliper measurement of the tumor width

(W) and tumor length (L). An ellipsoid shape is assumed, and the volume computed as V=1/2 (L x W^2). Using this technique, inter-observer variation is 15% [39]. Measurement of tumor volume using calipers is not possible in orthotopic animal models known to much closer resemble local and tumor vascular events seen in HCC patients relative to xenograft models [17]. Volume size estimates from a 3D ultrasound image set are more accurate due to the ability to account for non-ellipsoidal shapes. Currently, there are commercially available software that can view individual slices and manually outline the tumor on individual slices in both xenograft and orthotopic tumors in rats and mice. By interpolating between slices, an accurate representation of the 3D tumor shape is provided along with the volume estimation. For fine sweeps, not every slice needs to be evaluated. We have found that with a slice separation in the range of 100 to 300 μm, manual tumor delineation on every 10th slice provides accurate volume estimation (unpublished data).

Along with tumor delineation, ultrasound grayscale images can also allow for detection of change in tumor composition including tumor necrosis. Necrotic regions in tumor xenograft appear as fluid filled pockets within the tumor (Figure 6). By using the same techniques utilized to assess the tumor volume, the necrotic volume can also be estimated.

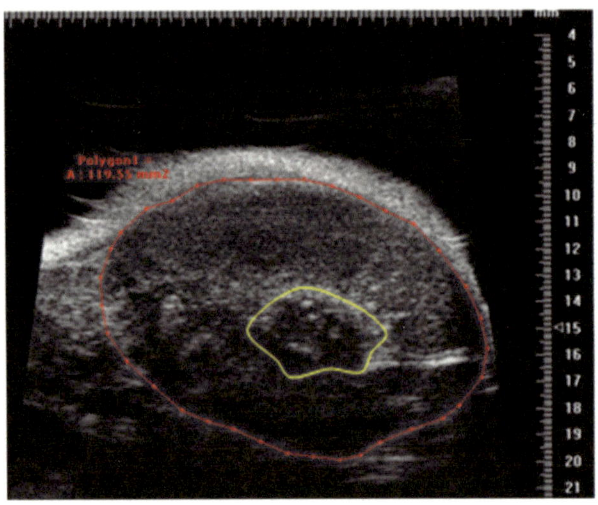

Fig. 6. Example-scan of a xenograft tumor composed of human Huh7.5 cell line outlined in red with necrotic core outlined in yellow.

4.2 Change of tumor vasculature following drug treatment

Dynamic contrast methods may present some difficulties in the rodent liver due to breathing motion. The high frequency ultrasound systems allow for respiratory gating, but the tumor bearing liver in rodents can still be difficult to image with sufficient accuracy. Early testing of anti-angiogenic compounds in both xenograft and orthotopic models have utilized US imaging in order to provide the proof of mechanism and facilitate design of follow-up clinical trials [40,41].

Ultrasound has been shown to help in quantifying changes in tumor perfusion in response to combination therapy [14]. In this study both, an anti-angiogenic mono-therapy and an anti-angiogenic plus a tyrosine kinase inhibitor combination were tested. Under approval of the IACUC, male nude rats (Taconic) were implanted with Huh7.5 human hepatocarcinoma cells suspended in Matrigel. During the first phase of the study (days 5 - 21 after cell inoculation) rats were treated with either vehicle, sunitinib (Sutent®, Pfizer Inc.) or sunitinib plus a FAK/Pyk2 tyrosine kinase inhibitor (PF-562,271). In the second phase of the study the rats switched treatments so that half of vehicle treated rats remained on vehicle, the other half of vehicle treated rats switched to sunitinib + FAK/Pyk2 compound, rats receiving sunitinib alone switched to vehicle while rats receiving sunitinib + FAK/Pyk2 switched to vehicle.

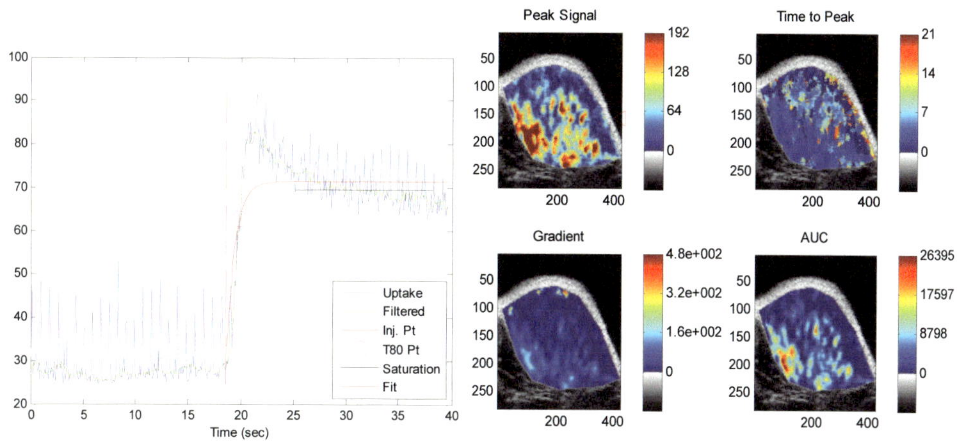

Fig. 7. Examples of parametric maps and uptake curves generated on HCC xenografts using contrast enhanced ultrasound imaging (CEUS).

Using the high-frequency Vevo770 (VisualSonics, Toronto, ON), 3D grayscale volumes were collected along with B-scan cineloops of the center slice of the tumor. These cineloops were collected at 50% power and 100 µl of contrast (MicroMarker, VisualSonics) was given as a slow bolus. Ultrasound imaging, blood and tumor measurements by caliper were collected on day 10, 14, 21, and 28 post cell injection, under isoflurane anesthesia. At the end of the study, day 36, the rats were euthanized and the livers were collected and processed for histology. Ultrasound images were analyzed using in house developed methods based in Matlab (Mathworks). Post processing involved both motion correction and filtering.

Temporal uptake curves were obtained for each pixel, and pseudo-colored parametric maps were created to reflect spatial variation. Regions where the peak signal was less than a predefined threshold were labeled non-perfused. Region averages were then computed to provide data on total peak signal and peak signal without necrosis/non-perfused (Figure 8). Therefore, early testing of anti-angiogenic compounds for proof of mechanism using xenograft model provide valuable data that can be used to improve the design of the studies using orthotopic models as well as to devise a better plan human trials. Non-imaging assessment in the study published by Bagi et al. [13] showed there was a good correlation between results obtained by CEUS and tumor size measured by caliper as well as with serum alpha-fetoprotein levels (tumor cell biomarker).

5. Summary

Preclinical experimentation allows for simultaneous longitudinal implementation of imaging techniques along with use of serum biomarkers to monitor the growth and

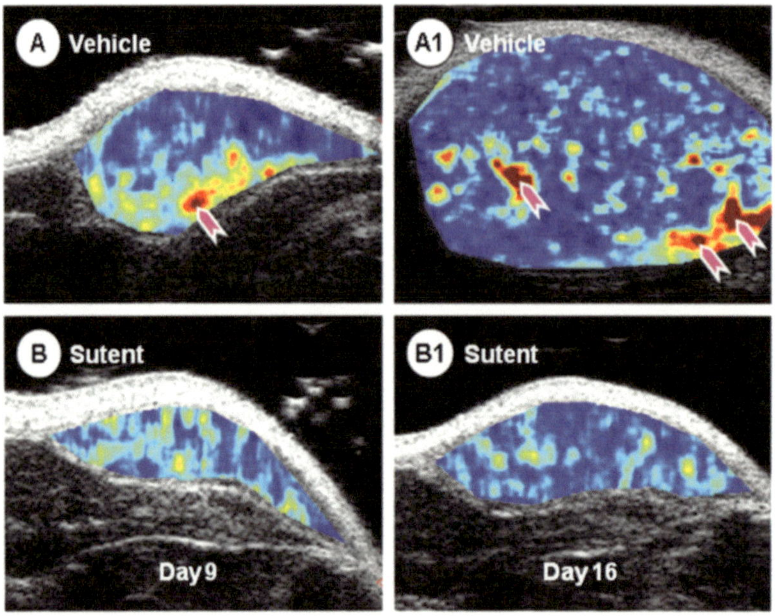

Fig. 8. Representative images obtained by CEUS depicting HCC xenograft treated with vehicle (A) or sunitinib (B) at 2 different time-points. There is a clear difference in tumor size and vascularity between control and treated tumor.

response to treatment of HCC tumors. Although, xenograft and orthotopic models are complementary, and both models have a place in the screening strategy of novel therapies based on the complex vascular events and microenvironment of the liver that plays a role in tumor growth and spreading, only orthotopic liver tumor models can provide the level of complexity that is needed to reliably evaluate the antitumor effects of compounds under investigation in preclinical studies.

The first step to establish the clinical diagnosis of HCC in patients consists of a blood test for elevated AFP concentrations followed by structural imaging utilizing one of several imaging modalities that are currently available including ultrasonography. Ultrasonography has been validated for preclinical and clinical use and it has been one of the most valuable translational tools to assess the efficacy of novel therapies in animal models of HCC as well as in the patients. Additional technological advances toward developing safe contrast agents continue to add value to current ultrasonography methods. Therefore, the thorough preclinical research of HCC should include both, predictive animal models and reliable technologies.

6. References

[1] Blomley MJ, Eckersley RJ (2002) Functional ultrasound methods in oncological imaging. Eur J Cancer 38:2108-21115.

[2] Ferrara KW, Merritt CR, Burns PN, et al. (2000) Evaluation of tumor angiogenesis with US: imaging, Doppler, and contrast agents. Acta Radiol 7:824-839.

[3] Colombo M (1992) Hepatocellular carcinoma. J Hepatol 15:225-236.

[4] Venook AP (1994) Treatment of hepatocellular carcinoma: too many options? J Clin Oncol 12:1323-1334.

[5] Bruix J (1997) Treatment of hepatocellular carcinoma. Hepatol 25:259-261.

[6] Folkman J (1995) Angiogenesis in cancer, vascular, rheumatoid and other diseases. Natl Med 1:27-31.
[7] Hurwitz H (2003) Antiangiogenic therapy plus IFL improves survival for patients with metastatic colorectal cancer. Proc Am Soc Clin Oncol 22:3646a.
[8] Kesisis G, Broxterman H, Giaccone E (2007) Angiogenesis inhibitors. Drug selectivity and target specificity. Current Pharmaceutical Design 13:2795-2809.
[9] Franco M, Man S, Chen L, Emmenegger U, Shaked Y, Cheung AM, Brown AS, Hicklin DJ, Foster FS, Karbel RS (2006) Targeted anti-vascular endothelial growth factor receptor-2 therapy leads to short-term and long-term impairment of vascular function and increase in tumor hypoxia. Cancer Res 66:3639-3648.
[10] Goertz DE, Christopher DA, Yu JL, et al.(2000) High-frequency color flow imaging of the microcirculation. Ultrasound Med Biol 26:63-71.
[11] Gee MS, Saunders HM, Lee JC et al. (2001) Doppler ultrasound imaging detects changes in tumor perfusion during antivascular therapy associated with anatomic alterations. Cancer Res 61:2974-2982.
[12] Rehman S, Jayson GC (2005) Molecular imaging of antiangiogenic agents. The Oncologist 10:92-103.
[13] Bagi C M, Christensen J, et al. (2009) Sunitinib and PF-562,271 (FAK/Pyk2 inhibitor) effectively block growth and recovery of human hepatocellular carcinoma in a rat xenograft model. Cancer Biol Ther 8:856-865.
[14] McCarville MB, Streck CJ, Dickson PV, Li C-S, Nathwani AC, Davidoff AM (2006) Angiogenesis inhibitors in a murine neuroblastoma model: Quantitative assessment of intratumoral blood flow with contrast-enhanced gray-scale US. Radiology 240:73-81.
[15] Lamuraglia M, Escudier B, Chami L, Schwartz B, Leclere J, Roche A, Lassau N (2006) To predict progression-free survival and overall survival in metastatic renal cancer treated with sorafenib: Pilot study using dynamic contrast-enhanced Doppler ultrasound. European J Cancer 42:2472-2479.
[16] Lassau N, Chebil M, Chami L, Roche A (2008) A new functional imaging technique for the early functional evaluation of antiangiogenic treatment: dynamic contrast-enhanced ultrasonography (DCE-US). Targ Oncol 3:111-117.
[17] Bagi CM, Andresen CJ (2010) Models of hepatocellular carcinoma and biomarker strategy. Cancers 2:1441-1452.
[18] Killion JJ, Radinsky R, Fidler IJ (1998) Orthotopic models are necessary to predict therapy of transplantable tumors in mice. Cancer Metastasis Rev 17:279-284.
[19] Frijhoff AF, Conti CJ, Sanderowicz AM (2004) Advances in molecular carcinogenesis: Current and future use of mouse models to screen and validate molecularly targeted anticancer drugs. Mol Carcinog 39:183-194.
[20] Barajas M, Mazzolini G, Genove G, Bilbao R, Narvaiza I, Schmitz V, Sangro B, Melero I, Qian C, Prieto J (2001) Gene therapy of orthotopic hepatocellular carcinoma in rats using adenovirus coding for interleukin 12. Hepatology 33:52-61.
[21] Wilmanns C, Fan D, O'Brian CA, Bucana CD, Fidler IJ (1992) Orthotopic and ectopic organ environments differentially influence the sensitivity of murine colon carcinoma cells to doxorubicin and 5-fluorouracil. Int J Cancer 52:98-104.
[22] Labonte P, Kadhim S, Bowlin T, Mounir S (2000) Inhibition of tumor growth with doxorubicin in a new orthotopically implanted human hepatocellular carcinoma model. Hepatology Res 18:72-85.
[23] Davis HC, Morse IS (1957) Segmental liver revascularization. Arch Surg 74:525-527.

[24] McCuskey RS (1994) The hepatic microvascular system. In *The Liver: Biology and pathology* Ed. Arias IM, Boyer JL, Fausto N, Jacoby BW, Schachter DA, Shafritz DA, New Yourk, Raven Press, pp. 1089-1106.
[25] Rubaltelly L, Del Maschio A, Candiani F, Miotto D (1980) The role of vascularization in the formation of echographic patterns of hepatic metastases: microangiographic and echographic study. Br J Radiology 53:1166-1168.
[26] Archer SG, Gray BN (1989) Vascularization of small liver metastases. Br J Surg 76:545-548.
[27] Nakashima Y, Nakashima O, Hsia CC, Kojiro M, Tabor E (1999) Vascularization of small hepatocellular carcinomas: correlation with differentiation. Liver 19:12-18.
[28] Matsui O, Kadoya M, Kameyama T, Yoshikawa J, Takashima T, Nakanuma Y, Unoura M, Kobayashi K, Izumi R, Ida M (1991)Benign and malignant nodulus in cirrhotic liver: distinction based on blood supply. Radiology 178:493-497.
[29] Foster FS, et al (2002) A new ultrasound instrument for in vivo microimaging of mice. Ultrasound Med Biol 28:1165-1172.
[30] Bekeredjian R, Kroll RD, Fein E, Tinkov S, Coester C, Winter G, Katus HA, Kulaksiz H (2007) Ultrasound targeted microbubble destruction increases capillary permeability in hepatomas. Ultrasound in Med Biol 33:1592-1598.
[31] Kang J, Wu X, Wang Z, Ran H, Xu C, Wu J, Wang Z, Zhang Y (2010) Antitumor effect of docetaxel-loaded lipid microbubbles combined with ultrasound-targeted microbubble activation on VX2 rabbit liver tumors. J Ultrasound Med 29:61-70.
[32] Hastie LC, Graham KC, Groom AC, MacDonald IC, Chambers AF, Fenster A, Lacefield JC (2004) Variability of three-dimensional high-frequency ultrasound measurements of small tumor volumes. Ultrasonics Symposium 3:2185-2188.
[33] Donnelly E F, Geng L, et al. (2001) Quantified power Doppler US of tumor blood flow correlates with microscopic quantification of tumor blood vessels. Radiology 219:66-170.
[34] Palmowski M, et al. 92008) Vessel fractions in tumor xenografts depicted by flow - or contrast-sensitive three-dimensional high-frequency Doppler ultrasound respond differently to antiangiogenic treatment. Cancer Res 68:7042-7049.
[35] Wei K, Jayaweera AR, et al. (1998) Quantification of myocardial blood flow with ultrasound-induced destruction of microbubbles administered as a constant venous infusion. Circulation 97:473-483.
[36] Pollard R E, Broumas AR, et al. (2007) Quantitative contrast enhanced ultrasound and CT assessment of tumor response to antiangiogenic therapy in rats. Ultrasound Med Biol 33: 35-245.
[37] Averkiou M, Lampaskis M, et al. (2010) Quantification of tumor microvascularity with respiratory gated contrast enhanced ultrasound for monitoring therapy. Ultrasound Med Biol 36:68-77.
[38] Hu-Lowe D D, Chen E, et al. (2011) Targeting activin receptor-like kinase 1 inhibits angiogenesis and tumorigenesis through a mechanism of action complementary to anti-VEGF therapies. Cancer Res 71:1362-1373.
[39] Euhus DM, Hudd C, et al. (1986) Tumor measurement in the nude mouse. J Surg Oncol 31:229-234.
[40] Goertz DE, Yu JL, Kerbel RS, Burns PN, Foster FS (2002) High frequency Doppler ultrasound monitors the effects of antivascular therapy on blood flow. Cancer Res 62:6371-6375.
[41] Peters-Engl C, Medl M, Mirau M et al. (1998) Color-coded and spectral Doppler flow in breast carcinomas - relationship with the tumor microvasculature. Breast Cancer Res Treat 47:83-89.

16

Feasibility of Clinical Application of Ultrasound Molecular Imaging

Kentaro Otani
Department of Regenerative Medicine and Tissue Engineering
National Cerebral and Cardiovascular Center Research Institute
Japan

1. Introduction

Ultrasound imaging has been utilized for the non-invasive and real-time observation of pathophysiological conditions in clinical settings. To enhance blood flow signals, microbubbles that are quite different in acoustic impedance from blood have been utilized as the contrast agent for ultrasound imaging. Unfortunately, the initial performance of intravenous contrast-enhanced ultrasound imaging was hampered by the pulmonary circulation due to the size of the microbubbles. Additionally, the detection of microbubbles was not easy because of the weak signals derived from the bubbles. However, recent improvements in the bubble physics and ultrasound imaging technologies have enabled non-invasive assessment of organ perfusion by intravenous administration of microbubbles (Chahal & Senior, 2010; Porter & Xie, 2010; Wilson & Burns, 2010). Of note, the fate of intravenously administrated microbubbles is similar to that of red blood cells (Keller et al., 1989; Jayaweera et al., 1994). Many contrast agents for contrast-enhanced ultrasound imaging are now clinically available all over the world (Table 1).

On the other hand, ultrasound molecular imaging, which visualizes molecular dynamics in situ by detecting the signals derived from retained microbubbles in the target regions, has been recently developed. As microbubbles are the intravascular blood flow tracer, ultrasound molecular imaging predominantly targets activated leukocytes and molecules expressed on endothelial cells. Many papers have been published regarding the diagnostic utility of ultrasound molecular imaging for the detection of inflammation, atherosclerosis and tumor angiogenesis (Villanueva & Wagner, 2008; Leong-Poi, 2009; Lindner, 2009; Chadderdon & Kaul, 2010; Deshpande et al., 2010).

The utility of molecular imaging has been demonstrated using several modalities, including positron emission tomography (PET), magnetic resonance imaging (MRI) and near-infrared fluorescence (NIRF) (Jaffer & Weissleder, 2005). Although PET and MRI provide accurate diagnostic information, the versatility of these two modalities is limited. On the other hand, ultrasound examination is cost effective and is able to be performed at the bedside. Therefore, the adaptation of ultrasound molecular imaging for clinical settings is desired.

For the clinical translation of ultrasound molecular imaging, however, some bottlenecks need to be overcome at the same time, including the development of clinically translatable targeted bubbles and the improvement of ultrasound imaging techniques. This chapter summarizes the recent advances in the preparation of targeted bubbles and ultrasound imaging technologies for realizing the clinical translation of ultrasound molecular imaging in the near future.

	Core gas	Shell composition	Mean diameter
Levovist *Bayer Yakuhin, Ltd.* *Osaka, Japan*	Air	Palmitic acid	2.0-3.0 μm
Optison *GE Healthcare* *Buckinghamshire, UK*	C_3F_8	Human serum albumin	3.0 – 4.5 μm
Definity *Lantheus Medical Imaging, Inc.* *N. Billerica, MA*	C_3F_8	Phospholipid	1.1-3.3 μm
Sonovue *Bracco Imaging SpA* *Milan, Italy*	SF_6	Phospholipid	2.5 μm
Sonazoid *Daiichi-Sankyo Co., Ltd.* *Tokyo, Japan*	C_4F_{10}	Hydrogenated egg phosphatidylserine	2.0-3.0 μm

Table 1. Commercially available ultrasound contrast agents

2. Recent progress in development of targeted bubbles

In the previously reported animal studies with ultrasound molecular imaging, various intravital molecules have served as target molecules (Chadderdon & Kaul, 2010; Hwang et al., 2010). In ultrasound molecular imaging, the methodology for accumulating bubbles at a specific target is a principal issue. Until now, two types of bubbles have been developed to achieve this purpose, including non-targeted and targeted bubbles (Dayton & Rychak, 2007; Deshpande et al., 2010) (Table 2).

	Method to modify bubbles	Application
Non-targeted bubbles	Incorporate phospholipids/lipids into bubble shell by sonication	Inflammation imaging, Kupffer imaging
Targeted bubbles	Attach ligands onto bubble surface via covalent/non-covalent coupling	Overall

Table 2. Two types of bubbles for ultrasound molecular imaging

Non-targeted bubbles contain phosphatidylserine (PS) or other lipids in their shell components, and have been utilized as the contrast agent for inflammation and Kupffer cell imaging (Lindner et al., 2000; Christiansen et al., 2002; Watanabe et al., 2007; Yanagisawa et al., 2007). On the other hand, targeted bubbles bear antibodies or peptides on the surface of the shell via chemical conjugation, including covalent or non-covalent coupling methods (Hernot & Klibanov, 2008; Deshpande et al., 2010). Several kinds of potential covalent coupling reaction have been considered for the attachment of ligands onto the surface of bubbles (Klibanov, 2005; Kiessling et al., 2009) (Table 3). However, the major method for ligand attachment in recent ultrasound molecular imaging studies was non-covalent avidin-biotin complex formation because of its versatility.

	Primary coupling reaction
Covalent coupling	Carboxylic Acid (-COOH) / Amine ($-NH_2$)
	Maleimide / Thiol (-SH)
	Aldehyde (-CHO) / Amine ($-NH_2$) etc.
Non-covalent coupling	Biotin / Avidin or Streptavidin

Table 3. Coupling strategies for attachment of ligands onto bubble shell

It is well known that the binding between biotin and streptavidin exhibits extremely high affinity (dissociation constant ~10^{-15}); however, at the same time, streptavidin is a major barrier for clinical translation of targeted bubbles. Because of the immunogenicity of streptavidin, repeated injection of streptavidin-containing bubbles is difficult in humans (Marshall et al., 1996; Carter, 2001). Therefore, the development of targeted bubbles that do not contain streptavidin is necessary for the clinical translation of ultrasound molecular imaging.

2.1 Commercially available targeted bubbles for basic research

Because of its difficulty, the preparation of targeted bubbles has been a principal issue in ultrasound molecular imaging. Fortunately, several targeted bubbles only for use in basic research have been developed recently; MicroMarker® (VisualSonics Inc., Toronto, Canada) and Targestar™/Visistar™ (Targeson Inc., San Diego, CA, USA). Because of their versatility, these bubbles have been well utilized in in vivo studies (Rychak et al., 2007; Willmann et al., 2008a, 2008b, 2010; Barreiro et al., 2009). However, the clinical application of these bubbles is difficult in the present condition because of the use of streptavidin as a mediator between bubbles and ligands.

2.2 Chemical modification to improve targetability of bubbles

For ultrasound molecular imaging, improvement of the targetability of ligand-bearing bubbles to the disease-related intravital molecule is a principal issue. To this end, several chemical modifications have been recently applied to targeted bubbles (Klibanov, 2009; Gessner & Dayton, 2010). Firstly, Klibanov et al. conjugated clustered polymeric forms of ligands onto the surface of the bubble shell to increase the surface density of ligands

(Klibanov et al., 2006b). Secondly, targeted bubbles for two intravital molecules have been developed by simultaneous conjugation of two kinds of ligands onto the bubble shell (Weller et al., 2005; Willmann et al., 2008b; Ferrante et al., 2009). However, dense ligands, especially antibodies on the bubble surface would increase the risk of non-specific binding and immunogenic responses at the same time. To overcome this issue, Borden et al. developed "stealth bubbles" those ligands were buried in a forest of long polyethylene glycol (PEG)-brushes (Borden et al., 2008). In this stealth bubble, a radiation force was required to induce emergence and activation of the buried ligands. Therefore, the utilization of buried ligands might enable the development of targeted bubbles with both low non-specific binding and low immunogenic response.

2.3 Streptavidin-free targeted ultrasound contrast agents

Recently, several approaches for the preparation of targeted bubbles without streptavidin have been demonstrated. Anderson et al. utilized covalent maleimide-thiol coupling for conjugating the targeting ligands onto the bubble shell (Anderson et al., 2010). As well as avidin-biotin binding, this covalent coupling approach would be applicable to a wide variety of ligands in the near future. Meanwhile, novel vascular endothelial growth factor 2 (VEGFR2)-specific bubbles; BR55, which contains a lipopeptide construct in the bubble shell, was recently developed (Pysz et al., 2010; Pochon et al., 2010; Tardy et al., 2010). Since BR55 contains neither antibodies nor biotin/streptavidin complex, the clinical translation of targeted bubbles for angiogenesis without an immunogenic response might be feasible by using BR55.

2.4 Preparation of targeted bubbles based on clinically available bubbles

To achieve easy translation of ultrasound molecular imaging in clinical settings, we considered that the easiest approach would be the preparation of targeted bubbles based on a clinically available ultrasound contrast agent. However, there have been no reports regarding the preparation of targeted bubbles based on a clinically available contrast agent.
Sonazoid, a clinically available ultrasound contrast agent in Japan, consists of perfluorobutane gas microbubbles stabilized by a membrane of hydrogenated egg PS (Sontum, 2008). Generally, PS is well known as an important molecule in the cellular apoptotic process, especially in the clearance of apoptotic cells (Wu et al., 2006; Nagata et al., 2010). Under normal physiological conditions, PS is sequestered from the cell surface by phospholipid translocators, known as flippases. However, this process is interrupted during apoptosis and PS translocates to the cell surface. This translocation of PS triggers the recognition and removal of apoptotic cells by phagocytes. In the field of apoptotic research, annexin V has been well utilized for detecting PS-expressing apoptotic cells (Vermes et al., 1995). Recently, the clinical availability of annexin V for the detection of apoptosis or plaque instability was demonstrated (Hofstra et al., 2000; Narula et al., 2001; Kietselaer et al., 2004).
In ultrasound molecular imaging, PS-containing bubbles have been utilized as targeted bubbles for activated leukocytes (Lindner et al., 2000; Christiansen et al., 2002). Interestingly, PS-containing bubbles were labeled with annexin V as well as apoptotic cells (Lindner et al., 2000). Based on this result, we hypothesized that preparation of antibody-carrying bubbles based on Sonazoid could be feasible by detecting PS in Sonazoid with annexin V and utilizing avidin-biotin complex formation (Figure 1).

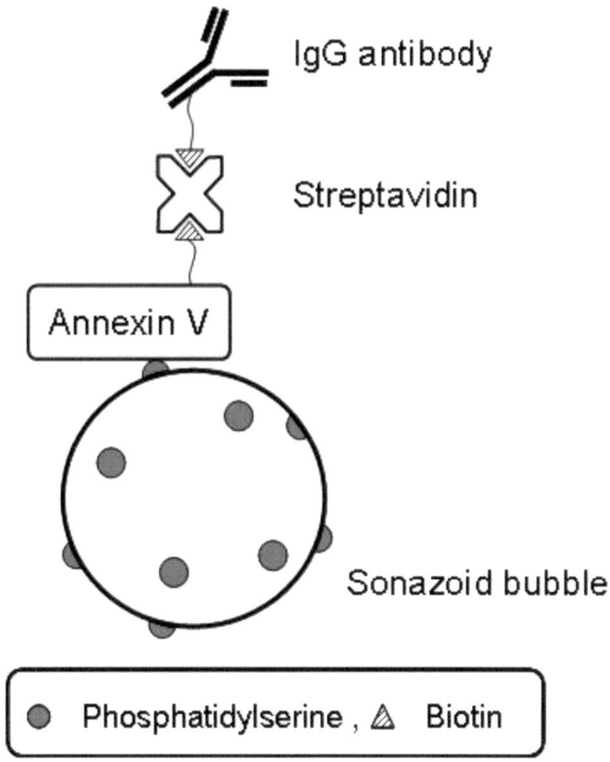

Fig. 1. Theoretical schema of IgG antibody-carrying bubbles based on Sonazoid through use of annexin V and avidin-biotin complex formation.

As annexin V is a well-known protein that detects PS in a Ca^{2+}-dependent manner, we firstly examined the effect of Ca^{2+} addition on Sonazoid bubbles. By adding a higher concentration of $CaCl_2$, obvious and significant aggregation of bubbles was observed (Figure 2A). The size distribution histogram was markedly smaller after the addition of 0.25 mmol/L $CaCl_2$ than that of naked Sonazoid bubbles (Figure 2B). Additionally, the bubble concentration was markedly reduced after the addition of 0.25 mmol/L $CaCl_2$ (naked Sonazoid: 5.3×10^8 bubbles/mL vs. 0.25 mmol/L $CaCl_2$: 7.0×10^7 bubbles/mL). This phenomenon was considered to result from neutralization of the surface charge of Sonazoid bubbles (Otani & Yamahara, 2011). However, bubble number was not decreased after the addition of 0.05 mmol/L $CaCl_2$ (5.8×10^8 bubbles/mL) (Figure 2B). Therefore, the following experiments were performed in the presence of 0.05 mmol/L $CaCl_2$, which did not induce obvious aggregation of Sonazoid bubbles.

Secondly, the attachment of annexin V to the PS in Sonazoid bubbles was examined using fluorescein isothiocianate (FITC)-conjugated annexin V. The fluorescent signal was determined by FACSCalibur (BD Bioscience, San Jose, CA, USA). Even in the condition with low Ca^{2+}, FITC-positive bubbles were observed after the conjugation of Sonazoid bubbles with FITC-annexin V (Figure 3). In contrast, the fluorescent signal derived from bubbles after conjugation in the absence of Ca^{2+} was significantly reduced. These results imply that the PS in Sonazoid could be detected by using annexin V even in the condition of 0.05 mmol/L $CaCl_2$ (Otani & Yamahara, 2011).

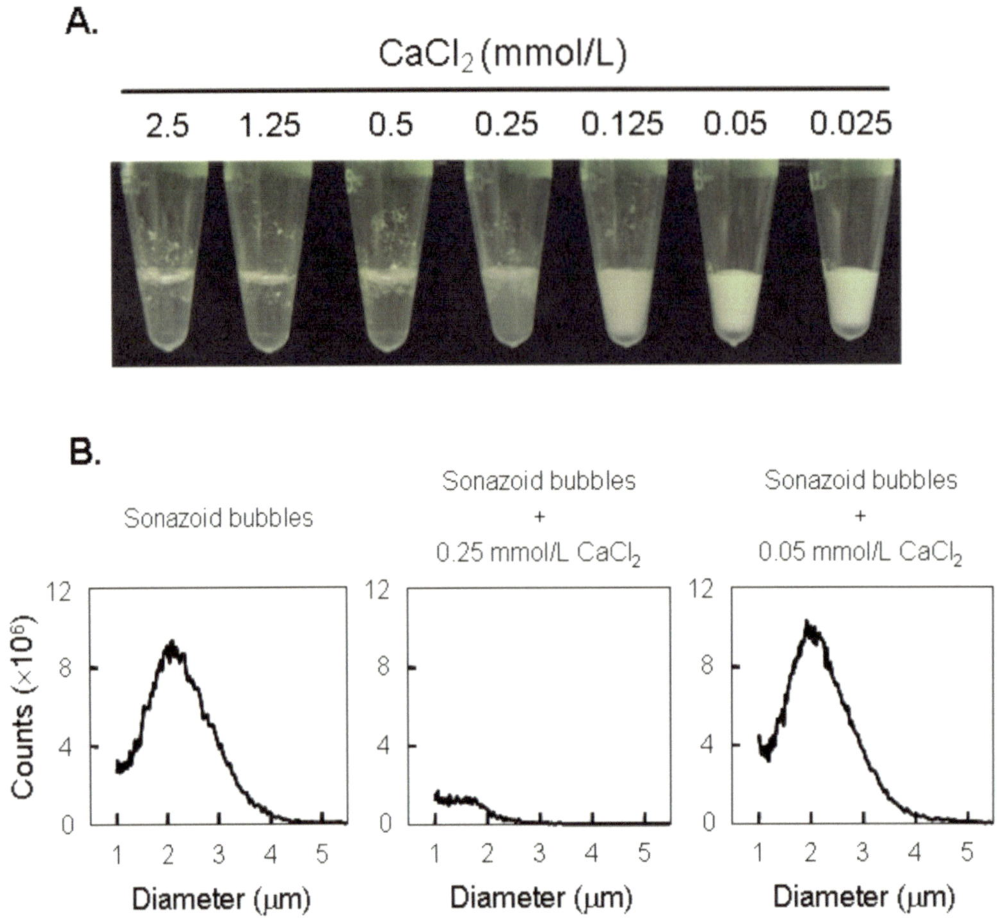

Fig. 2. Changes of Sonazoid bubbles after addition of $CaCl_2$. A) At 30 minutes after addition of $CaCl_2$, obvious bubble aggregation was observed when the concentration of $CaCl_2$ was 0.25 mmol/L or higher. B) The size distribution of Sonazoid bubbles was markedly altered at 45 minutes after 0.25 mmol/L $CaCl_2$ addition. (Reproduced from Otani et al. with permission)

Thirdly, we examined whether streptavidin could detect biotinylated-Sonazoid bubbles with annexin V. Sonazoid bubbles were conjugated with biotinylated-annexin V followed by R-phycoerythrin (PE)-conjugated streptavidin. A strong PE signal was detected from Sonazoid bubbles in the presence of biotinylated-annexin V (Figure 4). However, the PE signal was obviously weaker in the absence of biotinylated-annexin V. These results imply that streptavidn could attach to the surface of Sonazoid via avidin-biotin binding.

Finally, we examined whether the attachment of IgG antibodies onto the surface of Sonazoid bubbles is feasible via annexin V and avidin-biotin complex formation. Sonazoid bubbles were conjugated with biotinylated-annexin V followed by streptavidin and biotinylated-Alexa488-IgG. As shown in Figure 5A, Alexa488-positive bubbles were confirmed by FACS analysis (Otani & Yamahara, 2011). However, the suspension of targeted-Sonazoid bubbles was obviously thinner than that of naked Sonazoid bubbles (Figure 5B).

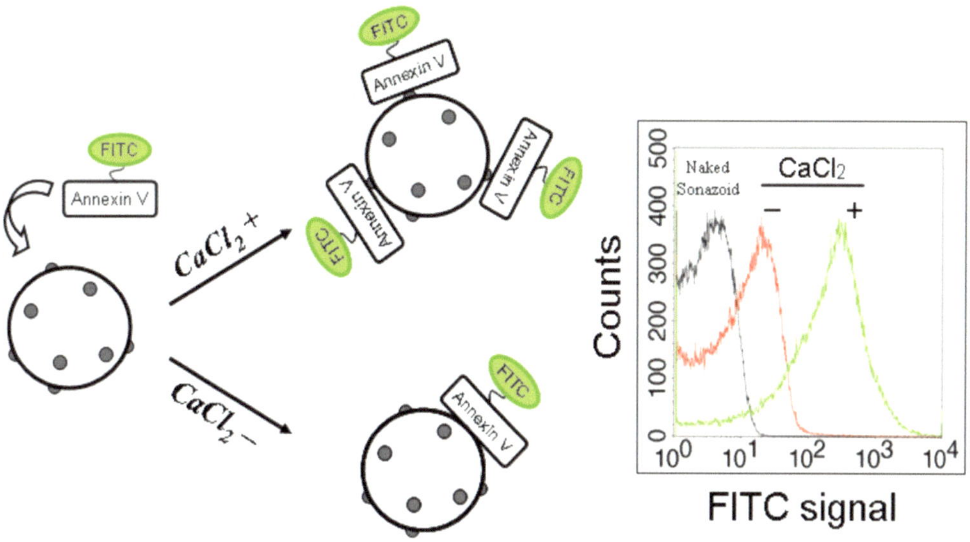

Fig. 3. Attachment of annexin V to PS on surface of Sonazoid bubble. In the presence of $CaCl_2$, FITC-positive bubbles were detected after the conjugation of Sonazoid bubbles with FITC-annexin V. In contrast, the FITC signal derived from Sonazoid bubbles was markedly reduced in the absence of $CaCl_2$. (Reproduced from Otani et al. with permission)

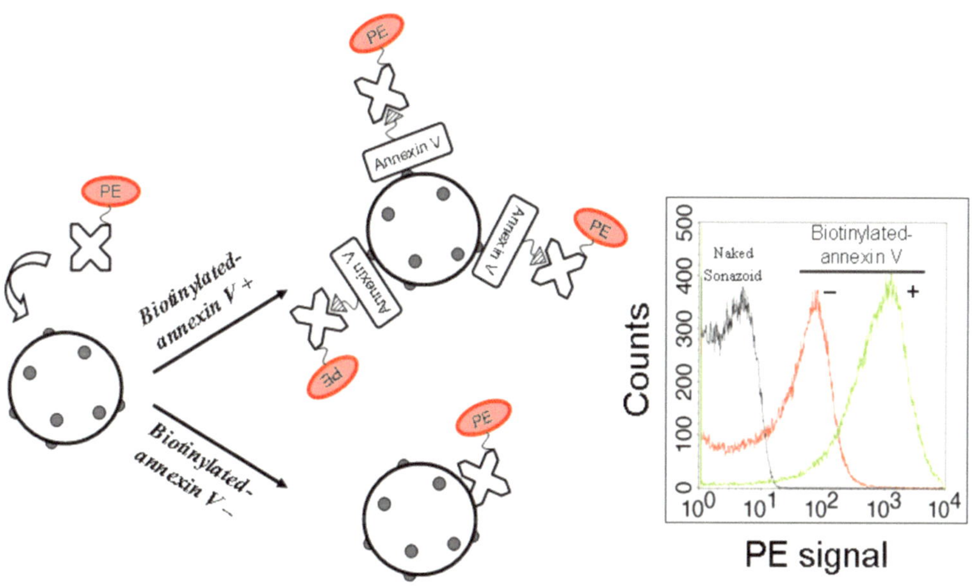

Fig. 4. Attachment of streptavidin to surface of Sonazoid bubble via avidin-biotin binding. PE-positive bubbles were detected after conjugation of Sonazoid bubbles with biotinylated-annexin V followed by PE-conjugated streptavidin. However, the PE signal was markedly reduced in the absence of biotinylated-annexin V. (Reproduced from Otani et al. with permission)

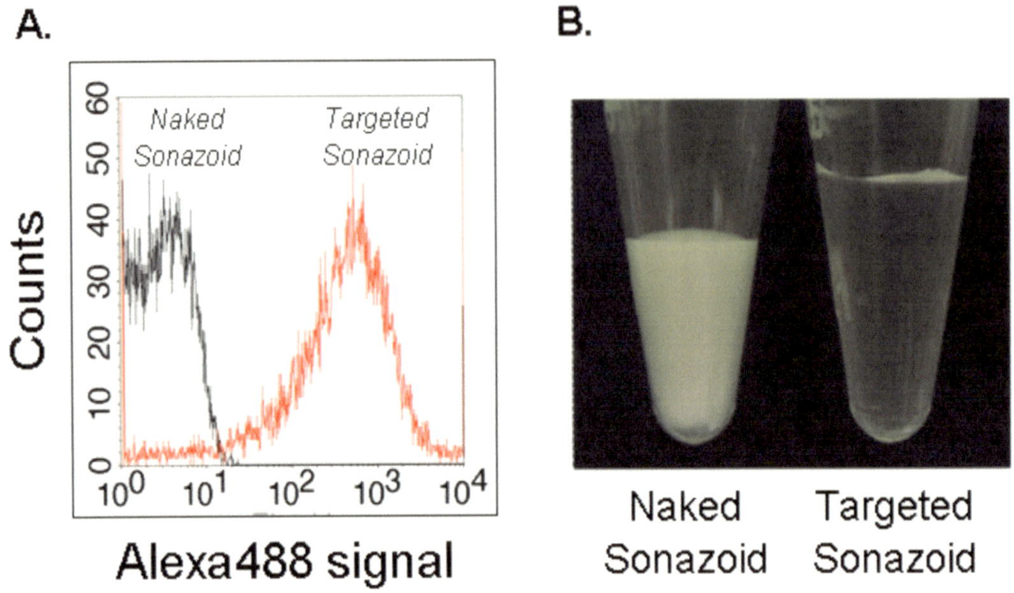

Fig. 5. IgG-carrying bubbles based on Sonazoid. A) Alexa488-positive Sonazoid bubbles were confirmed after conjugation with biotinylated-annexin V followed by streptavidin and biotinylated-Alexa488-IgG. B) The concentration of targeted bubbles based on Sonazoid was obviously lower than that of naked Sonazoid bubbles. (Reproduced from Otani et al. with permission)

Although our preliminary results demonstrated the feasibility of preparation of targeted bubbles based on clinically available microbubbles Sonazoid, the translation of targeted Sonazoid bubbles to in vivo settings would be difficult in the present circumstances because of the decrease of bubble number and the use of streptavidin. However, our results imply that PS in Sonazoid bubbles has the potential to be a mediator of targeted bubbles based on Sonazoid.

2.5 Improvement of targeted sonazoid by using lactadherin

PS is well known as an important molecule for the clearance of apoptotic cells, and several kinds of proteins that bind with PS have been discovered (Wu et al., 2006; Nagata et al., 2010). Milk fat globule epithelial growth factor 8 (MFG-E8)/lactadherin is a glycoprotein which was originally identified as a component of milk fat globules (Stubbs et al., 1990). Lactadherin contains a PS-binding C-domain and an RGD (arginine-glycine-aspartate)-motif present in the epidermal growth factor domain, which binds to integrins $\alpha v\beta 3$ and $\alpha v\beta 5$ (Andersen et al., 2000; Hanayama et al., 2002; Yamaguchi et al., 2008). It is well known that the recognition of PS by lactadherin is Ca^{2+}-independent (Shi et al., 2003; Dasgupta et al., 2006). Therefore, we examined whether PS in Sonazoid could be detected using PE-conjugated lactadherin instead of annexin V (Figure 6A). By conjugating Sonazoid bubbles with PE-labeled lactadherin, PE-positive bubbles were detected by FACS analysis (Figure 6B, *unpublished data*).

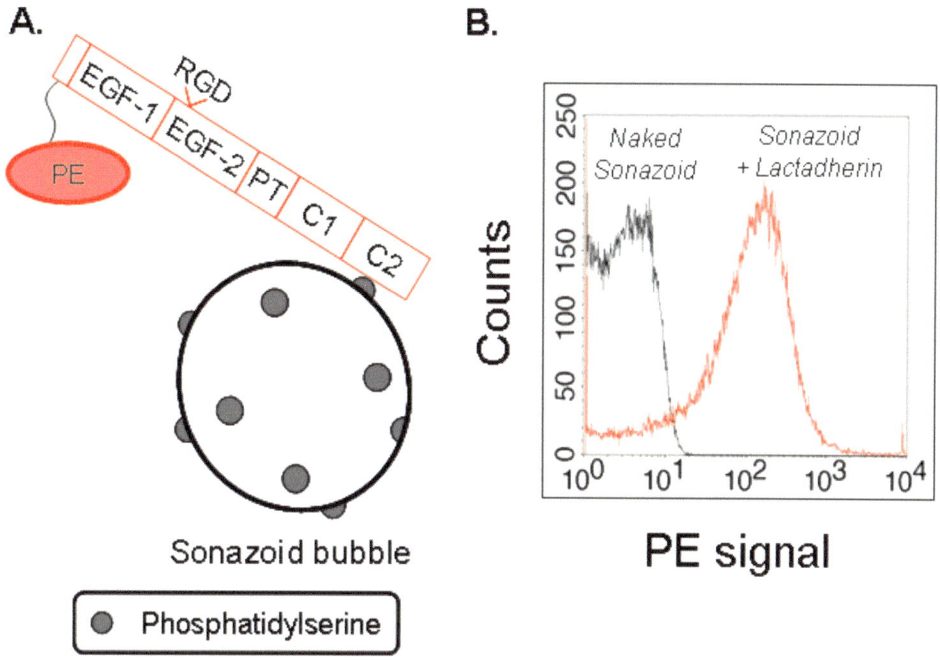

Fig. 6. Detection of PS in Sonazoid using lactadherin. A) Schema of expected binding between Sonazoid bubbles and PE-conjugated lactadherin. B) After conjugation with PE-lactadherin, the presence of PE-positive Sonazoid bubbles was confirmed.

Because of the unnecessity of Ca^{2+} addition in the case of lactadherin, no obvious aggregation or decrease in number of bubbles was observed during the preparation of lactadherin-bearing bubbles (data not shown). Although the binding between Sonazoid bubbles and annexin V was fragile, robust binding with PS in Sonazoid was achieved using lactadherin (Figure 7). These results imply that lactadherin is superior to annexin V in regard to the detection of PS in Sonazoid bubbles. As lactadherin has a RGD motif in its epidermal growth factor domain, lactadherin-bearing Sonazoid bubbles might have the potential to attach to integrin αvβ3-expressing cells. Furthermore, lactadherin-bearing Sonazoid bubbles might be a novel targeted bubble for angiogenesis, because the integrin αvβ3 is well known to play a key role in angiogenesis (Friedlander et al., 1995). Therefore, further study to examine the potential of lactadherin-bearing Sonazoid bubbles both in vitro and in vivo would be of benefit.

Although the feasibility of preparation of targeted bubbles based on a clinically available ultrasound contrast agent was demonstrated in our present study, there are some concerns with lactadherin-bearing Sonazoid bubbles at the present time. The most important issue is the direct conjugation of lactadherin onto the bubble shell. This might influence: 1) the efficiency of attachment to the target molecule (integrin αvβ3) both in vitro and in vivo studies, and 2) the surface density of ligands. The majority of recent targeted bubbles contain long PEG spacer arms on the bubble surface to project ligands away from the surface of the bubble shell (Klibanov, 2006a; Lindner, 2010). This projection of ligands resulted in improvement of flexibility and targetability of bubbles. Furthermore, the surface density of ligands would be lower in the case of direct conjugation of ligands to the bubble shell. In these regards, the efficiency of attachment of lactadherin-bearing Sonazoid bubbles to integrin αvβ3-expressing cells might be low. This concern should be clarified by further study.

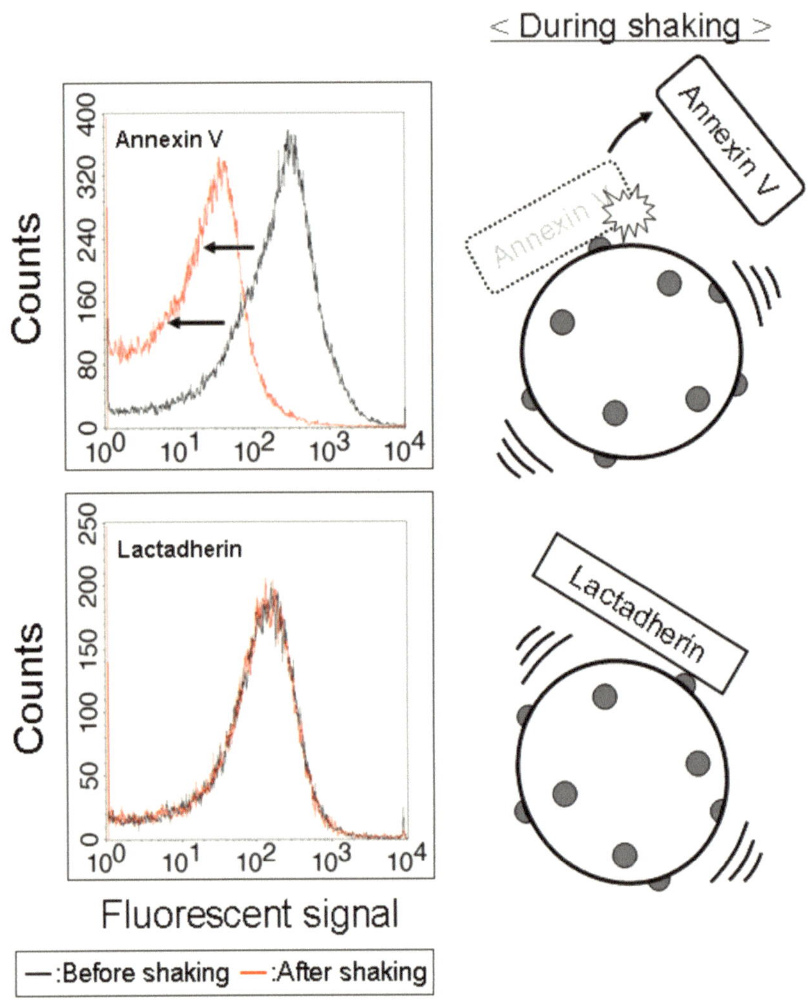

Fig. 7. Stability of annexin V- and lactadherin-bearing Sonazoid bubbles. Compared to annexin V-bearing Sonazoid bubbles, lactadherin-conjugated bubbles were more resistant to violent shaking. (Reproduced from Otani et al. with permission)

3. Improvement of ultrasound technology

In conjunction with the development of targeted bubbles, improvement of ultrasound technology is also an essential issue in ultrasound molecular imaging. Unlike conventional contrast-enhanced ultrasound imaging, the number of retained bubbles to the target region is quite small. Therefore, a more sensitive ultrasound detection technique would be required for the clinical translation of ultrasound molecular imaging. Additionally, a bubble-specific imaging method that suppresses signals from surrounding tissues, to emphasize the ultrasound signals derived from bubbles, would be a help for accurate observation of molecular dynamics.

3.1 Evolution of ultrasound detection techniques

Contrast-enhanced ultrasound imaging visualizes the signals derived from microbubbles. Under high mechanical index (MI) ultrasound exposure, bubbles exhibit unique scattering behavior. By utilizing this characteristic, harmonic imaging, especially second harmonic imaging, has been developed at an early stage of contrast-enhanced ultrasound imaging (Porter et al., 1996). In addition, the Doppler technique has been applied for sensitive detection of bubbles (harmonic power Doppler imaging). Until now, several harmonic imaging techniques including subharmonic, 1.5 harmonic and ultraharmonic imaging have been developed (Table 4). However, high MI ultrasound exposure resulted in the destruction of bubbles - the source of acoustic signals. Therefore, intermittent exposure is inevitable for acquiring contrast-enhanced images in high MI imaging. As a result, real-time observation of contrast enhancement has not been achieved in high MI imaging. To overcome this issue, real-time imaging which utilizes low power ultrasound has been developed in conjunction with high MI imaging techniques. Until now, several techniques that detect the bubble signal efficiently with multiple ultrasound pulses have been developed, including pulse inversion, power pulse inversion, power modulation, coherent contrast imaging and cadence pulse sequencing (Table 4).

	Imaging mode	References
High MI imaging techniques (for intermittent observation)	**Subharmonic imaging**	*Forsberg et al., 2000*
	1.5 harmonic imaging	*Toshida et al., 2005*
	Ultraharmonic imaging	*Kuersten et al., 2001*
	Harmonic power Doppler	*Heinle et al., 2000*
Low MI imaging techniques (for real-time observation)	**Pulse inversion**	*Burns et al., 2000*
	Power pulse inversion	*Tiemann et al., 1999*
	Power modulation	*Caiani et al., 2005*
	Coherent contrast imaging	*Otani et al., 2004*
	Cadence pulse sequencing	*Phillips, 2001*

Table 4. Imaging technologies for contrast-enhanced ultrasound imaging

Compared to conventional contrast-enhanced ultrasound imaging, the number of retained or attached bubbles to the target region in ultrasound molecular imaging is quite small. Additionally, the sensitivity for bubble detection in high MI imaging is higher than that in low MI real-time imaging. Therefore, early examination of ultrasound molecular imaging had been performed using high MI, intermittent imaging (Lindner et al., 2001; Leong-Poi et al., 2003). However, high MI imaging interferes with the continuous imaging of molecular dynamics, due to the destruction of retained or attached bubbles. Recently, low MI, real-time imaging has been applied in ultrasound molecular imaging (Kaufmann et al., 2007; Stieger et al., 2008). Although the acoustic signal derived from targeted bubbles in low MI real-time imaging was weaker than that in high MI imaging, real-time ultrasound molecular imaging would enable temporal and spatial recognition of molecular dynamics (Kaufmann et al., 2010). Additionally, Klibanov et al. reported the feasibility of individual bubble detection using low MI ultrasound imaging (Klibanov et al., 2004). This result implied that the sensitivity of low MI ultrasound techniques would be sufficient for application to ultrasound molecular imaging.

3.2 Specialized ultrasound machine for small animal research

In previous small animal studies on ultrasound perfusion and molecular imaging, the detection of bubbles has been performed using clinically available ultrasound imaging systems (Weller et al., 2003; Otani et al., 2008). Recently, high resolution ultrasound imaging systems specialized for small animal experiments have been developed (Vevo770 and Vevo2100; VisualSonics Inc., Toronto, Canada). Several recent basic research studies on ultrasound molecular imaging have utilized these machines (Rychak et al., 2007; Willmann et al., 2008a, 2008b, 2010). Because of the usage of too high frequency ultrasound (center frequency; ~ 55 MHz), this machine would not be suitable for clinical use. However, the accumulated results from genetically-modified animal studies using these instruments will be of much help for the clinical translation of ultrasound molecular imaging.

4. Conclusion and future direction

Contrast-enhanced ultrasound imaging has been applied in clinical settings, and its usability has also been demonstrated all over the world. On the other hand, the utility of ultrasound molecular imaging has been proved by many animal studies. Therefore, the development of clinically translatable targeted bubbles has potential for spreading ultrasound molecular imaging into clinical settings rapidly. In parallel with perfusion or molecular imaging, the potential of microbubbles as a carrier for drug or gene delivery into cells has been demonstrated recently in both in vitro and in vivo studies (Liu et al., 2006; Otani et al., 2009; Tinkov et al., 2009). The combination of these features might lead to the localized delivery of drugs or genes into target cells in vivo. Although further study is required, progress in targeted bubbles physics and ultrasound imaging technologies might realize the clinical application of ultrasound molecular imaging and the development of non-invasive localized drug/gene delivery systems in the near future.

5. Acknowledgement

This work was supported by a Grant-in-Aid for Young Scientists (B) from the Ministry of Education, Culture, Sports, Science and Technology (MEXT).

6. References

Andersen, MH., Graversen, H., Fedosov, SN., Petersen, TE., & Rasmussen, JT. (2000). Functional analysis of two cellular binding domains of bovine lactadherin. *Biochemistry*, 39, pp. 6200-6206, ISSN 0006-2960.

Anderson, CR., Rychak, JJ., Backer, M., Backer, J., Ley, K., & Klibanov, AL. (2011). scVEGF microbubble ultrasound contrast agents: a novel probe for ultrasound molecular imaging of tumor angiogenesis. *Invest Radiol*, 45, pp. 579-585, ISSN 0020-9996.

Barreiro, O., Aguilar, RJ., Tejera, E., Megías, D., de Torres-Alba, F., Evangelista, A., & Sánchez-Madrid, F. (2009). Specific targeting of human inflamed endothelium and in situ vascular tissue transfection by the use of ultrasound contrast agents. *J Am Coll Cardiol Img*, 2, pp. 997-1005, ISSN 1936-878X.

Borden, MA., Zhang, H., Gillies, RJ., Dayton, PA., & Ferrara, KW. (2008). A stimulus-responsive contrast agent for ultrasound molecular imaging. *Biomaterials*, 29, pp. 597-606, ISSN 0142-9612.

Burns, PN., Wilson, SR., & Simpson, DH. (2000). Pulse inversion imaging of liver blood flow: improved method for characterizing focal masses with microbubble contrast. *Invest Radiol*, 35, pp. 58-71, ISSN 0020-9996.

Caiani, EG., Lang, RM., DeCara, J., Bednarz, JE., Weinert, L., Korcarz, CE., Collins, KA., & Mor-Avi, V. (2005). Objective assessment of left ventricular wall motion from contrast-enhanced power modulation images. *J Am Soc Echocardiogr*, 15, pp. 118-128, ISSN 0894-7317.

Carter, P. (2001). Improving the efficacy of antibody-based cancer therapies. *Nat Rev Cancer*, 1, pp. 118-129, ISSN 1474-175X.

Chadderdon, SM., & Kaul, S. (2010). Molecular imaging with contrast enhanced ultrasound. *J Nucl Cardiol*, 17, pp. 667-677, ISSN 1071-3581.

Chahal, NS., & Senior, R. (2010). Clinical applications of left ventricular opacification. *J Am Coll Cardiol Img*, 3, pp. 188-196, ISSN 1936-878X.

Cristiansen, JP., Leong-Poi, H., Klibanov, AL., Kaul, S., & Lindner, JR. (2002). Noninvasive imaging of myocardial reperfusion injury using leukocyte-targeted contrast echocardiography. *Circulation*, 105, pp. 1764-1767, ISSN 0009-7322.

Dasgupta, SK., Guchhait, P., & Thiagarajan, P. (2006). Lactadherin binding and phosphatidylserine expression on cell surface-comparison with annexin A5. *Transl Res*, 148, pp. 19-25, ISSN 1931-5244.

Dayton, PA., & Rychak, JJ. (2007). Molecular ultrasound imaging using microbubble contrast agents. *Front Biosci*, 12, pp. 5124-5142. ISSN 1093-9946.

Deshpande, N., Pysz, MA., & Willmann, JK. (2010). Molecular ultrasound assessment of tumor angiogenesis. *Angiogenesis*, 13, pp. 175-188, ISSN 0969-6970.

Ferrante, EA., Pickard, JE., Rychak, J., Klibanov, A., & Ley, K. (2009). Dual targeting improves microbubble contrast agent adhesion to VCAM-1 and P-selectin under flow. *J Control Release*, 140, pp. 100-107, ISSN 0168-3659.

Forsberg, F., Shi, WT., & Goldberg, BB. (2000). Subharmonic imaging of contrast agents. *Ultrasonics*, 38, pp. 93-98, ISSN 0041-624X.

Friedlander, M., Brooks, PC., Shaffer, RW., Kincaid, CM., Varner, JA., & Cheresh, DA. (1995) Definition of two angiogenic pathways by distinct alpha v integrins. *Science*, 270, pp. 1500-1502, ISSN 0036-8075.

Gessner, R., & Dayton, PA. (2010). Advances in molecular imaging with ultrasound. *Mol Imaging*, 9, pp. 117-127, ISSN 1535-3508.

Hanayama, R., Tanaka, M., Miwa, K., Shinohara, A., Iwamatsu, A., & Nagata, S. (2002). Identification of a factor links apoptotic cells to phagocytes. *Nature*, 417, pp. 182-187, ISSN 0028-0836.

Heinle, SK., Noblin, J., Goree-Best, P., Mello, A., Ravad, G., Mull, S., Mammen, P., & Grayburn, PA. (2000). Assessment of myocardial perfusion by harmonic power Doppler imaging at rest and during adenosine stress: comparison with ^{99m}Tc-sestamibi SPECT imaging. *Circulation*, 102, pp. 55-60, ISSN 0009-7322.

Hernot, S., & Klibanov, AL. (2008). Microbubbles in ultrasound-triggered drug gene delivery. *Adv Drug Deliv Rev*, 60, pp. 1153-1166, ISSN 0169-409X.

Hofstra, L., Liem, IH., Dumont, EA., Boersma, HH., van Heerde, WL., Doevendans, PA., DeMuinck, E., Wellens, HJ., Kemerink, GJ., Reutelingsperger, CP., & Heidendal, GA. (2000). Visualisation of cell death in vivo in patients with acute myocardial infarction. *Lancet*, 356, pp. 209-212, ISSN 0140-6736.

Hwang, M., Lyshchik, A., & Fleischer, AC. (2010). Molecular sonography with targeted microbubbles: current investigations and potential applications. *Ultrasound Q*, 26, pp. 75-82, ISSN 0894-8771.

Jaffer, FA., & Weissleder, R. (2005). Molecular imaging in the clinical arena. *JAMA*, 293, pp. 855-862, ISSN 0098-7484.

Jayaweera, AR., Edwards, N., Glasheen, WP., Villanueva, FS., Abbott, RD., & Kaul, S. (1994). In vivo myocardial kinetics of air-filled albumin microbubbles during myocardial contrast echocardiography: comparison with radiolabeled red blood cells. *Circ Res*, 74, pp. 1157-1165, ISSN 0009-7300.

Kaufmann, BA., Sanders, JM., Davis, C., Xie, A., Aldred, P., Sarembock, IJ., & Lindner, JR. (2007). Molecular imaging of inflammation in atherosclerosis with targeted ultrasound detection of vascular cell adhesion molecule-1. *Circulation*, 116, pp. 276-284, ISSN 0009-7322

Kaufmann, BA., Carr, CL., Belcik, T., Xie, A., Kron, B., Yue, Q., & Lindner, JR. (2010). Effect of acoustic power on in vivo molecular imaging with targeted microbubbles: implication for low-mechanical index real-time imaging. *J Am Soc Echocardiogr*, 23, pp. 79-85, ISSN 0894-7317.

Keller, MW., Segal, SS., Kaul, S., & Duling, B. (1989). The behavior of sonicated albumin microbubbles within the microcirculation: a basis for their use during myocardial contrast echocardiography. *Circ Res*, 65, pp. 458-467, ISSN 0009-7300.

Kiessling, F., Huppert, J., & Palmowski, M. (2009). Functional and molecular ultrasound imaging: concepts and contrast agents. *Curr Med Chem*, 16, pp. 627-642, ISSN 0929-8673.

Kietselaer, BL., Reutelingsperger, CP., Heidendal, GA., Daemen, MJ., Mess, WH., Hofstra, L., & Narula, J. (2004). Noninvasive detection of plaque instability with use of radiolabeled annexin A5 in patients with carotid-artery atherosclerosis. *N Engl J Med*, 350, pp. 1472-1473, ISSN 0028-4793.

Klibanov, AL., Rasche, PT., Hughes, MS., Wojdyla, JK., Galen, KP., Wible, JH., & Brandenburger, GH. (2004). Detection of individual microbubbles of ultrasound contrast agents: imaging of free-floating and targeted bubbles. *Invest Radiol*, 39, pp. 187-195, ISSN 0020-9996.

Klibanov, AL. (2005). Ligand-carrying gas-filled microbubbles: ultrasound contrast agents for targeted molecular imaging. *Bioconjugate Chem*, 16, pp. 9-17, ISSN 1043-1802.

Klibanov, AL. (2006). Microbubble contrast agents: targeted ultrasound imaging and ultrasound assisted drug-delivery application. *Invest Radiol*, 41, pp. 354-362, ISSN 0020-9996.

Klibanov, AL., Rychak, JJ., Yang, WC., Alikhani, S., Acton, S., Lindner, JR., Ley, K., & Kaul, S. (2006). Targeted ultrasound contrast agent for molecular imaging of inflammation in high-shear flow. *Contrast Media Mol Imaging*, 1, pp. 259-266, ISSN 1555-4309.

Klibanov, AL. (2009). Preparation of targeted microbubbles: ultrasound contrast agents for molecular imaging. *Med Biol Eng Comput*, 47, pp. 875-882, ISSN 0140-0118.

Kuersten, B., Murthy, TH., Li, P., Liu, Z., Locricchio, E., Baisch, C., Rafter, P., & Vannan, M. (2001). Ultraharmonic myocardial contrast imaging: in vivo experimental and clinical data from a novel technique. *J Am Soc Echocardiogr*, 14, pp. 910-916, ISSN 0894-7317.

Leong-Poi, H., Christiansen, J., Klibanov, AL., Kaul, S., & Lindner, JR. (2003). Noninvasive assessment of angiogenesis by ultrasound and microbubbles targeted to α_v-integrins. *Circulation*, 107, pp. 455-460, ISSN 0009-7322.

Leong-Poi, H. (2009). Molecular imaging using contrast-enhanced ultrasound: evaluation of angiogenesis and cell therapy. *Cardiovasc Res*, 84, pp. 190-200, ISSN 0008-6363.

Lindner, JR., Song, J., Xu. F., Klibanov, AL., Singbartl, K., Ley, K., & Kaul, S. (2000). Noninvasive ultrasound imaging of inflammation using microbubbles targeted to activated leukocytes. *Circulation*, 102, pp. 2745-2750, ISSN 0009-7322.

Lindner, JR., Song, J., Christiansen, J., Klibanov, AL., Xu, F., & Ley, K. (2001). Ultrasound assessment of inflammation and renal tissue injury with microbubbles targeted to P-selectin. *Circulation*, 104, pp. 2107-2112, ISSN 0009-7322.

Lindner, JR. (2009). Contrast ultrasound molecular imaging of inflammation in cardiovascular disease. *Cardiovasc Res*, 84, pp. 182-189, ISSN 0008-6363.

Lindner, JR. (2010). Molecular imaging of vascular phenotype in cardiovascular disease: new diagnostic opportunities on the horizon. *J Am Soc Echocardiogr*, 23, pp. 343-350, ISSN 0894-7317.

Liu, Y., Miyoshi, H., & Nakamura, M. (2006). Encapsulated ultrasound microbubbles: therapeutic application in drug/gene delivery. *J Control Release*, 114, pp. 89-99, ISSN 0168-3659.

Marshall, D., Pedley, RB., Boden, JA., Boden, R., Melton, RG., & Begent, RHJ. (1996). Polyethylene glycol modification of a galactosylated streptavidin clearing agent: effects on immunogenicity and clearance of a biotinylated anti-tumour antibody. *Br J Cancer*, 73, pp. 565-572, ISSN 0007-0920.

Nagata, S., Hanayama, R., & Kawane, K. (2010). Autoimmunity and the clearance of dead cells. *Cell*, 140, pp. 619-630, ISSN 0092-8674.

Narula, J., Acio, ER., Narula, N., Samuels, LE., Fyfe, B., Wood, D., Fitzpatrick, JM., Raghunath, PN., Tomaszewski, JE., Kelly, C., Steinmetz, N., Green, A., Tait, JF., Leppo, J., Blankenberg, FG., Jain, D., & Strauss, HW. (2001). Annexin-V imaging for noninvasive detection of cardiac allograft rejection. *Nat Med*, 7, pp. 1347-1352, ISSN 1078-8956.

Otani, K., Toshida, T., Iwata, A., Asanuma, T., Ishikura, F., & Beppu, S. (2004). Adenosine triphosphate stress myocardial contrast echocardiography detects coronary artery stenosis with greater sensitivity than wall-motion abnormality measurements. *J Am Soc Echocardiogr*, 17, pp. 1275-1280, ISSN 0894-7317.

Otani, K., Ohnishi, S., Obata, H., Ishida, O., Kitamura, S., & Nagaya, N. (2008). Contrast sonography enables noninvasive and quantitative assessment of neovascularization after stem cell transplantation. *Ultrasound Med Biol*, 34, pp. 1893-1900, ISSN 0301-5629.

Otani, K., Yamahara, K., Ohnishi, S., Obata, H., Kitamura, S., & Nagaya, N. (2009). Nonviral delivery of siRNA into mesenchymal stem cells by a combination of ultrasound and microbubbles. *J Control Release*, 133, pp. 146-153, ISSN 0168-3659.

Otani, K., & Yamahara, K. (2011). Development of antibody-carrying microbubbles based on clinically available ultrasound contrast agent for targeted molecular imaging: a preliminary chemical study. *Mol Imaging Biol*, 13, pp. 250-256, ISSN 1536-1632.

Phillips, PJ. (2001). Contrast pulse sequences (CPS): imaging nonlinear microbubbles. *Proceedings of the Institute of Electrical and Electronics Engineers (IEEE) Ultrasonics Symposium*, 2, pp. 1739-1745, ISSN 1051-0117.

Pysz, MA., Foygel, K., Rosenberg, J., Gambhir, SS., Schneider, M., & Willmann, JK. (2010). Antiangiogenic cancer therapy: monitoring with molecular US and a clinically translatable contrast agent (BR55). *Radiology*, 256, pp. 519-527, ISSN 0033-8419.

Pochon, S., Tardy, I., Bussat, P., Bettinger, T., Brochot, J., von Wronski, M., Passantino, L., & Schneider, M. (2010). BR55: a lipopeptide-based VEGFR2-targeted ultrasound contrast agent for molecular imaging of angiogenesis. *Invest Radiol*, 45, pp. 89-95, ISSN 0020-9996.

Porter, TR., Xie, F., Kricsfeld, D., & Armbruster, RW. (1996). Improved myocardial contrast with second harmonic transient ultrasound response imaging in humans using intravenous perfluorocarbon-exposed sonicated dextrose albumin. *J Am Coll Cardiol*, 27, pp. 1497-1501, ISSN 0735-1097.

Porter, TR., & Xie, F. (2010). Myocardial perfusion imaging with contrast ultrasound. *J Am Coll Cardiol Img*, 3, pp. 176-187, ISSN 1936-878X.

Rychak, JJ., Graba, J., Cheung, AM., Mystry, BS., Lindner, JR., Kerbel, RS., & Foster, FS. (2007). Microultrasound molecular imaging of vascular endothelial growth factor receptor 2 in a mouse model of tumor angiogenesis. *Mol Imaging*, 6, pp. 289-296, ISSN 1535-3508.

Shi, J., & Gilbert, GE. (2003). Lactadherin inhibits enzyme complexes of blood coagulation by competing for phospholipid-binding sites. *Blood*, 101, pp. 2628-2636, ISSN 0006-4971.

Sontum, PC. (2008). Physicochemical characteristics of Sonazoid, a new contrast agent for ultrasound imaging. *Ultrasound Med Biol*, 34, pp. 824-833, ISSN 0301-5629.

Stieger, SM., Dayton, PA., Borden, MA., Caskey, CF., Griffey, SM., Wisner, ER., & Ferrara, KW. (2008). Imaging of angiogenesis using Cadence™ contrast pulse sequencing and targeted contrast agents. *Contrast Media Mol Imaging*, 3, pp. 9-18, ISSN 1555-4309.

Stubbs, JD., Lekutis, C., Singer, KL., Bui, A., Yuzuki, D., Srinivasan, U., & Parry, G. (1990). cDNA cloning of a mouse mammary epithelial cell surface protein reveals the existence of epidermal growth factor-like domains linked to factor VIII-like sequences. *Proc Natl Acad Sci USA*, 87, pp. 8417-8421, ISSN 0027-8424.

Tardy, I., Pochon, S., Theraulaz, M., Emmel, P., Passantino, L., Tranquart, F., & Schneider, M. (2010) Ultrasound molecular imaging of VEGFR2 in a rat prostate tumor model using BR55. *Invest Radiol*, 45, pp. 573-578, ISSN 0020-9996.

Tiemann, K., Lohmeier, S., Kuntz, S., Köster, J., Pohl, C., Burns, P., Porter, TR., Nanda, NC., Lüderitz, B., & Becher, H. (1999). Real-time contrast echo assessment of myocardial perfusion at low emission power: first experimental and clinical results using power pulse inversion imaging. *Echocardiography*, 16, pp. 799-809, ISSN 0742-2822.

Tinkov, S., Bekeredjian, R., Winter, G., & Coester, C. (2009). Microbubbles as ultrasound triggered drug carries. *J Pharm Sci*, 98, pp. 1935-1961, ISSN 0022-3549.

Toshida, T., Ishikura, F., Asanuma, T., Iwata, A., Miki, A., Otani, K., & Beppu, S. (2005). Efficacy of 1.5 harmonic imaging for intravenous myocardial contrast echocardiography. *J Echocardiogr*, 3, pp. 104-108, ISSN 1349-0222.

Vermes, I., Haanen, C., Steffen-Nakken, H., & Reutelingsperger, H. (1995). A novel assay for apoptosis. Flow cytometric detection of phosphatidylserine expression on early apoptotic cells using fluorecein labeled annexin V. *J Immunol Methods*, 184, pp. 39-51, ISSN 0022-1759.

Villanueva, FS., & Wagner, WR. (2008). Ultrasound molecular imaging of cardiovascular disease. *Nat Clin Pract Cardiovasc Med*, 5, pp. S26-32, ISSN 1743-4297.

Watanabe, R., Matsumura, M., Munemasa, T., Fujimaki, M., & Suematsu, M. (2007). Mechanism of hepatic parenchyma-specific contrast of microbubble-based contrast agent for ultrasonography: microscopic studies in rat liver. *Invest Radiol*, 42, pp. 643-651, ISSN 0020-9996.

Weller, GER., Lu, E, Csikari, MM, Klibanov, AL., Fischer, D., Wagner, WR., & Villanueva, FS. (2003). Ultrasound imaging of acute cardiac transplant rejection with microbubbles targeted to intercellular adhesion molecule-1. *Circulation*, 108, pp. 218-224, ISSN 0009-7322.

Weller, GER., Villanueva, FS., Tom, EM., & Wagner, WR. (2005). Targeted ultrasound contrast agents: in vitro assessment of endothelial dysfunction and multi-targeting to ICAM-1 and Sialyl Lewis^x. *Biotechnol Bioeng*, 92, pp. 780-788, ISSN 0006-3592.

Willmann, JK., Paulmurugan, R., Chen, K., Gheysens, O., Rodriguez-Porcel, M., Lutz, AM., Chen, IY., Chen, X., & Gambhir, SS. (2008). US imaging of tumor angiogenesis with microbubbles targeted to vascular endothelial growth factor receptor type 2 in mice. *Radiology*, 246, pp. 508-518, ISSN 0033-8419.

Willmann, JK., Lutz, AM., Paulmurugan, R., Patel, MR., Chu, P., Rosenberg, J., & Gambhir, SS. (2008). Dual-targeted contrast agent for US assessment of tumor angiogenesis in vivo. *Radiology*, 248, pp. 936-944, ISSN 0033-8419.

Willmann, JK., Kimura, RH., Deshpande, N., Lutz, AM., Cochran, JR., & Gambhir, SS. (2010). Targeted contrast-enhanced ultrasound imaging of tumor angiogenesis with contrast microbubbles conjugated to integrin-binding knottin peptides. *J Nucl Med*, 51, pp. 433-440, ISSN 0161-5505.

Wilson, SR., & Burns, PN. (2010). Microbubble-enhanced US in body imaging: what role? *Radiology*, 257, pp. 24-39, ISSN 0033-8419.

Wu, Y., Tibrewal, N., & Birge, RB. (2006). Phosphatidylserine recognition by phagocytes: a view to a kill. *Trends Cell Biol*, 16, pp. 189-197, ISSN 0962-8924.

Yamaguchi, H., Takagi, J., Miyamae, T., Yokota, S., Fujimoto, T., Nakamura, S., Ohshima, S., Naka, T., & Nagata, S. (2008). Milk fat globule EGF factor 8 in the serum of human patients of systemic lupus erythematosus. *J Leukoc Biol*, 83, pp. 1300-1307, ISSN 0741-5400.

Yanagisawa, K., Moriyasu, F., Miyahara, T., Yuki, M., & Iijima, H. (2007). Phagocytosis of ultrasound contrast agent microbubbles by Kupffer cells. *Ultrasound Med Biol*, 33, pp. 318-325, ISSN 0301-5629.

17

Clinical Application of Ultrasound Imaging in Radiation Therapy

Hayeon Kim, Edward Brandner, M. Saiful Huq and Sushil Beriwal
University of Pittsburgh Cancer Institute
USA

1. Introduction

Radiation therapy plays an important role in cancer treatment. It is well known that good local control is achieved when planned dose of radiation is delivered to the target.
Recent advances in technology, in particular in image guided radiation therapy (IGRT), has significantly improved the accuracy of target localization for daily radiation treatment. Daily localization of the target is critical to the delivery of the prescription dose to the target. Thus, to achieve accurate targeting and reduce the irradiation of normal tissues and to potentially escalate dose to target volumes, IGRT needs to be implemented for daily use in the clinic.
Various IGRT techniques are currently available. One of the techniques integrates an On Board low kilovoltage imaging capability into the linear accelerator that produces diagnostic quality images. However, this imaging technique requires that extra radiation dose be delivered to the patient. Another IGRT imaging system that has been integrated recently with the linear accelerator is 3D ultrasound imaging. This technique is non invasive, requires no extra radiation to a patient and provides capabilities for daily target localization and verification prior to the delivery of radiation treatment.
Currently, 3D ultrasound imaging is used for target localization and verification of prostate, gynecological and breast cancers. Since the late nineties, 2D ultrasound imaging has been used for prostate localization only, but only recently has 3D ultrasound localization been available. This has also led to the use of 3D ultrasound for localizing other treatment sites as well; although, each site requires unique methods.
For the prostate cancer treatment, the prostate can move daily compared to the reference planning CT (radiation therapy planning and dose calculation for all disease sites is done with CT image based)due to bladder and rectal filling. Ultrasound imaging can be used to image and localize the prostate target daily. The prostate and bladder can all typically be well visualized and compared to the reference ultrasound image or CT image. Shifts are then identified and made to reposition the patient to the point that the treatment volumes identified each day are aligned with where they were on the planning CT images relative to the linear accelerator's isocenter. This isocenter is the point in space about which the linear accelerator rotates and all planning and radiation beam delivery for a daily treatment is performed relative to it.
For gynecological cancer treatment, the ultrasound image does not show the entire target because target definition is complex and composed of multiple structures. The purpose of

ultrasound is to visualize the vaginal canal (for hysterectomy patients) or uterus and cervix motion with respect to change in bladder filling volume and rectal motion. Daily changes of these organs relative to their planned locations can be found by ultrasound localization and treatment margins for organ motions can be adjusted accordingly to avoid geographical miss especially when patients are being treated with Intensity Modulated Radiation Therapy (IMRT).

For breast cancer treatment, ultrasound is used to image the lumpectomy cavity daily with each radiation treatment. This provides an actual visual image and location of the tumor cavity. The standard way to treat lumpectomy cavities is based on a reference CT scan before the radiation treatment course starts. Using 3D ultrasound, daily tumor bed is visualized with the excellent soft tissue imaging and shifts can be made to align the planned and treatment locations relative to the isocenter for the boost or partial breast treatments.

Ultrasound image use is user dependent and requires special skills to acquire good quality images compared to other imaging systems used in radiation therapy. This includes techniques for acquiring good images and evaluation of the images acquired.

In this chapter, we will review the application of 3D ultrasound imaging as a tool for daily image guidance in radiation therapy. Application of this imaging technique will be discussed for various tumor sites such as prostate, gynecological and breast cancers. We will also report on the findings of our clinical investigations for these disease sites. Quality assurance of the equipment and process, detailed scan acquisition techniques and steps for the use of ultrasound for the visualization of various tumors will also be provided based on our clinical experiences with the Resonant/Clarity system. Other ultrasound systems are commercially available, and they use similar techniques to visualize and localize targets. Finally, we will also provide a brief review of other imaging modalities that are used for target localization in radiation therapy and a comparison of each of these modalities as well.

2. Basic concepts for treatment planning and delivery in external beam radiation therapy

2.1 Linear accelerator

In radiation therapy, a beam (typically photons and/or electrons) is delivered from the linear accelerator toward a single point in space—the isocenter. The linear accelerator is a device that uses high-frequency electromagnetic waves to accelerate charged particles such as electrons to high energies (Mega voltage level) through a linear tube. High -energy electron beam or photon beam (electrons can be made to strike a target to produce X-rays) can be used for treating cancers. The linear accelerator rotates around the isocenter so that at every angle the central axis of the beam is directed through the isocenter. Therefore, within the patient, the target to be treated must be precisely placed relative to isocenter.

2.2 Target definition and prescription for treatment planning

The treatment target volume is initially identified and outlined by a radiation oncologist on a computed tomographic (CT) image. CT scan is the standard method for creating image based plans in radiation oncology. The visualized tumor is outlined as the gross tumor volume (GTV). A margin or shell is added to this GTV to include volumes that may be expected to contain cancerous cells that are too small to be visualized. This larger volume is the clinical target volume (CTV). An additional margin is added to the CTV to account for uncertainties due to day to day variations such as internal organ motions and setup of a patient. This larger volume is the planning target volume (PTV) and is planned to receive the prescribed dose of radiation. The radiation oncologist's prescription defines the target, the type of radiation to be used, the total dose to be delivered to the target, the daily radiation dose per fraction to the target, the total number of fractions to deliver that dose, and any special instructions regarding how the dose is to be delivered. Typical radiation treatments are delivered daily for five to six weeks.

If imaging is to be used to localize the target, the special instructions will include the type and frequency of imaging to be done for this purpose.

2.3 Process of generating treatment plan

Once the target has been outlined and a prescription is written, a plan for delivering the prescription dose is developed by physicists/dosimetrists with treatment planning software. Planning software needs CT scan images for dose calculations and simulation. The plan determines the angles from which the linear accelerator will deliver a radiation beam for selected beam energy (within the parameters of the prescription), the shape of treatment fields (or portals) for each beam angle, and any special devices in the path of the beams to further tailor them. The portals are shaped using blocks or a series of thin leaves collectively referred to as a multi-leaf collimator (MLC). The blocks or MLCs must be sufficiently thick (parallel to the beam direction) to block nearly all of the radiation outside of the block or MLC opening so that it can attenuate the beam to an intensity of less than 5.0 percent, and each leaf of the MLC must be thin enough, typically 5.0mm or 10.0mm at the level of isocenter, and perpendicular to the beam direction to conform to the PTV shape.

In addition to covering the PTV with the prescription dose, the treatment plan must limit dose to nearby critical structures. All tissues within the human body have tolerances of radiation dose that they can receive before the risk of radiation damage becomes significant. Conventionally generous margins are applied around the target to incorporate uncertainties due to organ motion and setup error. This ensures that the PTV receives the prescription dose. However, this can result in an increased dose to the normal tissues thus increasing risks of normal tissue complications. Maximizing setup accuracy is one of the most important ways to reduce the margin added to the CTV and thus reduce risks of normal tissues complications.

Daily imaging of the target on the linear accelerator is an accurate way to localize it relative to the isocenter and a key factor in aligning the patient so that the planned dose is delivered to the target and critical structures are spared.

2.4 Verification and confirmation of daily patient setup

Once the plan is completed, the radiation oncologist will review it and subsequently approve the final plan. The patient will then be scheduled for a confirmation simulation by radiation therapists. During confirmatory simulation, the patient is setup on a special table that is used to move the patient so that the target is aligned to the isocenter as planned. Images are taken to confirm isocenter location and shape of beam portals if necessary. Once in the final position, the patient's skin is marked at the points where the central axis of the beam enters the skin directly from above and from both sides (these are orthogonal angles). The radiation oncologist reviews and approves these images before the patient is treated.

Each day the patient is setup using the skin marks placed during the confirmatory simulation to align the target to the isocenter. Room lasers, sagittal, vertical and lateral are used for this setup. The margins in the PTV must account for the uncertainties of where the target is relative to the skin marks. Daily imaging reduces much of this uncertainty by directly viewing internal soft tissues or fiducial markers placed inside the tumor. Small (e.g. 1 mm diameter and 5 mm long) fiducial markers are radio-opaque to kilovoltage radiation and are therefore well visualized in kilovoltage images. They can be implanted into soft tissues to assist with comparing daily images to reference images. These images can be reviewed daily by the radiation oncologist before treatment is delivered.

Several types of daily imaging are now used in radiation oncology to aid in Image Guided Radiation Therapy (IGRT). These new innovative technologies include megavoltage (MV) and kilovoltage (KV) X-ray energies to acquire individual radiographs or cone beam CT (CBCT). Also, ultrasound images—either planar or volume images—can be used for daily localization of certain targets such as gynaecological, prostate, or breast.

In next couple of sections, 3D ultrasound application as an IGRT in radiation oncology will be reviewed.

3. Applications of ultrasound imaging in prostate cancer

The prostate location is particularly conducive to ultrasound imaging in that it is located beneath the bladder which when full creates a favourable ultrasound path from the skin surface of the lower abdomen to the prostate. The bladder-prostate interface is well visualized.

In addition, the prostate is displaced by rectal and bladder filling. This displacement is unpredictable and can approach 2 cm (Scarborough et al., 2006). Such a large displacement is rare (typically less than 7 % of the time). A few millimetres are more typical on a daily basis, and it is less than 1 cm (0.8 - 0.9 mm) with a 95 % confidence interval (Scarborough et al., 2006; Serago et al., 2006). Therefore, 1 cm is a typical expansion around the prostate CTV to create the PTV without imaging (Hanks et al., 2000; Boersma et al., 1998). With daily ultrasound imaging, we have found that the 95 % confidence interval is reduced to 0.7 cm which agrees with Serago et al (Serago et al., 2006). Boda-Heggemann et al and Langen et al also demonstrated that ultrasound imaging improves prostate localization (Boda-Heggemann et al., 2008; Langen et al., 2003). Serago et al and Langen et al identified a significant improvement in localization in the anterior-posterior direction which is the direction of largest prostate displacement because of rectal filling (Serago et al., 2006; Langen et al., 2003). Further, the rectum and bladder are adjacent to the prostate, but are critical structures that should be spared as much dose as is possible without compromising the delivery of the prescribed dose to the prostate.

Prescribed total doses of 70 to 78 Gy to the entire prostate at 1.8 Gy per daily fraction are common for treating prostate cancer (Pollack et al., 2002). Because of the proximity of the bladder and rectum to the prostate, a portion of each of these organs typically receives the entire dose. In order to avoid serious toxicities to these organs, their volumes receiving such large doses of radiation must be limited. A recent review of the literature evaluating bladder and rectal tolerances to radiation has suggested the following dose constraints (Michalski et al., 2010; Viswanathan et al., 2010): (Table 1)

Toxic effects are graded using one a few standardized criteria including the Common Terminology Criteria for Adverse Events version 3.0 (CTCAE 3.0) and Radiation Therapy Oncology Group (RTOG) scoring criteria. Long term toxic effects can include rectal stricture, rectal bleeding, diminished rectal compliance, decreased storage capacity with resultant small and frequent bowel movements, urgency to empty the bladder frequently, incontinence, reduced flow, bladder spasms, hematuria, fistula, obstruction, ulceration, and necrosis (Michalski et al., 2010; Viswanathan et al., 2010). The tabulated limits are expected to avoid these serious long term toxic effects in 90% or more of patients (Michalski et al., 2010; Viswanathan et al., 2010). These criteria were developed over many years without the benefits of daily localization; however, daily localization can be expected to help reduce the doses to these critical structures (Michalski et al., 2010; Viswanathan et al., 2010) by helping us treat with smaller margins thereby reducing toxic effects of radiation.

Specified Dose	Percentage of Organ Volume Receiving Greater than Specified Dose (%)	
(Gy)	Bladder	Rectum
50		50
60		35
65	50	25
70	35	20
75	25	15
80	15	

Table 1. Summary of critical organ and dose volume limits in prostate cancer treatment

Each day the new ultrasound image is aligned to the reference image right before a treatment starts. Our technique included acquiring a reference ultrasound image at the time of initial CT scan for the planning.

At this time, positioning reference volume (PRV) of prostate from ultrasound scan (US) is created and this PRV is compared to daily US image during radiation treatment. The reference ultrasound image is aligned to the planning CT image with the co-registration of the planning CT and PRV to confirm that the prostate, bladder, and rectum are well localized and readily visible on both images near the prostate. It is not necessary to visualize the entire bladder or rectum in order to localize the prostate in US image. However, patient positioning is critical. Ultrasound image is acquired by pressing the ultrasound probe against the patient's lower abdomen and rolling it in the sagittal plane while continuously acquiring ultrasound image slices. These slices are then reconstructed based on the position and tilt of the ultrasound probe relative to the reference point to create a 3D image of the patient.

The images are acquired through the bladder which serves as a high transmission interface between the skin and the prostate. It is therefore necessary that the bladder be relatively full. In order to accomplish this, patients are asked to drink 16 ounces of fluid 30 minutes before the simulation and every day of treatment. Each day the patient's skin marks are used to align the patient to isocenter. An ultrasound is acquired in the same way that it was acquired at the time of the planning CT. The newly acquired image is then compared to the PRV and the images of the prostates are aligned Fig 1. This alignment requires a directional couch shift which is then made. The treatment is then delivered.

Other localization techniques exist such as kilovoltage and megavoltage imaging, and fiducial markers implanted into the prostate can be used. Studies have demonstrated that ultrasound localization is not as precise as these other localization techniques particularly when implanted fiducial markers are used where it is possible to align the prostate to within 4mm at the 95% confidence interval (Moseley et al, 2007). However, kilovoltage and megavoltage imaging use ionizing radiation which may have long term radiation effects, and implanting fiducial markers is an invasive procedure. Ultrasound can therefore be considered an alternative localization method.

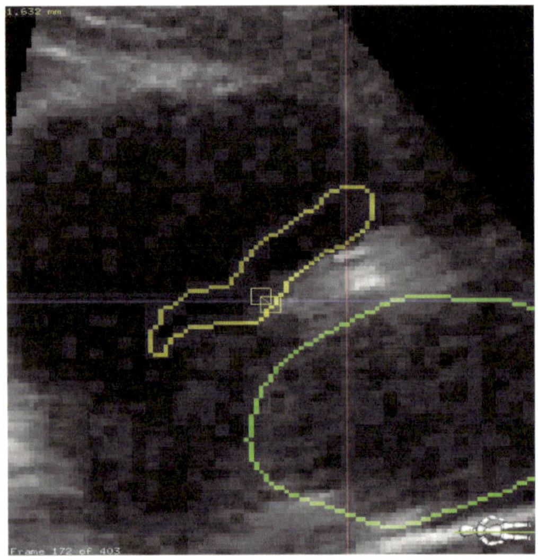

Fig. 1. Contour of the PRV and inferior bladder wall aligned on a daily ultrasound in the sagittal view.

4. Applications in gynaecological cancers

For gynaecological cancers (endometrial cancer or cervical cancer), clinical target volume (CTV) definition for external beam radiation therapy is more complex compared to other cancer sites. It has been challenging to create accurate PTV margins because the CTV is composed of multiple structures and they move relative to each other as well as deform during the radiation therapy course. Also adjacent normal tissues move randomly daily. In order to reproduce a daily consistent setup, patients are instructed to empty their rectum and have a full bladder before the acquisition of planning CT and radiation treatment.

4.1 Anatomy and organ motions

Pelvic anatomy consists of movable organs such as small bowel, sigmoid, bladder, rectum, and cervix/uterus. With radiation therapy for gynaecological cancer treatment, there are risks of small bowel and bladder complications due to anatomical close relationship. A full bladder can push away small bowel out of the radiation field and reduce target motion (cervix/uterus) variability. Therefore, it is important to have a full bladder prior to the acquisition of planning CT and the daily radiation treatments. This also ensures consistency and reproducibility of target positioning daily during radiation treatment. All patients who undergo radiation treatments are given guidelines for bladder filling.

4.2 Ultrasound images with full bladder for daily treatment

Patients are instructed to drink 24-32oz of water or fluids 30 minutes prior to scanning for daily treatment. Bladder is an easy structure to identify in ultrasound image and full bladder impacts the ultrasound image quality by enhancing the image and sharpening the edge between bladder and uterus/cervix/vaginal canal. (Fig.2) For cervical cancer patients with an intact uterus, the vaginal canal, cervix and uterus are posterior to the bladder (Fig.3). For patients who had a hysterectomy, only the vaginal canal is seen posterior to the bladder.

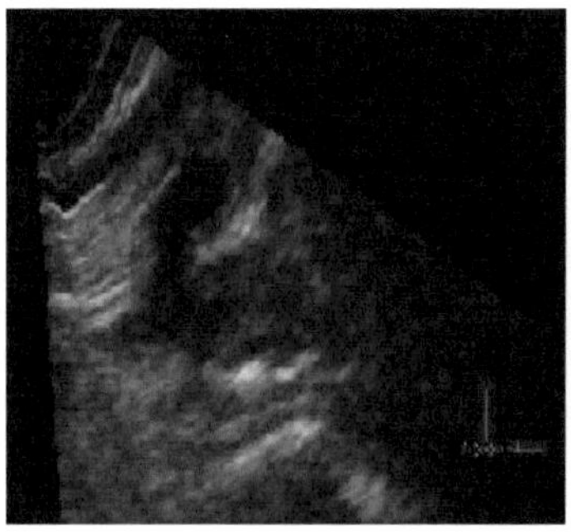
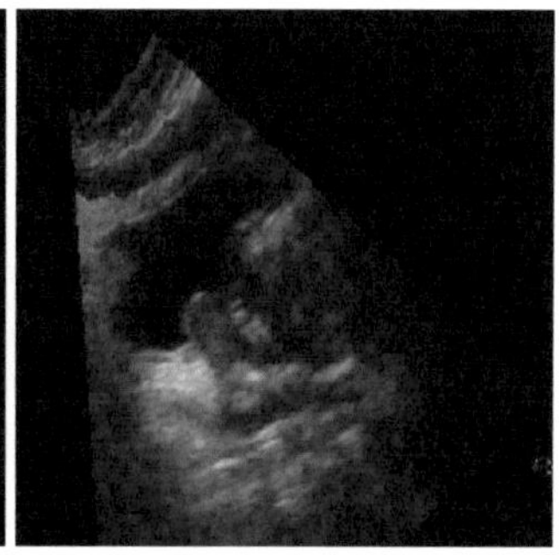

(a) (b)

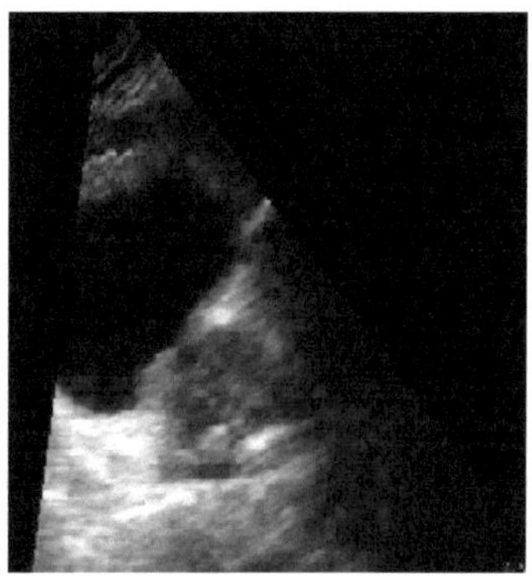

(c)

Fig. 2. a. Empty bladder, b. Partially filled and c. Full bladder in ultrasound images. Used with permission of the Resonant/Clarity.

Before radiation therapy is started for each patient, a treatment planning CT scan is done with a full bladder followed by acquisition of an ultrasound scan. The reference ultrasound image is aligned to the CT image. At this time, a positioning reference volume (PRV) of the bladder from the ultrasound scan (US) are created and this PRV are compared to the daily US images taken during radiation treatment course.

The US image is acquired as follows. The US probe is placed with firm pressure on the pubic symphysis and slowly rotated. The probe is then swept across the abdomen toward the patient's head. Since a full bladder provides good propagation of the sound waves, the uterus/cervix/vagina images are acquired by scanning through the bladder. As seen from Fig. 4, the outline of bladder and other organs such as the uterus, cervix and vaginal canal can be drawn on the US image directly, and their volumes can be measured too. After acquisition of the daily US image, 3D reconstructions of the images are made. These 3D images are then used for the calculation of any directional shift that are necessary for target alignment prior to radiation treatment (Fig.5) Also, with the co-registration of the planning

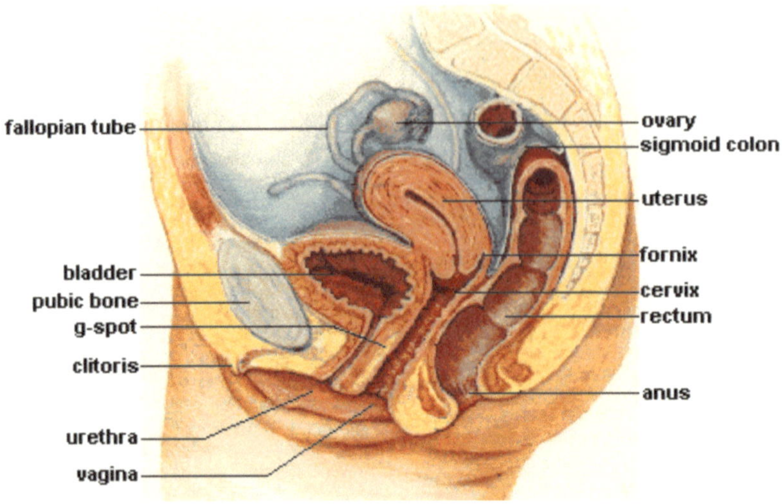

Fig. 3. Anatomy location of bladder, vaginal canal, cervix and uterus.

CT and the reference US image, the radiation treatment fields (each portal) and target contours can be overlaid on the daily US images as a verification of the setup of the patient prior to daily treatment (Fig. 6). However, patient repositioning solely by daily US imaging for gynaecological cancers is questionable because the target is of complicated shape and is composed of multiple other structures such as the common iliac, external iliac, and internal iliac with inguinofemoral and periaortic nodes as well as the uterus, cervix, parametrium and vagina. As mentioned before, ultrasound can only image the vaginal canal and uterus in the target. In our clinic, as shown in Fig 6, daily US image is compared to the PTV contour from the planning CT and verified if the uterus/cervix or vaginal canal is still within the PTV. This is a major difference in using US images as an IGRT method between gynecological use and other disease sites use such as prostate and breast.

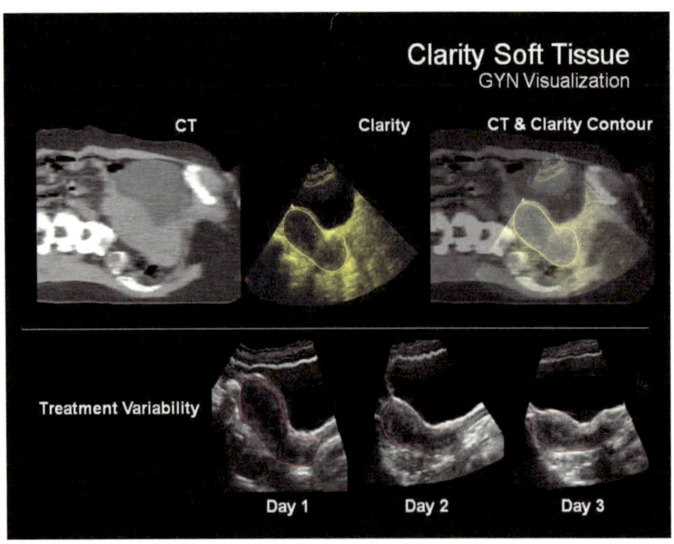

Fig. 4. Daily US image. Used with permission of the Resonant/Clarity.

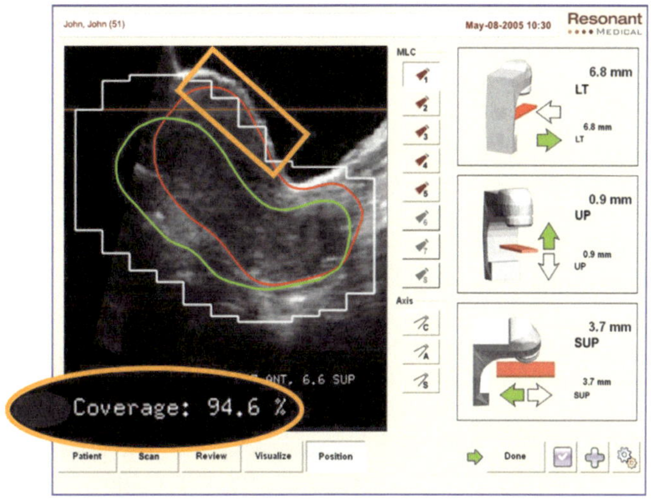

Fig. 5. Daily US image and PRV comparison and calculated positional shift. Used with permission of the Resonant/Clarity.

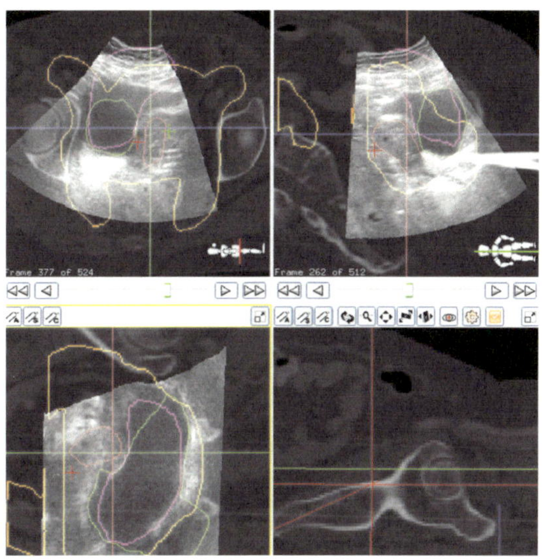

Fig. 6. Image co-registration of planning CT and US PRV with PTV contours from CT overlaid to daily US. Orange colored shape is PTV defined in CT image. Pink shows bladder on reference CT and green for bladder with daily US.

4.3 Clinical data for bladder and target motion during radiation treatment course

Data quantifying bladder motion during radiation therapy have been published in the literature (Ahmad et al., 2008; Jhingran et al., 2010; Jurgenliemk-Schulz et al., 2011; Lim et al., 2009; McBain et al., 2009; Thawani et al, 2008; Yee et al., 2010). From the experiences gained with US imaging at our institution we found that inter-fraction bladder volume variations are prominent for gynaecological cancer treatments. Mean bladder volume was 254.2 cc with a standard deviation of 138.5 cc for 202 fractions with 11 patients.

From these patients, it was found to be a bladder volume change more than 30% compared to their PRV in 40%-94% of total treatment fractions.
A US study of 24 cervical patients by Ahmad et al. (2008) found that bladder volume decreases dramatically during the treatment course compared to the planning CT scan (mean total reduction of 71%). Using US imaging, McBain et al. (2009) investigated bladder volume change during the treatment course. Of the 24 patients studied, they found that seven patients had more than a 50 % volume change during the treatment course. Lim et al. (2009) assessed bladder volume change using weekly MRI scan for twenty cervical patients. They found bladder volume change of 7- 450% relative to baseline volumes.
Studies have shown that inter-fraction changes in bladder volume are unpredictable and it is very difficult to reproduce the daily bladder filling even though written and verbal instructions are given to patients. Because target location depends on the fullness of the bladder, the reproducibility of the target location daily cannot be guaranteed. Daily ultrasound imaging can help ensure that the change in target volume with respect to bladder filling is accounted for by PTV margin and if not then the margins should be adjusted for individual patient to avoid geographical miss.
Although many published data show that uterus/cervix positions can be at different locations depending on bladder filling (Ahmad et al., 2011; Buchali et al., 1999; Chan et al., 2004; Han et al., 2006; Huh et al., 2004; Jhingran et al., 2010; Kerkhof et al., 2009; Taylor & Powell, 2008; Van de Bunt et al., 2008), one study reported recently that motion of the vagina after the hysterectomy varies in a random manner daily and found no correlation with changes in bladder and rectum volumes (Jurgenliemk- Schulz et al. ,2011). Also some studies claimed that uterus and cervix motion are weakly correlated with bladder and rectum filling status because change in target motion not only depends on adjacent bladder and rectal filling but also depends on tumor regression and deformation with a patient-specific correlation (Huh et al., 2004; Van de Bunt et al., 2008).
On the contrary, consistent clinical investigations with prostate demonstrate that the prostate motion strongly depends on bladder and rectum filling (Pinkawa et al., 2006; Schild et al.,1993; Stam et al, 2006; Ten Haken et al., 1991; Thawani et al, 2008; Van Herk et al., 1995)

5. Image guidance to minimize dosimetric impact on target and organs at risk

IMRT[1] has been proven to be beneficial and superior to conform the dose distribution to targets and spare critical organs reducing morbidity and toxicity by using sharp dose gradient compared to other conventional radiation therapy techniques. Thus IMRT is more attractive for the treatment of gynaecological and prostate cancer because of better tumor control and sparing critical organs thereby reducing the organ toxicity (Beriwal et al., 2006; Cahlon et al., 2008). As dose distribution has sharp gradient with IMRT, it is important to localize the target daily in order to reproduce the dose to critical organs and target as

[1] Intensity-modulated radiation therapy (IMRT) is an advanced mode of high-precision radiotherapy that utilizes computer-controlled linear accelerators to deliver precise radiation doses to a malignant tumor or specific areas within the tumor. IMRT allows for the radiation dose to conform more precisely to the three-dimensional (3-D) shape of the tumor by modulating the intensity of the radiation beam . IMRT also allows higher radiation doses to be focused to regions within the tumor while minimizing the dose to surrounding normal critical structures.

planned from the initial planning CT. The use of IGRT is critical to accomplish this goal because it enables localization of the target prior to treatment and thus account for inter-fraction motion.

6. Applications in partial breast irradiation or electron boost treatment

Standard of care for early stage breast cancer is to deliver photon radiation to the whole breast after segmental mastectomy (lumpectomy) as a breast conserving surgery. The photon radiation is followed by the electron radiation as a boost to the tumor bed (surgical cavity). The total treatment period is about 6-7 weeks of which whole breast radiation takes 5-6 weeks in 25-28 fractions and the boost is delivered in 4-8 fractions. This approach is well tolerated and has good cosmetic result with local control rates comparable to a mastectomy (Fisher et al., 1994, 2002; Holland et al., 1985; Veronesi et al., 2002).

An alternative technique to this standard approach is the APBI (accelerated partial breast irradiation) technique. In this technique radiation targeting is to the tumor bed area only instead of the whole breast. The reason is that high local recurrence of the tumor occurs at the primary tumor sites after the lumpectomy (Clark et al., 1987; Liljegren et al., 1999; Veronesi et al., 2002). APBI helps to avoid radiating normal tissue unnecessarily which will reduce the morbidity. Also, APBI offers a shorter treatment course (one week with twice daily treatments in contrast to 6-8 weeks for whole breast radiation therapy) which may be favourable over the conventional whole breast treatment technique.

6.1 Ultrasound imaging for tumor bed delineation

Historically, the palpable tumor bed predicted from the scar position on the skin with a clinical margin was the clinical description of the boost volume. This method has shown to inaccurately define the tumor bed and dosimetry is poor (Benda et al., 2003; Landis et al., 2007; Ringash et al. 2004) .An ideal method for the delineation of the surgical cavity for the boost volume has not been established (Landis et al., 2007; Ringash et al., 2004). Ultrasound, MRI and CT scans with or without surgical clips are the currently available techniques for identifying the boost volume. Various studies reported difficulties in contouring the boost volume in CT images because of poor seroma clarity from the surrounding tissue specifically in patients with dense breast parenchyma (Berrang et al. , 2009; Landis et al., 2007; Petersen et al., 2007) . This can lead to high inter-observer variability. 3D US for defining the breast boost volume has been introduced recently. Unlike CT images, US can differentiate fluid-filled cavity (which is the lumpectomy cavity) from the surrounding tissue with high specificity because of excellent soft tissue imaging characteristics (Smitt et al., 2001; Yang & Dempsey, 2007 ; Weinstein et al., 2006). This helps to identify the tumor bed volume more accurately and has an improved inter-observer consistency.

6.2 Tumor bed volume localization between US and CT

Before daily treatment, the US probe is swept over the area near the surgical scar in one direction until the lumpectomy cavity is located. After the cavity is identified, it is compared to the PRV which is created at the time of the planning CT and directional shifts are made based on the comparison. Procedures for the CT and US scans at the time of planning CT are explained in previous sections.

Fig 7. shows a comparison of US to CT for tumor bed volume.

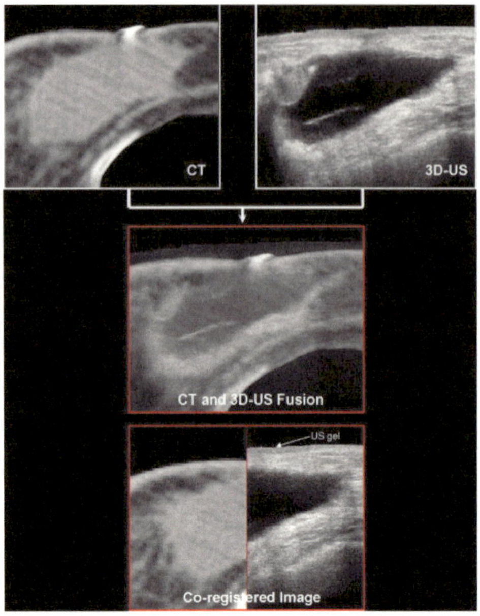

Fig. 7. Co-registered images of US and CT for a tumor bed. Used with permission of the Elsevier (International Journal of Radiation Oncology, Biology, Physics., vol. 73, No.2, pp 375-383,2009)

CT overestimates the true tumor bed volume compared to US images. One study (Wong et al., 2011) reported that the average difference of the tumor bed volume between US and CT is 55% because the seroma or fluid cavity is well visualized in US, but not as well in CT. On a CT scan, the fluid cavity plus the fibrotic tissue surrounding the cavity are drawn as the cavity/seroma. Fig.8 is one example.

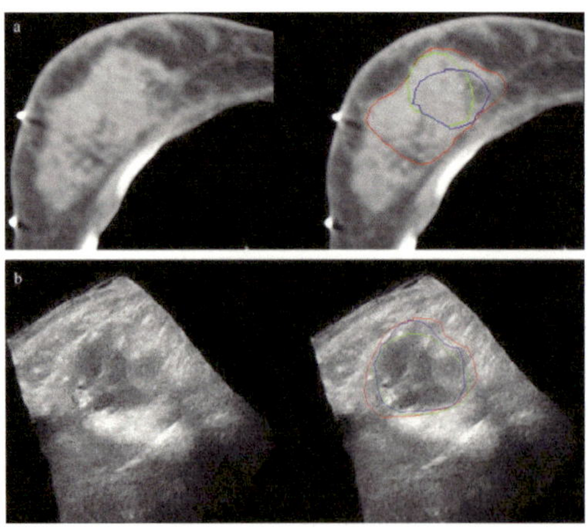

Fig. 8. Poor correlation between US and CT for the low seroma clarity from the CT. Upper: On CT image there are three different tumor bed drawn (low interobserver corformity index). Lower: improved interobserver conformity index with US guidance. Used with permission of the Elsevier (International Journal of Radiation Oncology, Biology, Physics., vol. 73, No.2, pp 375-383,2009)

6.3 Inter-fractional changes in tumor bed volume and position with US study

By the use of 3D US, daily localization of the tumor bed becomes viable. Few studies have quantified tumor bed volume changes during the course of treatment (Prendergast et al., 2009). Redefining the tumor bed right before the boost treatment will give a better assessment for the boost volume, and the ultrasound image provides a convenient method for this without giving extra dose to the patient. Wong et al., (2011) reported that the average tumor bed displacement in the radial direction was 10.8 mm with a standard deviation of 6.3 mm, and 50% of the time the fractions had displacements. Other study (Weed et al., 2004) using surgical clips or CT images identified average displacements of 3mm in the radial direction. This suggests that tumor bed localization is important and 3D US scans can play an important role in an assessment of surgical bed and localization before treatment. This is particularly important for 3D conformal or IMRT for accelerated partial breast radiation (APBI techniques) where better daily targeting becomes critical.

7. Technical issues

Acquiring ultrasound images requires special skill in the radiation oncology department because technicians, physicists, and physicians are not typically trained to scan and review ultrasound images. Traditionally ultrasound images have been reviewed by radiologists/radiology technicians. Technical skills for acquiring US images for different body sites by the radiation oncology staff can be highly user dependent thus affecting acquired image quality. In the absence of proper training, the interpretation of US images by the radiation staff can also be highly user dependent. Special consultation by a radiologist is thus needed until the radiation oncology staff is properly trained with this imaging modality.

The Resonant/Clarity ultrasound system for IGRT requires establishment of correspondence between the planning CT, acquired ultrasound images in the CT room and the treatment images acquired at the treatment vault. This is done by establishing an appropriate calibration procedure. In this way, the US workstations can create and save the PRV as a reference image by the image co-registration process, sharing the same coordinates with the treatment machine from the fusion of CT and the US images. MR and CT images are fused by mathematical methods such as pixel data or bony anatomy matching, and PET and CT images are fused by the automatic dicom match method. However, fusion of US and CT images is more challenging if it is done with manual registration, and it needs more careful consideration to achieve an accurate image co-registration if the images do not share a common reference point.

8. Quality assurance

As explained in previous sections, the US system is used for daily verification of the patient position as well as creating a reference volume for the target localization when fused with the CT images for a treatment plan. A calibration phantom is used to check the performance of the system which is referred to as a Quality Assurance (QA). QA for the Ultrasound system consists of the system integrity check (mechanical function), isocenter verification, directional shift calculation, imaging quality check and software performance check. Daily QA and monthly QA are routine check-ups for the system.

8.1 Daily QA

As a daily check, isocenter accuracy verification and directional shift calculations are performed by a therapist. The linear accelerator beam is calibrated at the isocenter and

intersections of the CT room lasers and treatment room lasers are referenced to the isocenter. The calibration phantom that contains a positional guidance volume (PGV) is used for QA. The phantom is calibrated at the isocenter by using the optical tracking camera in the system. The PGV has a known 3D coordinate position shared with the treatment room and CT unit lasers, and it can be verified with daily US scans. The calibration phantom is set up with the room lasers (at the isocenter) and scanned with the US probe. After the PGV is reconstructed, a 3D view of the US shows the isocenter coordinate. It is then compared to the known coordinates (reference value) by image co-registration between the reference PGV of the phantom and the daily PGV. Directional shifts and offsets are calculated (Fig 9). Tolerance level in isocenter position is 2.0mm in radiation therapy. Isonceter verification is done at CT room and treatment room both.
As for directional shifts calculations, it is performed at the treatment room after the isocenter accuracy is checked. The couch is moved from isocenter by a known amount of offset in all three directions (anterior-posterior, superior-inferior, medial-lateral), and the phantom is scanned. After reconstruction of the PGV is done, 3D coordinates are calculated and checked if the offset is correctly calculated.

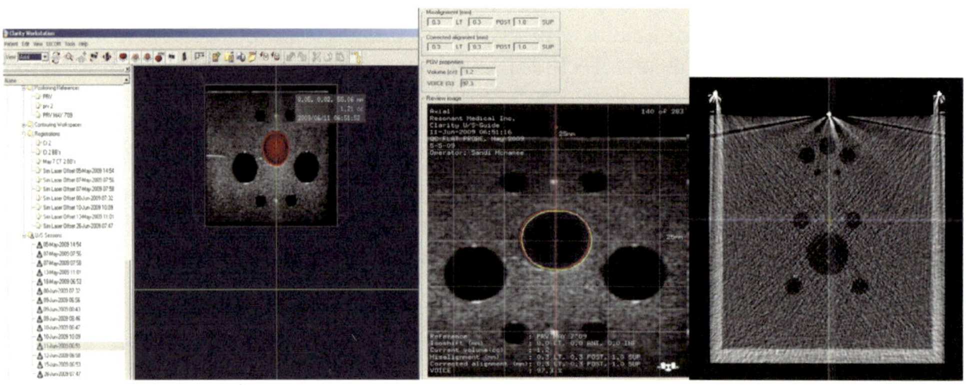

Fig. 9. Daily QA : Green circle is the reference PGV and red one is daily scan image of PGV: left image shows 3D coordinates of daily scan, middle image for comparison and directional shift between reference and daily PGV, right image is the QA phantom.

8.2 Monthly QA

The physicist performs monthly QA. For monthly QA, daily QA is repeated along with additional checks such as verification of the phantom PGV image in the US and CT images, registration of US and CT images, image reconstruction, and system integrity tests. A CT scan of the calibration phantom is performed and an US scan follows. Image co-registration is performed by fusing both images, the PGV is contoured, and the size of the PGV is measured and compared in both images. After that, the phantom is placed in the treatment room and the daily QA is performed. System functionality is checked for the each part of the system.

9. Other image modalities in radiation therapy

KV/MV verification imaging systems for patient set up such as kV planar images, kV CBCT, MV CBCT and MV portal images have been accepted more widely in radiation oncology community for IGRT than US systems. In contrast to US systems, these other IGRT systems are integrated with the linear accelerator (Fig 10.) making data transfer and connectivity between treatment machine and imaging device easier. MV portal images have the oldest history for patient setup verification and renders verification only of bony anatomy because of the poor image quality from the MV photon beams. In addition, MV portal imaging can't be taken on a daily basis because of the extra dose from the high energy therapeutic MV beams. Traditionally portal images are taken once a week. kV x-ray based OBI (2D planner images) provides better image quality. It allows verifying the bony anatomy as well as soft tissues, and daily imaging can be acceptable because of low extra doses. CBCT can provide 3D volumetric images and renders visualization of soft tissue targets as well as adjacent organs. Although doses from kV imaging are low it still gives extra daily dose to a patient and careful consideration for the daily extra dose needs to be investigated.

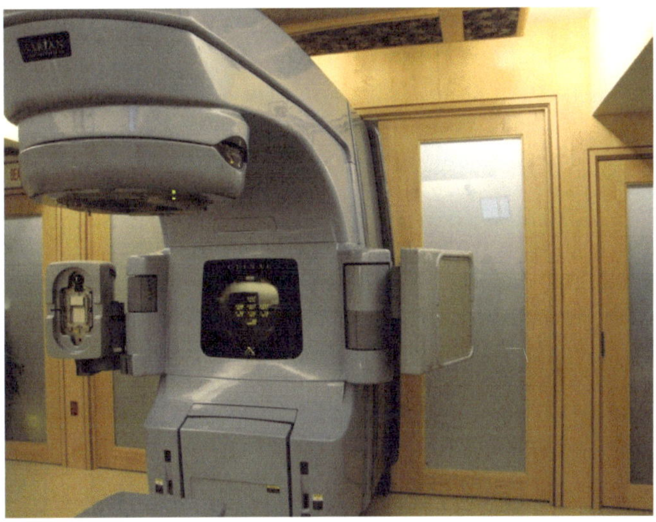

Fig. 10. Linear Accelerator with kV imaging arms attached. VARIAN 23 iX with OBI (On Board Imager).

10. Conclusion

Ultrasound application as IGRT in radiation therapy has been established. Because it is non-ionizing, provides excellent soft tissue image quality and non invasive in nature, it can be beneficial as an IGRT tool for radiation patients. The drawback of this technique is user dependence, challenging learning curve for radiation oncology staff and applicability to few disease sites only. Besides, it also doesn't account for intrafraction motion which is also important for daliy target localization. Nevertheless, ultrasound guidance has been useful for daily localization in target position such as prostate, breast and gynaecological cancers as well as for monitoring inter-fractional bladder filling status and organ motion.

11. References

Ahmad, R et al (2008) Inter-fraction bladder filling variation and time trends for cervical cancer patients assessed with a portable 3-dimensional ultrasound bladder scanner.

Radiotherapy and Oncology,Vol. 89, No.2, (November 2008), pp. 172-179, ISSN 0167-8140

Ahmad, R et al (2011) Increasing treatment accuracy for cervical cancer patients using correlations between bladder-filling change and cervix-uterus displacements: Proof of principle. *Radiotherapy and Oncology*, In Press, (n.d.2011), ISSN 0167-8140

Benda, RK et al (2003) Breast boost:Are we missing the target? *Cancer*, Vol. 97, No. 4, (February 2003), pp. 905-909, ISSN 1097-0142

Beriwal, S et al (2006) Clinical outcome with adjuvant treatment of endometrial carcinoma using IMRT. *Gynecologic Oncology*, Vol. 102, No.2, (August 2006), pp. 195-199, ISSN 0090-8258

Berrang,T et al (2009) 3D ultrasound can contribute to planning CT to define the target for partial breast radiotherapy. *International Journal of Radiation Oncology, Biology, Physics*, Vol. 73, No.2, (February 2009), pp. 375-383, ISSN 0360-3016

Boda-Heggemann, J et al (2008) Accuracy of Ultrasound-Based (BAT) Prostate-Repositioning: A Three-Dimensional On-Line Fiducial-Based Assessment with Cone-Beam Computed Tomography. *International Journal of Radiation Oncology, Biology, Physics*, Vol. 70, No. 4, (2008), pp. 1247-1255, ISSN 0360-3016

Boersma, L et al (1998) Estimation of the Incidense of Late Bladder and Rectum

Complications after High-Dose (70-78 Gy) Conformal Radiotherapy for Prostate Cancer, Using Dose-Volume Histograms. *International Journal of Radiation Oncology, Biology, Physics*, Vol. 41, No. 1, (1998), pp. 83-92, ISSN 0360-3016

Buchali, A et al (1999) Impact of the filling status of the bladder and rectum on their integral dose distribution and the movement of the uterus in the treatment planning of gynaecological cancer. *Radiotherapy and Oncology* , Vol. 52, No.1, (January 1999), pp. 29-34, ISSN 0167-8140

Cahlon, O et al (2008) Ultra high dose IMRT for localized prostate cancer :Toxicity and biochemical outcomes. *International Journal of Radiation Oncology, Biology, Physics*, Vol. 71, No.2, (June 2008), pp. 330-337, ISSN 0360-3016

Chan, P et al (2008) Inter and intrafractional tumor and organ movement in patients with cervical cancer undergoing radiotherapy: A cinematic MRI point of interest study. *International Journal of Radiation Oncology, Biology, Physics*, Vol. 70, No.5, (April 2008), pp. 1507-1515, ISSN 0360-3016

Clark, RM et al (1987) Breast cancer. Experiences with conservation therapy. *Am J Clin Oncol*. Vol. 10, No. 6, (December 1987), pp. 461-468, ISSN 0277-3732

Fisher, B et al (1994) Conservative surgery for the management of invasive and non invasive carcinoma of the breast: NSABP trials. National Surgical Adjuvant Breast and Bowel Project. *World J Surg*, Vol. 18 , No.1 , (January 1994), pp. 63-69, ISSN 0364-2313

Fisher, B et al (2002) Twenty year follow up of a randomized trial comparing total mastectomy, lumpectomy, and lumpectomy plus irradiation for the treatment of invasive breast cancer. *N Engl J Med*, Vol. 347, No.16, (October 2002), pp. 1233-1241, ISSN 0028-4793

Han, Y et al (2006) Interfractional dose variation during intensity-modulated radiation therapy for cervical cancer assessed by weekly CT evaluation. *International Journal of Radiation Oncology, Biology, Physics*, Vol. 65, No.2, (June 2006), pp. 617-623, ISSN 0360-3016

Hanks, G et a1 (2000) Dose Selection for Prostate Cancer patients Based on Dose Comparison and Dose Response Studies. *International Journal of Radiation Oncology, Biology, Physics,* Vol. 46, No. 4, (2000), pp. 823-832, ISSN 0360-3016

Holland, R et al (1985) Histologic multifocality of Tis, T1-2 breast carcinomas. Implications for clinical trials of breast conserving surgery. *Cancer,* Vol. 56, No. 5, (September 1985), pp. 979-990, ISSN 1097-0142

Huh, SJ et al (2004) Interfractional variation in position of the uterus during radical radiotherapy for cervical cancer. *Radiotherapy and Oncology,* Vol. 71, No. 1, (April 2004), pp. 73-79, ISSN 0167-8140

Jhingran, A et al (2010) Vaginal motion and bladder and rectal volumes during pelvic intensity modulated radiation therapy after hysterectomy. *International Journal of Radiation Oncology, Biology, Physics,* In Press, (n.d. 2010), ISSN 0360-3016

Jürgenliemk-Schulz, I et al (2011) Internal motion of the vagina after hysterectomy for gynaecological cancer. *Radiotherapy and Oncology,* Vol. 98, No.2, (February 2011), pp. 244-248, ISSN 0167-8140

Kerkhof, E et al (2009) Intrafraction motion in patients with cervical cancer: The benefit of soft tissue registration using MRI. *Radiotherapy and Oncology* , Vol. 93, No.1, (October 2009), pp. 115-121, ISSN 0167-8140

Landis, DM et al (2007) Variability among breast radiation oncologists in delineation of the postsurgical lumpectomy cavity. *International Journal of Radiation Oncology, Biology, Physics,* Vol. 67, No.5, (April 2007), pp. 1299-1308, ISSN 0360-3016

Langen, K et al (2003) Evaluation of Ultrasound-Based Prostate Localization for Image-Guided Radiotherapy. *International Journal of Radiation Oncology, Biology, Physics,* Vol. 57, No. 3, (2003), pp. 635-644, ISSN 0360-3016

Liljegren, G et al (1999) 10 year results after sector resection with or without postoperative radiotherapy for stage 1 breast cancer. A randomized trial. *J Clin Oncol.* Vol. 17, No. 8, (August 1999), pp. 2326-2333, ISSN 0732-183X

Lim, K et al (2009) Pelvic radiotherapy for cancer of the cervix:Is what you plan actually what you deliver? *International Journal of Radiation Oncology, Biology, Physics,* Vol. 74, No.1, (May 2009), pp. 304-312, ISSN 0360-3016

McBain, C.A. et al (2009) Ultrasound imaging to assess inter and intra fraction motion during bladder radiotherapy and its potential as a verification tool. *Clinical Oncology,* Vol. 21, No.5, (June 2009), pp. 385-393, ISSN 0936-6555

Michalski, J et al (2010) Radiation Dose-Volume Effects in Radiation-Induced Rectal Injury. *International Journal of Radiation Oncology, Biology, Physics,* Vol. 76, No. 3, Supplement, (2010), pp. S123-S129, ISSN 0360-3016

Moseley, D et al (2007) Comparison of Localization Performance with Implanted Fiducial Markers and Cone-Beam Computed Tomography for On-Line Image-Guided Radiotherapy of the Prostate. *International Journal of Radiation Oncology, Biology, Physics,* Vol. 67, No. 3, pp. 952-953, ISSN 0360-3016

Petersen, RP et al (2007) Target volume delineation for partial breast radiotherapy planning: Clinical characteristics associated with low interobserver concordance. *International Journal of Radiation Oncology, Biology, Physics,* Vol. 69, No.1, (September 2007), pp. 41-48, ISSN 0360-3016

Pinkawa, M et al (2006) Prostate position variability and dose- volume histograms in radiotherapy for prostate cancer with full and empty bladder. *International Journal of Radiation Oncology, Biology, Physics,* Vol. 64, No.3, (March 2006), pp. 856-861, ISSN 0360-3016

Pollack, A et al (2002) Prostate Cancer Radiation Dose Response: Results of the M. D. Anderson Phase III Randomized Trial. *International Journal of Radiation Oncology, Biology, Physics,* Vol. 53, No. 5, (2002), pp. 1097-1105, ISSN 0360-3016

Prendergast, B et al (2009) The dynamic tumor bed : Volumetric changes in the lumpectomy cavity during breast conserving therapy. *International Journal of Radiation Oncology, Biology, Physics,* Vol. 74, No.3, (July 2009), pp. 695-701, ISSN 0360-3016

Ringash,J et al (2004) Accuracy of ultrasound in localization of breast boost field. *Radiotherapy and Oncology,* Vol. 72, No. 1, (July 2004), pp. 61-66, ISSN 0167-8140

Scarborough, T et al (2006) Comparison of Ultrasound and Implanted Seed Marker Prostate Localization Methods: Implications for Image-Guided Radiotherapy. *International Journal of Radiation Oncology, Biology, Physics,* Vol. 65, No. 2, (2006), pp. 378-387, ISSN 0360-3016

Schild, SE et al (1993) Movements of the prostate due to rectal and bladder distension: implications for radiotherapy. *Med Dosim,* Vol. 18, No. 1, (Spring 1993), pp. 13-15, ISSN 0958-3947

Serago, C et al (2006) Comparison of Daily Megavoltage Electronic Portal Imaging or Kilovoltage Imaging with Marker Seeds to Ultrasound Imaging or Skin Marks for Prostate Localization and Treatment Positioning in Patients with Prostate Cancer. *International Journal of Radiation Oncology, Biology, Physics,* Vol. 65, No. 5, (2006), pp. 1585-1592, ISSN 0360-3016

Smitt, MC et al (2001) Breast electron boost planning: Comparison of CT and US. *Radiology,* Vol. 219, No.1, (April 2001), pp. 203-206, ISSN 0033-8419

Stam, MR et al (2006) Bladder filling variation during radiation treatment of prostate cancer: can the use of a bladder ultrasound scanner and biofeedback optimize bladder filling? *International Journal of Radiation Oncology, Biology, Physics,* Vol. 65, No.2, (June 2006), pp. 371-377, ISSN 0360-3016

Taylor,A & Powell, M (2008) An assessment of interfractional uterine and cervical motion: Implications for radiotherapy target volume definition in gynaecological cancer. *Radiotherapy and Oncology,* Vol. 88, No. 2, (August 2008), pp. 250-257, ISSN 0167-8140